CLINICAL PHARMACOLOGY

ENCYCLOPAEDIA OF BIOPHARMACEUTICAL

Vol. 3

CLINICAL PHARMACOLOGY

By

Dr. S.K. Prasad

School of Studies of Zoology & Biotechnology
Vikram University
Ujjain

DISCOVERY PUBLISHING HOUSE PVT. LTD.
NEW DELHI-110 002

First Published – 2011

Reprinted – 2025

ISBN: 978-81-8356-735-0

Clinical Pharmacology

Published by:

DISCOVERY PUBLISHING HOUSE

4383/4B, Ansari Road, Darya Ganj

New Delhi-110 002 (India)

Phone: +91-11-23279245; 23253475; 43596065

Mobile: +91 9811179893 / +91 9871656464

E-mail: discoverybooksindia@gmail.com

orderdphbooks@gmail.com

namitwasan9@gmail.com

web: www.discoverypublishinggroup.com

Printed at:

Infinity Imaging Systems

Delhi

Preface

The present title "Encyclopaedia of Biopharmaceutical" has been written for those in the pharmaceutical research and those responsible for the education and training in pharmaceutical science and technology of graduate and undergraduate students. Medicine is an ever changing science. As new research and clinical experience broaden our knowledge, changes in treatment and drug therapy are required. This branch of life science has progressed enormously in recent years and the significant advances in therapeutics and an understanding of the need to optimize during delivery in the body have brought about an increased awareness of the valuable role played by the dosage forms. This statement is as true as it was back in ninteenth century and perhaps more so, given the increasing emphasis being placed on discovery, development, and use of large molecular entities as therapeutic and diagnostic agents. Development of these abilities requires an integration of knowledge, skills, attitudes, and values that can be acquired only through structured learning process including independent study, hands on practice and the availability of advanced literature. This tittle has designed to meet such needs of learners in the health professions.

In the last two decades, the pharmaceutical industry has experimented and successfully adopted several integrated and multidisciplinary approaches in the research areas of dring compound screening, toxicological evaluation, and pharmaceutical product development. The book is written in a concise style that facilitates an in-depth level of understanding of the essential concepts. The objectives of the present title are three folds: (i) to serve as a useful tool to help guide scientists in research and development by out-lining the theory and successful practice of in vitro - in vivo correlation, (ii) to help formulators apply the tool in designing and developing prototypes that enable selection of clinical formulations, and (iii) to help formulate strategy(ies) for product life-cycle management.

To make the work more comprehensive and informative, the author has consulted many authoritative books, research journals, abstracts, monographs etc., so there can be no claim to originality except in the manner of treatment.

The author expresses his thanks to his friends and colleagues whose continue inspirations have initiated him to bring out this book.

The author expresses his gratitude to Mr. Wasan and staff of M/s Discovery Publishing House Pvt. Ltd. for their whole hearted co-operation in the publication of this book.

Author

CONTENTS

1

INTRODUCTION

Ancient civilisations, like modern society, had a keen interest in the health of man and other animals. Continuation of this interest over a period of time led to the discovery of a large number of therapeutic agents primarily from natural sources. In more recent times (about 50 years), with the involvement of a large number of pharmaceutical companies and many academic institutions, progress in the understanding of disease processes and mechanisms to control or eliminate the disease has accelerated. However, despite the advances and achievements of the last 50 years, the need to discover treatments for existing and evolving diseases has not decreased. This is primarily because of the inadequacies of current medicines. In many cases the treatment only leads to symptom relief and in various other cases the cure is associated with undesirable side-effects. In some cases (for example infectious diseases like tuberculosis, malaria and HIV), resistance/tolerance may develop to the existing treatments, thus making them ineffective against the infecting bacteria, parasite or virus. In addition, with the changing lifestyle and increasing life span, more and more pathological abnormalities that require entirely new treatments are being identified. For example, obesity and a number of cardiovascular diseases may have their origins in altered (more prosperous?) lifestyle habits, including environmental and psychosocial factors and diet. Changing social attitudes are also creating markets for the so called "lifestyle" drugs. Increasing knowledge about the underlying causes of diseases is enabling the discovery of more selective and less toxic drugs.

Progress in molecular biology (for example sequencing of human genome, proteomics, pharmacogenomics and protein engineering) is creating new avenues for the understanding of the precise disease mechanisms (biochemical pathways) and the discovery of new targets. Advances in this field are expected to lead to highly selective and efficacious medicines. Recombinant technologies are enabling the synthesis of larger biologically active proteins in sufficient quantities. Proteins and monoclonal antibodies are therefore becoming more important and common as therapeutic agents. Equally important is the progress being made in the fields of combinatorial chemistry, enabling the synthesis of millions of compounds, high-throughput screening technologies and other automation techniques facilitating more rapid drug discovery. In the longer run, a combination of all the new developments is likely to generate safer and more effective medicines, not only for the existing diseases but also for the diseases of the future which may become more important as a consequence of changes in lifestyle, and increasing age.

Malaria (caused in humans by single-celled *Plasmodium* protozoa parasites) can be considered an example of an "older" disease still in need of effective and cheaper treatments. Each year, 300–500 million people contract malaria and about 2–3 million die. A number of medicines, including chloroquine,

4-aminoquinolines, atovaquone, malarone, halofantrine, mefloquine, proguanil and artemisinin derivatives, are available. Three main types of vaccines, based on the three major phases of the parasite life cycle, are being developed: antisporozoite vaccines designed to prevent infection, anti-asexual blood-stage vaccines designed to reduce severe and complicated manifestations of the disease, and transmission blocking vaccines aimed at arresting the development of the parasite in the mosquito itself. Monoclonal antibodies against specific malarial antigens are being explored for diagnostic and potential therapeutic purposes. In addition, efforts are beginning to be made to shed light on the origin of the development of resistance in specific cases. Finally, with the availability of the malaria parasite genome map, researchers will be able to identify and validate good drug targets much more rapidly, leading to effective new therapies and vaccines.

Bone disorders like arthritis and osteoporosis are examples of diseases that are becoming increasingly important with the ageing population. Anti-inflammatory glucocorticoids like prednisolone and methylprednisolone, and immunosuppressants such as cyclosporin A and dexamethasone are used for the treatment. Although the treatment options have increased recently, most of these therapies, focus on addressing the symptoms rather than the underlying causes, of the disease. For example, cyclooxygenase (COX) 2 inhibitors like celecoxib and rofecoxib are being marketed as safer non-steroidal anti-inflammatory drugs (NSAIDs). Although the older NSAIDs are highly effective as analgesic, antipyretic and anti-inflammatory agents, long term ingestion causes gastric lesions. The discovery that the COX enzyme exists in two isoforms, with COX-2 being the primary isoform at sites of inflammation, led to a suggestion that inhibition of this isoform accounts for the therapeutic benefit of NSAIDs whereas inhibition of COX-1 results in adverse effects. The newer COX-2 selective agents appear to have a superior gastrointestinal safety profile. In addition to COX-2 inhibitors, inhibitors of matrix metalloproteinases (MMPs) are emerging for the treatment of many diseases, including arthritis. Enzymes that degrade the extracellular MMPs, are normally controlled by a set of tissue inhibitors that, if disrupted, will allow the enzymes to work unchecked, degrading the matrix and promoting not only arthritis but also tumour growth and metastasis. Another treatment option is inhibition of tumour necrosis factor (TNF)α, an inflammation promoting cytokine associated with multiple inflammatory events, including arthritis. Anti-TNFα therapies are already on the market. Finally, a variety of genes that code for antiarthritic proteins are under investigation, including interleukin (IL)-1Ra, IL-1sR, TNFsR, transforming growth factor β (TGFβ), IL-13, IL-10, and vIL-10, as are the vectors that will carry them to arthritic tissues.

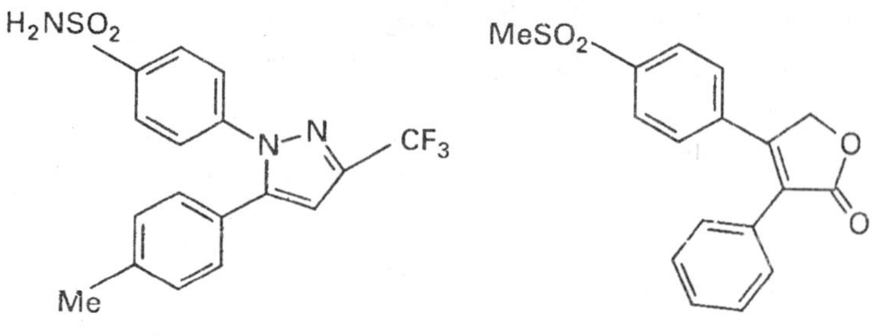

H_2NSO_2 N–N CF_3 Me

Celecoxib

$MeSO_2$ O O

Rofecoxib

Recently, the process of drug discovery has been expanded to cover a range of molecular biology, biotechnology and medicinal chemistry (including combinatorial chemistry) techniques. The newer disciplines like genome analysis, proteomics, and bioinformatics are likely to lead to many new targets (receptors, enzymes, etc.) and therapeutically important proteins. Techniques like combinatorial chemistry and high-throughput screening are expected to identify hits/leads against various therapeutically important receptors and enzymes. Depending on the knowledge available on the receptor or the enzyme of interest, the hits/leads can then be modified in a random "*semi-rational*" or "*rational*" manner to generate the drug candidates. This chapter includes a short account of the historical aspects and a short introduction to some of the newer disciplines. The main theme/objective of the chapter is to give examples of receptor agonists and antagonists, enzyme inhibitors, including signal transduction inhibitors, and inhibitors of protein–protein interactions that have been discovered by random and semi-rational/rational approaches. This enables one to understand actual drug discovery procedures and the science that has led to many drugs currently on the market. Examples include:

1. COX inhibitors
2. Angiotensin converting enzyme (ACE) inhibitors, for example, antihypertensives such as captopril and lisinopril
3. Histamine H_1 receptor antagonists, for example antiallergy compounds such as fexofenadine
4. Histamine H_2 receptor antagonists – inhibitors of gastric acid secretion, such as cimetidine and ranitidine
5. Proton pump inhibitors – inhibitors of gastric acid secretion, such as omeprazole and esomeprazole
6. Activators of nuclear peroxisome proliferator activated receptor-γ, for example pioglitazone and troglitazone, used to treat type 2 diabetes
7. Lipid-lowering agents such as atorvastatin and cerivastatin
8. Anti-influenza treatments like zanamivir
9. Acetylcholinesterase inhibitors like donepezil for the treatment of Alzheimer's disease
10. Selective and competitive inhibitors of the cysteinyl leukotrienes (LTC_4, LTD_4 and LTE_4) such as zafirlukast and montelukast for the treatment of asthma
11. Sildenafil, an inhibitor of phosphodiesterase type 5 used to treat erectile dysfunction
12. Orlistat, an antiobesity compound
13. Atypical antipsychotic agents such as quetiapine and olanzapine for the treatment of schizophrenia.

It may be useful to mention at this stage that many of the highly successful drugs launched in the last 25 years were discovered in the pregenomic era and the real contribution of all the new technologies mentioned above remains to be proven. In some cases the drug was initially investigated for different indications. For example, sildenafil was being investigated in the clinic as an antianginal drug when its beneficial effects in improving erectile function were observed.

Historical Aspects

Early Discoveries

A number of early medicines, including morphine (analgesic) and quinine (antimalarial), were isolated from plants. Over the years the search for therapeutic agents has widened to isolate products from living agents such as bacteria, fungi, sea animals and even human beings. The important discoveries from this research not only include antibiotics such as penicillin but also many hormones and transmitters. Ivermectin (a drug used to treat tropical filariasis), lovastatin (HMG CoA reductase inhibitor), insulin, and cyclosporin A and FK 506 (immunosuppressants) are other examples of drugs originating from natural sources. Many of the biologically active peptides such as oxytocin, vasopressin, adrenocorticotropic hormone (ACTH), insulin, calcitonin, luteinising hormone releasing hormone (LHRH), growth hormone and erythropoietin are important examples of compounds isolated from humans and other animals that have led to medicines currently used in clinical practice. In addition, discoveries of many other agents like adrenaline, histamine and tryptamine and their receptors have led to extremely important medicines.

Many other early discoveries were primarily based on low-throughput random screening approaches. The mechanism of action was later rationalised when additional biochemical and pharmacological information became available. Examples of early drugs include sulfa drugs which led to the discoveries of several other classes of drugs. For example, the active metabolite of the sulfonamide prontosil inhibits the enzyme carbonic anhydrase, leading to an increase in natriuresis and the excretion of water. Sulfanilamide gave rise to better carbonic anhydrase inhibitors such as acetazolamide and later led to more effective diuretics such as hydrochlorothiazide and furosemide. Further chemistry in the field led to development of the sulfonylureas such as tolbutamide, used in the treatment of type 2 diabetes.

Impact of New Technology on Drug Discovery

Receptor Subtypes

Since the idea of a receptor as a selective binding site for chemotherapeutic agents was developed, huge progress has been made in the identification, characterisation and classification of receptors and receptor subtypes. In addition, knowledge has been gained about the downstream signalling pathways, most often involving transcription factors, that ultimately act on DNA and result in altered gene expression. Mapping the key signalling molecules in biochemical pathways and attempting to modulate their effects is resulting in new areas of drug discovery. The early assumption that a ligand acts at one receptor is no longer tenable and it is now well established that many endogenous ligands act at different receptor subtypes. The availability of more selective synthetic ligands, and cloning and amino acid sequencing technologies, has shown that different receptor subtypes exist for most of the receptors. The situation is further complicated by the existence of different receptor subtypes in different tissues in the same species, and by structural differences in receptor subtypes in different species of animals. Thus, the accumulated knowledge has not only provided many challenges for the drug discovery process but has also opened a way to many new drug discovery targets and much more selective treatments. From the point of view of drug discovery, ligands acting at the G-protein coupled receptors have resulted in the most successful drug candidates. Some of the examples illustrating how receptor research has led to more selective drugs and enhanced our understanding of the roles played by various receptor subtypes in disease processes are mentioned below. Early examples of different receptor subtypes that led to clinically useful drugs include α and β adrenoceptors and histamine H_1 and H_2 receptor subtypes. One of the more complicated and extensively studied area of receptor subtypes is the field of 5-hydroxytryptamine (5-HT; serotonin) receptors. The seven receptor subtypes, 5-HT_1 to 5-HT_7, have been characterised using selective ligands (agonists and antagonists); cloning and amino acid sequencing techniques have been used to define the molecular structures and intracellular transduction mechanisms. Several of the more selective compounds have reached the market for the treatment of various disorders of the nervous system (for example, antiemetics). Tryptamine 5-$HT_{1B/1D}$ receptor agonists like zolmitriptan, naratriptan and rizatriptan are marketed for the treatment of migraine.

Other more recent examples of new receptor subtypes include neurokinin, melanocortin and somatostatin receptor subtypes. Neurokinins (substance P, neurokinin A and neurokinin B) act at three receptor subtypes: NK_1, NK_2 and NK_3. Selective ligands are being explored for the treatment of pain, asthma, depression, etc. The natural melanocortic peptides are derived from the precursor peptide pro-opiomelanocortin (expressed in the pituitary) by proteolytic cleavage in three regions of the protein, generating ACTH, and α-, β- and γ-melanocyte stimulating hormone (MSH) peptides. Pro-opiomelanocortin also generates a number of other peptides including enkephalin and β-endorphin. Five melanocortin receptor subtypes (MC_1–MC_5) belonging to the G-protein coupled receptor family have been cloned (40–60% sequence identities), and selective ligands for the receptor subtypes have been synthesised. Early pharmacological studies have indicated that drugs selective for the MC_1 receptor may be useful for the treatment of inflammatory conditions, whereas compounds selective for the MC_4 receptor may be useful for controlling eating behaviour and body weight. These biological effects are very different to the involvement of MSH and ACTH in skin pigmentation and secretion of corticosteroids, respectively. Cloning studies have also identified five receptor subtypes of somatostatin (Ala-Gly-Cys-Lys-Asn-Phe-Phe-Trp-Lys-Thr-Phe-Thr-Ser-Cys, a cyclic peptide with a disulphide bridge),

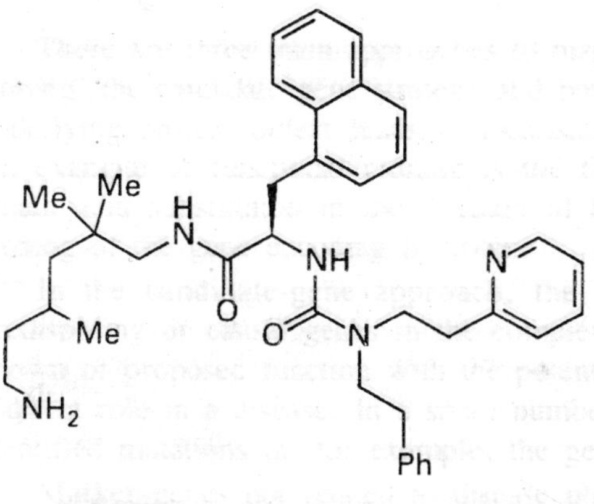

(hSSTR$_1$ selective)

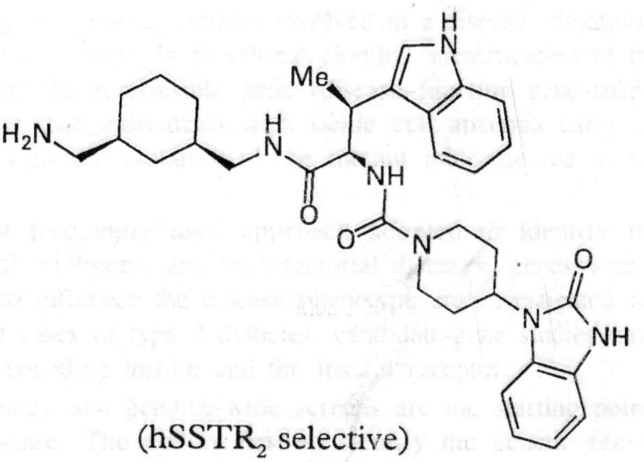

(hSSTR$_2$ selective)

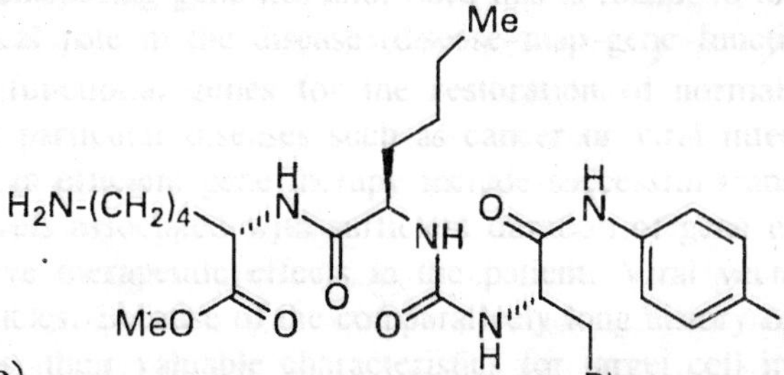

(hSSTR$_3$ selective)

a peptide discovered in 1971–72 and shown to be an inhibitor of growth hormone, insulin, glucagon and gastric acid secretion. Screening of heterocyclic β-turn mimetic libraries (based upon the Trp-Lys motif found in the turn region of somatostatin) against a panel of the five cloned human somatostatin receptors (hSSTR$_1$–hSSTR$_5$) led to the development of somatostatin receptor ligands that bind to the five receptor subtypes. Compound is relatively more selective for the hSSTR$_2$ receptor subtype and shows higher affinity against hSSTR$_3$ and hSSTR$_5$ subtypes. The turn mimetic is more potent at the hSSTR$_5$ receptor subtype. In another series of compounds, library screening followed by studies of structure–activity relationships (SAR) lead to the development of compounds selective for the hSST receptor subtypes. *In vitro* experiments using these selective compounds demonstrated the role of the hSST$_2$ receptor in inhibition of glucagon release from mouse pancreatic α cells and the hSST$_5$ receptor as a mediator of insulin secretion from pancreatic β cells. Both subtypes of receptor regulate release of growth hormone from the rat anterior pituitary gland. Some of the recent information has shown that the five receptor subtypes may fall into two classes or groups. One class (SRIF$_1$) appears to comprise SST$_2$, SST$_3$ and SST$_5$ and the other class (SRIF$_2$) consists of the other two recombinant receptor subtypes (SST$_1$ and SST$_4$).

More recently, attention has also been focused on orphan G-protein coupled receptors, a family of plasma membrane proteins involved in a broad array of signalling pathways. Novel orphan G-protein coupled receptors have continued to emerge through cloning activities as well as through bioinformatic analysis of sequence databases. Their ligands are unidentified and their physiological relevance remains to be defined. Methods are being developed to identify ligands acting at these receptors. One of these approaches identifies ligands by purification from biological fluids, cell supernatants or tissue extracts. The discoveries of endothelin (a vasoconstrictor peptide) and nociceptin (an orphan opioid-like receptor ligand) are examples of this type. Ligands can also be identified by screening the orphan receptor against a number of diverse chemical libraries. Once identified, the ligand is used to characterise physiological and pathological roles of the receptor, followed by the discovery of other agonist and antagonist analogues by medicinal chemistry approaches.

Currently the drug discovery process has progressed beyond the receptor stage and various steps that result from the interaction of the receptor with a specific ligand have been characterised. One of the more important processes, signal transduction, converts the external signals induced by hormones, growth factors, neurotransmitters and cytokines into specific internal cellular responses (for example, gene expression, cell division, or even cell suicide). The process involves a cascade of enzyme-mediated reactions inside the cell that typically includes phosphorylation and dephosphorylation of proteins (kinases and phosphatases) as mediators of downstream processes. Signal transduction inhibitors are currently being developed for the treatment of a number of diseases, including cancer and inflammation.

Genomics

Genetic factors influence virtually every human disorder (for example, Alzheimer's and Parkinson's diseases, diabetes, asthma and rheumatoid arthritis) by determining disease susceptibility or resistance and interactions with environmental factors. Gene transfer research ("*gene therapy*") holds promise for treating disorders through the transfer and expression of DNA in the cells of patients. Although some clinical trials have started, several important issues, including efficient delivery of the genetic material to the required sites, along with other chemical, biological, safety, toxicity and ethical issues, have not yet been fully resolved. From the point of view of drug discovery, mapping of the human genome is only the first step. It is likely that even when the human genomic sequencing has been fully completed and all genes have been identified, a substantial fraction of these, possibly up to 50%, will have complex biochemical or physiological functions. Therefore, only a proportion (about 20% of the genome) will be amenable to pharmacological exploitation. Another major problem is the involvement of many genes and environmental factors in various diseases. For example, with the exception of some diseases or traits resulting principally from specific and relatively rare mutations (for example, cystic fibrosis), most of the genetic disorders (for example, cardiovascular diseases, diabetes, rheumatoid arthritis and schizophrenia) develop as a result of a network of genes failing to perform correctly, some of which might have a major disease effect but many of which have a relatively minor effect. Complex diseases and traits result principally from genetic variation that is relatively common in the general population. Thus, completion of the human genome will not provide an immediate solution to the genetics of complex diseases. This can only be achieved by documenting the genetic variation of human genomes at the population level within and across ethnic groups and by characterising mutant genes. For further progress it is therefore essential to identify the function of each gene in the normal and disease situations and establish a link with the expressed protein (before and after post-translational modification) and its role in a disease pathway.

Since the complete genome of *Haemophilus influenzae* was published, sequencing of genomes from a wide range of organisms, from bacteria to man, has continued apace. Initial sequencing and analysis of the human genome has been published. Another more recent example is the genome sequence of *Escherichia coli* O157:H7, implicated in many outbreaks of haemorrhagic colitis. The functional characterisation of microbial genomics will have a significant impact on genomic medicine (new antimicrobial targets and vaccine candidates) and on environmental (waste management, recycling), food, and industrial biotechnology. In addition to the work on human and microbial genomes, progress is also being made on the sequencing of the mouse and rat genomes. Data from rodent species should speed the discovery of genes and regulatory regions in the human genome and make it easier to determine their functions. In addition, these sequences may have a significant impact on the disease models because these animal are most often used in the early discovery and preclinical testing of new drugs.

There are three main approaches to mapping the genetic variants involved in a disease: functional cloning, the candidate gene strategy and positional cloning. In functional cloning, identification of the underlying protein defect leads to localisation of the responsible gene (disease–function–gene–map). An example of functional cloning is the finding that individuals with sickle cell anaemia carry an amino acid substitution in the β chain of haemoglobin. Isolation of the mutant molecule led to the cloning of the gene encoding β globin.

In the candidate-gene approach, the most frequently used approach adopted to identify the predisposing or causal genes in the complex and multigenic and multifactorial diseases, genes with a known or proposed function with the potential to influence the disease phenotype are investigated for a direct role in a disease. In a small number of cases of type 2 diabetes, candidate-gene studies have identified mutations in, for example, the genes encoding insulin and the insulin receptor.

Marker genes not related to disease physiology and genome-wide screens are the starting points for mapping the genetic components of the disease. The aim is first to identify the genetic region within which a disease-predisposing gene lies and, once this is found, to localise the gene and determine its functional and biological role in the disease (disease–map–gene–function).

The introduction of functional genes for the restoration of normal function or the transfer of therapeutic genes to treat particular diseases such as cancer or viral infections is of growing interest. The hurdles to overcome in efficient gene therapy include successful transfer of the therapeutic genes, appropriate expression levels associated with sufficient duration of gene expression, and the specificity of gene transfer to achieve therapeutic effects in the patient. Viral vectors are still among the most efficient gene transfer vehicles. Because of the comparatively long history of characterisation of particular viruses and their genomes, their valuable characteristics for target cell infectivity, transgene capacity, and accessibility of established helper cell lines for the production of recombinant virus stocks to infect target cells, the most commonly used vectors are developed from retroviruses, lentiviruses, adenovirus, herpes simplex virus and adeno-associated virus. The advantages of retroviral vectors (stable integration into the host genome, generation of viral titres sufficient for efficient gene transfer, infectivity of the recombinant viral particles for a broad variety of target cell types, and the ability to carry foreign genes of reasonable size) are accompanied by several disadvantages, for example, instability of some retroviral vectors, possible insertional mutagenesis by random viral integration into host DNA, the requirement of cell division for integration of Moloney murine leukaemia virus-derived retroviral vectors, and targeting of retroviral infection and/or therapeutic gene expression. In addition to the viral transfection procedures, non-viral transfection procedures are also being developed. In a recent example, human monocyte-derived dendritic cells were transfected with genes encoding tumour-associated antigens. The transfection was achieved by dimerisation of a 35 amino acid cationic peptide (Lys-Lys-Lys-Lys-Lys-Lys-Gly-Gly-Phe-Leu-Gly-Phe-Trp-Arg-Gly-Glu-Asn-Gly-Arg-Lys-Thr-Arg-Ser-Ala-Tyr-Glu-Arg-Met-Cys-Asn-Ile-Leu-Lys-Gly-Lys) and then using a complex of this dimeric peptide with plasmid DNA expression constructs. Injection of transfected dendritic cells expressing a tumour-associated antigen protected mice from lethal challenge with tumour cells in a model of melanoma.

Identification of the genes that provide structural and regulatory functions in an organism are likely to be useful in obtaining genetically modified (transgenic) animals using gene knockout or knockin strategies. The transgenic animals are useful in the identification and validation of molecular drug targets, generation of animal models of disease for the testing of novel therapeutic strategies, and early recognition of toxicological effects.

Pharmacogenomics

Because different patients with the same disease symptoms may respond differently to the same drug, both in terms of therapeutic benefits and side-effects, understanding of the relationships between gene variation and the effect of such variation on drug responses within individuals is likely to lead to tailor made therapies for specific populations of patients. For example, a variety of antihypertensive drugs and drugs for congestive heart failure are now available, including calcium antagonists, ACE inhibitors, β-blockers, diuretics, α-blockers, centrally acting antihypertensives, and, more recently, angiotensin $(AT)_1$ receptor antagonists. Although all of these agents are effective in lowering blood pressure in most cases, there are significant differences between their therapeutic and side-effect profiles. A better knowledge of the mechanisms that influence the efficacy of the drugs in different individuals and understanding why some patients can tolerate the drug better than others may lead to more efficacious drugs with a better side-effect profile. The variation of the individual's response to such drugs may be caused by the heterogeneity of the mechanisms underlying hypertension, interindividual variation in the pharmacokinetics of the drug, or a combination of both.

The likely benefit of more efficacious tailormade drugs with fewer side-effects has led to the development of the science of pharmacogenomics, a name given to any drug-discovery platform that attempts to address the issues of efficacy and toxicity in individuals. The concept of individual variation at the molecular level is not new. Protein obtained from different individuals has been known to have different amino acid sequences. These protein isoforms originate either by genomic variation at the level of the actual gene sequence, or by variation in expression which results from changes in the promoter and control elements that regulate expression. Alleles differ from each other by structural features, such as single base-pair changes, or as the result of rearrangements or deletions of entire gene portions. Depending on the structure of regulatory sequences, some alleles may be expressed at very high levels, while others may be repressed. Similarly, depending on variation at the critical points in the assembly of genes, splicing variants may result from alternative arrangements of building blocks. Technologies that enable the monitoring of gene expression under different circumstances (based on high-throughput sequencing and screening approaches) are currently being developed and will enable systematic investigation of the patterns of gene expression between normal and disease states in a statistically meaningful way, along with the expression of the relevant proteins in different individuals. In addition, the potential of using single-nucleotide polymorphisms to correlate drug regimens and responses is also being investigated. The availability of precisely located single-nucleotide polymorphic sites spanning the genome holds promise for the association of particular genetic loci with disease states. This information, together with high-throughput gene-chip technologies, will offer new opportunities for molecular diagnostics and monitoring of disease predisposition in large sections of the population. It will also allow much earlier preventive treatment in many slowly evolving diseases.

Proteomics

The control mechanisms in health and disease are found at the protein level and, as mentioned above, genome sequencing does not provide sufficient information at the protein level. The tertiary structure and the type and extent of post-translational modifications (for example, glycosylation and phosphorylation) of a protein are critical to its function and cellular localisation but this information is not encoded in the protein's corresponding DNA. An additional complication between genes and proteins is the existence of alternative splice variants of messenger RNA which give rise to isomeric proteins that might contribute to regulatory processes in the cell. The processing of proteins may also be different in various tissues under different conditions. Some proteins may give rise to biologically active fragments and some may exert diverse functions in collaboration with other proteins. Therefore, the complete structure and function of an individual protein can not be determined by reference to its gene sequence alone. Thus, beyond genomics it is essential to compare the protein content of cells/tissues/organs in the normal and disease states and to generate the functional information on proteins required for various drug discovery processes. Proteomics is any protein-based approach that provides new information about proteins on a genome-wide scale, and addresses these difficulties by enabling the protein levels of cellular organisation to be screened and characterised. In a high-throughput manner, a large number of proteins from normal and disease samples (cells and tissue extracts) are separated on the basis of their charge and molecular weight by two-dimensional electrophoresis, and the amino acid sequences of proteins and their post-translational modifications are identified by mass spectrometry. The separated proteins are then stained and the maps of protein expression are digitally scanned into databases. These protein expression maps can be used to study cellular pathways and the perturbation of these pathways by disease and by drug action. Thus, an understanding of cellular pathways and protein changes resulting from the disease and from drug actions can not only lead to new drug targets but can also provide early markers for diseases and early indications of drug toxicity. It should be emphasised, however, that characterisation of a different protein in a disease state does not necessarily means that it plays a causal role or represents a potential therapeutic target. In many cases, the new protein may be a consequence of the disease rather than the cause. Further studies are required to check whether the activity of a candidate target eliminated by molecular/cellular techniques could reverse the disease phenotype. Moreover, even when a potential therapeutic target has been identified and a molecule capable of disrupting it has been obtained, we cannot assume that it will constitute an effective treatment for the disease under investigation. Alternative metabolic routes may provide cells with ways of circumventing blocked pathways.

The potential benefit of proteomics in predicting toxicity at an early stage may lead to accelerated drug discovery programmes. A comparison of the protein profiles of normal tissue with those of tissue treated with the known toxic agent might give an indication of the drug's toxic activity. Similarly, identification of a known toxic protein in drug-treated tissues may give an idea about the toxicity of the drug. As a first approach, an examination of liver and kidney, which are the major sites for metabolism and excretion of most drugs, before and after the drug administration may provide early indications about events that might result in toxicity. Proteomic analysis of the serum, where the majority of toxicity markers released from susceptible organs and tissues throughout the entire body collect, can be utilised to identify serum markers (and clusters thereof) as indicators of toxicity. The serum markers could subsequently be used to predict the response of each individual and allow tailoring of therapy whereby optimal efficacy is achieved whilst minimising adverse effects. Surrogate markers for drug efficacy could also be detected by this procedure and could be used to identify classes of patients who will respond favourably to a drug.

There is currently some debate about the ability of the techniques being used to detect all the proteins present in a given sample. It is possible that global proteome displays based on two-dimensional gel electrophoresis are largely limited to the more abundantly expressed and stable proteins. Thus, important classes of regulatory proteins involved in signal transduction and gene expression, for example, and other proteins of lower abundance remain undetected by current methodologies. Proteins of lower abundance are more likely to be detected by separating these from highly abundant proteins. The disadvantage of this strategy, however, is that it requires much larger amounts of protein, and many additional separations, and therefore may be impractical for studies of small cell populations or tissue samples. Efforts are underway to develop advanced proteomic technologies that do not rely on two-dimensional gel electrophoresis.

After the discovery of protein maps and characterisation of individual proteins, the most important aspect of proteomics is to define protein function. Although new proteins are likely to include receptors, ligands, enzymes, enzyme inhibitors, signalling molecules and pathways that may be therapeutic targets, precise functions of the individual proteins have to be identified. To discover and monitor the relevance of a protein to a disease-related process, it is important to find where, when and to what extent a protein is expressed. Many approaches are being used to discover protein function. Structural homology methods may be used to ascribe function to some proteins, since it is known that proteins of similar function often share structural homology (tertiary structure). Another approach to defining protein function is chemical proteomics, the identification of small molecules that interact with the proteins by screening new proteins against diverse chemical libraries using methods such as nuclear magnetic resonance (NMR) spectroscopy, microcalorimetry and microarrays. Another method for identifying ligand binding sites involves scanning the surface of a protein molecule for clefts. In many cases the largest cleft is the known primary binding site for small ligands. Further information about the ligand structures that can be accommodated in the binding site can be obtained by various computational programs like DOCK or HOOK.

Some of the proteins likely to have known enzyme activity or enzyme inhibition properties can be identified using screens for generic enzyme activities. Along with the structural and chemical library methods, several "*non-homology*" methods are being developed to identify protein functions. These are computational methods, and take advantage of the many properties shared among functionally related proteins, such as patterns of domain fusion, evolutionary co-inheritance, conservation of relative gene position, and correlated expression patterns. Protein function is defined by these methods in terms of context, that is, which cellular pathways or complexes the protein participates in, rather than by suggesting a specific biochemical activity. Large-scale functional analysis of new proteins can be accomplished by using peptide or protein arrays, ranging from synthetic peptide arrays to whole proteins expressed in living cells. Comprehensive sets of purified peptides and proteins permit high-throughput screening for discrete biochemical properties, whereas formats involving living cells facilitate large-scale genetic screening for novel biological activities. Protein arrays can be engineered to suit the aims of a particular experiment. Thus, an array might contain all the combinatorial variants of a bioactive peptide or specific variants of a single protein species (splice variants, domains or mutants), a family of protein orthologs from different species, a protein pathway, or even the entire protein complement of an organism.

Access to structural information on a proteome-wide scale is not only important for ascribing protein function but may also be useful in target validation and medicinal chemistry on hits/leads that require structural information for rational design processes. The most straightforward strategy for predicting structure is to search for sequence similarity to a protein with known three-dimensional structure. Additional information can be obtained by identifying known and novel folds in a protein. There are databases of structural motifs in proteins which contain data relevant to helices, β-turns, γ-turns, β-hairpins, ψ-loops, β-α-β motifs, β-sheets, β-strands and disulphide bridges extracted from proteins, which can be used for comparison. Novel folds can be identified by employing *ab initio* approaches used for prediction of protein structure. With the aim of extracting further information from protein sequences, sequence motif libraries have been developed. Advances in *x* ray crystallography, particularly the use of synchrotron radiation sources, and NMR spectroscopy also allow rapid determination of protein structures. Using protein crystals in which methionine residues are replaced by selenomethionine, and multiwavelength synchrotron experiments, electron-density maps for proteins can be generated in less than an hour instead of the weeks of experimental time required for a conventional structure determination by crystallography. Despite great improvements in *x* ray crystallography techniques, the rate-limiting step in structure determination remains the expression, purification and crystallisation of the target protein.

Many problems still remain to be solved before protein function can be confidently assigned by using the above techniques. For example, the idea of "one gene one protein one function" is not valid in many cases and increasing numbers of proteins are found to have two or more different functions.

The multiple functions of such moonlighting proteins can vary as a consequence of changes in cellular localisation, cell type, oligomeric state, or the cellular concentration of a ligand, substrate, cofactor or product. Multidrug transporter P-glycoprotein (a large 170 kD cell-surface molecule encoded by the human *MDR1* gene) is an example of a protein with multiple functions. It is well established that P-glycoprotein can efflux xenobiotics from cells and is one mechanism that tumour cells use to escape death induced by chemotherapeutic drugs. Recent observations have raised the possibility that P-glycoprotein and related transporter molecules may play a fundamental role in regulating cell differentiation, proliferation and survival. P-glycoprotein encoded by *MDR1* in humans and *Mdr1a* in mice can regulate an endogenous chloride channel. This activity of P-glycoprotein can be inhibited by phosphorylation by protein kinase C. MDR1 P-glycoprotein has also been proposed to play roles in phospholipid translocation and cholesterol esterification. Functional P-glycoprotein has also been suggested to play a role in regulating programmed cell death (apoptosis).

Bioinformatics and Data Mining Technologies

The availability of genomic data and the corresponding protein sequences from humans and other organisms, together with structure– function annotations, disease correlation and population variations, requires sophisticated data management systems (databases) for analytical purposes. Proteomics-oriented databases include data on the two-dimensional gel electrophoresis maps of proteins from a variety of healthy and disease tissues. Bioinformatic systems (computer-assisted data management and analysis) are used to gather and analyse this information in order to attach biological knowledge to genes, assign genes to biological pathways, compare the gene sets of different species, understand processes in healthy and disease states, and find new or better drugs. The currently available techniques have the capability to translate a given gene sequence into a protein structure, complete with predictions of secondary structure, and database comparisons. Progress is being made in devising systems that provide information on biological function derived from sequencing and functional analysis. In addition to the gene–function analysis studies, the need for data mining techniques (defined as "the non-trivial extraction of implicit, previously unknown, and potentially useful information from data") is becoming necessary in order to deal with the enormous amounts of information that the industry collects in individual databases (ranging, from, for example, databases of disease profiles and molecular pathways to sequences, chemical and biological screening data, including SAR, chemical structures of combinatorial libraries of compounds, individual and population clinical trial results and so on).

A large number of companies are developing data mining applications (software) which can identify cause–effect relationships between data sets and group together data points or sets based on different criteria. A time-delay data mining approach is used when a complete data set is not available immediately and in complete form, but is collected over time. The systems designed to handle such data look for patterns, which are confirmed or rejected as the data set increases and becomes more robust. This approach is geared towards analysis of long-term clinical trials and studies of multicomponent modes of action. It is also possible to overlay large and complex data sets that are similar to each other and compare them. This is particularly useful in all forms of clinical trial meta-analyses, where data collected at different sites over different time periods, and perhaps under similar but not always identical conditions, need to be compared. Here, the emphasis is on finding dissimilarities, not similarities. Predictive data mining programmes are available for making simulations, predictions and forecasts based on the data sets analysed.

Combinatorial Chemistry and High-throughput Screening

One of the earliest approaches to drug discovery was the random screening process. More recently, significant efforts were directed towards rational/semi-rational approaches. However, recent advances in high-throughput screening and synthesis techniques, coupled with large-scale data analysis and data management methods, have shifted the balance towards testing libraries of "diverse" chemical compounds in multiple screens (>20 000 compounds in a week) in the shortest possible time. This approach is expected to provide leads much more quickly for optimisation using combinatorial synthesis methods (targeted libraries) to generate drug candidates. Starting from the solid-phase peptide synthesis in the early sixties, which opened the way to chemical synthesis on solid supports, automated synthesis of diverse organic compounds has now become routine in many laboratories. Assays have been developed that make use of fluorescently labelled reagents (for example, receptors, ligands and enzyme substrates), allowing the rapid optical screening of large collections of compounds. Assays using microtitre plates (96–384 wells in each plate) have been designed to enable small quantities of compounds to be tested at a much reduced cost in terms of reagent use.

Combinatorial synthesis

Combinatorial chemistry is having a major impact in generating libraries containing large numbers of compounds in a relatively short period of time using solid phase-synthesis technologies. In addition, it is possible to buy readymade libraries built around specific molecular themes and consisting of many thousands of compounds, and to test these libraries in high-throughput screening systems using automated off-the-shelf instrumentation and reagents. The technique of combinatorial biocatalysis is also used to obtain diverse libraries. This approach takes advantage of natural catalysts (enzymes and whole cells), as well as the rapidly growing supply of recombinant and engineered enzymes, for the direct derivatisation of many different synthetic compounds and natural products. The types of reactions catalysed by enzymes and micro-organisms include reactions that can introduce functional groups (for example, carbon–carbon bond formation, hydroxylation, halogenation, cyclo additions, addition of amines), modify the existing functionalities (oxidation of alcohols to aldehydes and ketones, reduction of aldehydes or ketones to alcohols, oxidation of sulphides to sulphoxides, oxidation of amino groups to nitro groups, hydrolysis of nitriles to amides and carboxylic acids, replacements of amino groups by hydroxyl groups, lactonisation, isomerisation, epimerisation, dealkylation and methyl transfer) or addition onto functional groups (esterification, carbonate formation, carbamate formation, glycosylation, amidation and phosphorylation). Currently available technologies allow these biocatalysis reactions to be carried out in aqueous and non-aqueous solvents.

Techniques are available to screen individual compounds or mixtures in solution or still attached to the solid support. The main advantage of screening single compounds in solution (the technique most commonly used in the past) is that activity can be directly correlated with chemical structure. Screening mixtures of compounds has the advantage that fewer assays need to be performed and at the same time fewer synthetic steps are required to generate mixtures. However, it is not possible to synthesise mixtures that contain entirely different structures. Screening of mixtures can lead to false positives resulting from additive or cooperative effects of weakly active compounds. Thus, the most active mixture may not contain the most potent compound. An additional disadvantage of testing mixtures is that once an active mixture has been identified, the exact structure of the active compound, in most cases, can only be obtained by extensive deconvolution studies. There are some procedures like positional scanning approach which enable the active compound to be identified directly from screening. This method depends on the synthesis of a series of subset mixtures that contain a single building block (substituent) at one position and all the building blocks at the other positions. The structure of the most active compound is then assigned by selecting the building block from the most active subset at each position. The structure is confirmed by synthesis.

The most widely used solid phase method for the synthesis of libraries (originally used for peptides) has been termed the "*split-mix*", "divide, couple and recombine" and "one bead one compound" method. The resin beads display a linker to which building blocks are sequentially attached, to effectively grow molecules. As a first step, different batches of resin are reacted individually with a unique set of reagents (first set of building blocks); the resins are then combined and deprotected to liberate another reactive group. The resin is then divided into several components and each component is reacted individually by the second building block. This "divide, couple, recombine" strategy is continued until all the building blocks have been added. The resin batches are not combined after the final building blocks have been added. This strategy results in a resin library in which a single compound is attached to an individual bead. When a synthesis is complete, cleavage at the linker releases the molecule(s) from the bead(s). The screening of single beads, or the compounds derived from single beads, corresponds to screening of single compounds. Screening of these libraries can quickly identify the preferred last building block in the most active set. The subset library is then resynthesised by keeping this preferred final building block constant and screened to identify the penultimate preferred building block in each set. This deconvolution process, or iterative re-synthesis and screening, is repeated in order to define all the positions. The deconvolution process has to be repeated each time the library is tested in a new screen. Several different approaches have been investigated to avoid this inconvenient and time-consuming deconvolution method. One of these, using tagging/encoding strategies, involves the introduction of chemical tags at each stage of the "*split-mix*" synthesis either before the addition of each building block during the synthesis or before the subsequent mixing step. At the end of the synthesis any individual bead will possess a compound made up of a single combination of building blocks and an associated tag sequence with a specific tag corresponding to each specific building block. The identity of the compound on a single bead can be determined simply by analysing the tagging sequence. The original tagging methods, oligonucleotides (read by polymerase chain reaction (PCR) amplification and DNA sequencing) and peptides have now been replaced by using binary coding with chemical tags. This tagging strategy increases the number of steps in the synthesis of each library but allows more rapid identification of the active hits.

Library design

The design strategy may vary according to the information available on the target and the purpose of the library. For example, when the class of target is known (for example, an enzyme with a known mechanism of action and/or structural information or a known or similar receptor type/subtype), library design may be started from a known pharmacophore. For example, aspartyl proteinases like renin, HIV and cathepsin D proteases are inhibited by compounds containing a statine residue, a known transition-state analogue. Several libraries based on statine or a hydroxyethylamine core have been prepared and investigated against other aspartyl proteinases. The use of synthetic positional-scanning combinatorial libraries offers the ability to rapidly test and evaluate the extended substrate specificities of proteases. For example, a fluorogenic tetrapeptide positional-scanning library (containing a 7-amino-4-methylcoumarin-derivatised lysine) in which the P_1 amino acid was held constant as a lysine and the P_4-P_3-P_2 positions were positionally randomised was used to investigate extended substrate specificities of plasmin and thrombin, two of the enzymes involved in the blood coagulation cascade. The optimal P_4 to P_2 substrate specificity for plasmin was P_4-Lys/Nle/Val/Ile/Phe, P_3-Xaa, and P_2-Tyr/Phe/Trp. The optimal P_4 to P_2 extended substrate sequence determined for thrombin was P_4-Nle/Leu/Ile/Phe/Val, P_3-Xaa, and P_2-Pro. By three-dimensional structural modelling of the substrates into the active sites of plasmin and thrombin, it was possible to identify potential determinants of the defined substrate specificity. This method is amenable to the incorporation of diverse substituents at the P_1 position (all 20 proteinogenic and other non-proteinogenic amino acids) for exploring molecular recognition elements in various new uncharacterised proteolytic enzymes.

A similar approach can be adopted when a lead ligand has been identified by random screening. The structural template in the lead is modified to generate a targeted library. Many libraries have been synthesised around the so-called "*privileged structures*" which have shown activity against various targets. For example, compounds based on a benzodiazepine core have shown activity against a number of G-protein coupled receptors. However, when there is little information, or when entirely different structural leads are required, a larger diverse library is likely to be more suitable to increase the chance of success. The chemical diversity between the different members of the library is also very important to cover a wide chemical area and increase chances of success. In addition to some simple rules like incorporating acidic, basic, hydrophilic and hydrophobic groups of different sizes, a large number of computer-based methods are available for diversity analysis. Information is also available on the so-called "*drug-like molecules*" that tend to have certain properties. For example, log P, molecular weight, and the number of hydrogen bonding groups have been correlated with oral bioavailability. Analysis of a large number of compounds from the World Drug Index establishment resulted in the "rule of five" based on the assumption that compounds meeting these criteria have entered human clinical trials, and therefore must possess many of the desirable characteristics of drugs. A high percentage of compounds contained ≤ five hydrogen bond donors (expressed as the sum of OHs and NHs), ≤ 10 hydrogen bond acceptors, ≤ 500 relative molecular weight and log P of ≤ 5. Along with these measures, it is also desirable to exclude functional groups that tend to be undesirable because of chemical reactivity for example alkylating and acylating groups, and other unstable groups that lead to metabolism (solvolysis or hydrolysis).

The availability of complex large and diverse chemical libraries and ultra high-throughput screening technologies also provides an option whereby the biological pathways and proteins do not have to be fully characterised before starting the screening process. A number of preselected, incompletely characterised, disease-associated protein targets can be screened against many different libraries. Using the whole-cell systems and libraries containing membrane-permeable compounds, it is possible to identify compounds that perturb a cellular process or system, followed by identification of proteins required in cell function. From the perspective of drug discovery, this approach offers the means for the simultaneous identification of proteins that can serve as targets for therapeutic intervention ("*therapeutic target validation*") and small molecules that can modulate the functions of these therapeutic targets ("*chemical target validation*"). The overall process differs from the traditional methods of drug discovery in which biological methods are first used to select and characterise protein targets for therapeutic intervention, followed by chemical efforts to determine whether the protein target can be modulated by small molecules.

Structure-based Drug Design

The entire process of structure-based drug design requires identification and characterisation of a suitable protein target, determination of the structure of the target protein, the availability of an easy and reliable high-throughput screening assay, identification of a lead compound, development of computer-assisted methods for estimating the affinity of new compounds, and access to a synthetic route to produce the designed compounds. Progress has been made on many of these aspects. For example, expression systems are now available that allow the production of large amounts of naturally occurring proteins and modified proteins like isotope-labelled proteins required for NMR studies and proteins containing residues like selenomethionine (in place of methionine) that simplify determination of *x* ray structure. Advances in automation technologies have resulted in increased synthesis and screening capabilities. From the point of view of design, more important aspects of "*rational design*" strategy involve methods for using the information contained in the three-dimensional structure of a macromolecular target and of related ligand–target complexes, and predicting novel lead compounds. A variety of "docking" programmes now exist that can select from a large database of compounds a subset of molecules that usually includes some compounds that bind to the selected target protein. One such programme, DOCK, systematically attempts to fit each compound from a database into the binding site of the target structure, such that three or more of the atoms in the database molecule overlap with a set of predefined site points in the target binding site. The newer computational methods are aimed at using the information contained in the three-dimensional structure of the unligated target to design entirely new lead compounds *de novo*, as well as to construct large virtual combinatorial libraries of compounds that can be screened computationally (virtual screening) before going to the effort and expense of actually synthesising and testing them.

The *de novo* design of structure-based ligands involves fragment positioning methods, molecule growth methods, and fragment methods coupled to database searches. The fragment positioning methods determine energetically favourable binding site positions for various functional group types or chemical fragments. In the molecule growth methods, a seed atom (or fragment) is first placed in the binding site of the target structure. A ligand molecule is successively built by bonding another atom (or fragment) to it. Fragment positioning methods can also be coupled to database searching techniques either to extract from a database existing molecules that can be docked into the binding site with the desired fragments in their optimal positions or for *de novo* design.

Once a lead compound has been found by some means, an iterative process begins that involves solving the three-dimensional structure of the lead compound bound to the target, examining that structure, characterising the types of interactions the bound ligand makes, and using the computational methods to design improvements to the compound. A large number of examples that demonstrate the utility of this approach exist in the literature. Many inhibitors of enzymes, for example renin, HIV protease and thrombin, have been optimised using this approach.

Virtual screening

The virtual screening strategy involves construction or "synthesis" of molecules on the computer. The number of "synthesised" compounds is limited by synthesising focused libraries (for example, a hydroxamate library of MMP inhibitors) and concentrating on reactions that will work in high yield with reagents that are easily accessible, and incorporating "drug like" properties. Synthetic accessibility can be checked using programs such as computer-aided organic synthesis or computer-aided estimation of synthetic accessibility. As molecules are constructed, a variety of filters are applied to "weed out" compounds that do not meet certain criteria (for example, similarity and diversity analysis, presence of undesirable functional groups, molecular weight and lipophilicity). Once a virtual library has been created and the undesirable compounds removed, the next step is to generate three-dimensional conformations for each molecule. Since most molecules are quite flexible, a multiconformer docking approach is adopted. In this strategy, a set of conformations (typically 10–50) is generated and then each conformer is docked as a rigid molecule into the target enzyme or receptor, which is held fixed throughout. None of the docking approaches can take into account the important conformational changes that take place during the binding process of the ligand to its receptor. Before the three-dimensional conformational analysis, it is useful to get two-dimensional "shape" and "distance" information, to remove molecules that cannot possibly match the active site.

The factors taken into account for searching the virtual library include:

1. Knowledge about compounds that interact with the target, for example substrates, known classes of inhibitors, antagonists and agonists, SAR within various series, pharmacophores deduced from compound classes
2. Knowledge about receptor structure and receptor–ligand interactions, for example homology models, *x* ray and/or NMR structures, thermodynamics of ligand binding, effect of point mutations and dynamic motions of receptor and ligands

3. Knowledge about drugs in general, for example chemical structures and properties of known drugs, rules of conformational analysis and thermodynamics of receptor–ligand interactions.

In the early stages of the project when leads do not exist, computational methods can be used to select a diverse set of compounds from a large virtual library. If a compound shows activity, then other similar compounds from the library are synthesised and tested. If a lead already exists at the start of the programme, the size of the virtual library can be reduced by selecting a subset of compounds that are similar to the lead.

NMR, x ray and mass spectroscopic techniques

As a first step in structure-based design, the three-dimensional structure of the target macromolecule (protein or nucleic acid) is determined by *x* ray crystallography, NMR spectroscopy or homology modelling. Many examples of this type of research are well known in the literature. However, it should be emphasised that even after many cycles of the structure-based design process, when a compound that binds to the target with high affinity has been developed, it is still a long way from being a drug on the market. The compound may still fail in animal and clinical trials because of factors such as toxicity, bioavailability, poor pharmacokinetics (absorption, metabolism and half-life) and lack of efficacy.

In the lead generation phase, NMR methods are first used to detect weak binding of small molecule scaffolds to a target. The binding information is subsequently used to design much tighter binding inhibitors, or drug leads. SAR by NMR was the first NMR screening method disclosed in the literature. This is a fragment-based approach wherein a large library of small molecules is screened using two-dimensional ^{1}H or ^{15}N spectra of the target protein as a readout. From spectral changes one can identify the compounds that bind to the target. After deconvolution and identification of the active compound(s), a second screen of close analogues of the first "hit" is performed to optimise binding affinity to the first subsite. In order to identify small molecules that bind to another site on the target molecule, the screen is then repeated with the first site saturated. If small molecule fragments are identified that occupy several neighbouring subsites, one can then, based on the known structure, synthesise compounds that incorporate the small molecule fragments with various linking groups. If linked effectively, resulting compounds may have affinities for the target that are even stronger than the products of the binding constants of the individual unlinked fragments. As an example of the approach, several small fragments were discovered as ligands for the FK506 binding protein (K_i values 2–9500 μM). Linking these fragments led to more potent compounds like (K_i 49 nM).

The SHAPES strategy technique, like the above methods, relies on monitoring of ligand signals to determine which compounds in a mixture bind a drug target. The method uses standard one-dimensional line broadening and measurements of two-dimensional transferred nuclear Overhauser effect to detect binding of a limited ($<$ 200) but diverse library of soluble low molecular weight scaffolds to a potential drug target. The scaffolds are derived largely from shapes or frameworks, most commonly found in known therapeutic agents, and as such represent approximations to "successful" regions of diversity space. This approach was used to identify p38 inhibitors. In the initial screen, the simple imidazole core did not appear to bind to p38. However, several tethered bicyclic compounds containing an imidazole (or close derivative) and an aryl moiety (pyridyl, phenyl or benzoic acid) exhibited weak binding (200 μM–2 mM). Since imidazole by itself did not bind, it was used as a core to fuse two of the tethered bicyclics or their derivatives, creating tricyclic molecules

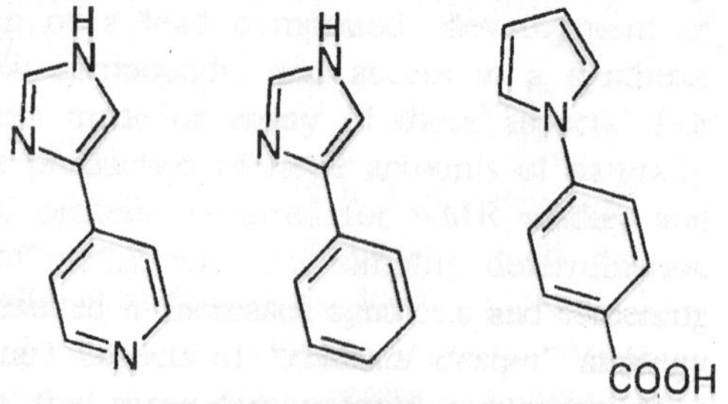

Tethered bicyclic compounds

with aryl derivatives as side chains and the imidazole as the binding core. Two such compounds showed improved binding. Further modifications resulted in more potent trisubstituted imidazoles like (K_i approximately 200 nM in a p38 enzyme assay).

Unlike in the past when *x* ray crystallography was used solely to study the structures of proteins and ligands, the technique is now being incorporated in all aspects of drug discovery, including lead identification, structural assessment, and optimisation. Crystallographic screening methods are being developed that enable experimental "*high-throughput*" sampling of up to thousands of compounds per day. One such technique, CrystaLEAD, has been used to sample large (≥ 10 000) compound libraries and detect ligands by monitoring changes in the electron density map relative to the unbound form. By careful design of the library, the technique leads to identification of the bound molecule from the primary data (electron density map) and eliminates the need for the deconvolution process. The electron density map yields a high-resolution picture of the ligand–protein complex and the resulting information on the ligand–target interactions can be used for structure-directed optimisation. As an example, the method was used for the discovery and optimisation of an orally active series of urokinase inhibitors for the treatment of cancer. The initially identified weaker 5-aminoindole and 2-aminoquinoline leads (K_i values 50–200 μM) were optimised. One of the 2-aminoquinoline inhibitors (K_i 0.37 μM) demonstrated oral bioavailability (38%). The 2-naphthamidine derivative did not show oral bioavailability.

H
N
N
N
NH_2
HN
2-naphthamidine derivative

In addition to its application in drug discovery, crystallographic screening may also be applied in the structural genomics field, where crystal structures become available even in the absence of functional characterisation of the protein. In such cases, the ligands discovered could facilitate target validation, assay development, and the assignment of function.

Pharmacokinetics

The issues related to pharmacokinetics - drug absorption, distribution, metabolism, and excretion (ADME) - have always been important to the success of the drug discovery process. In many cases, not enough attention was paid to these factors in the early stages of the discovery process, leading to failures in the late stages of development. To avoid expensive late-stage failures and to cope with the high-throughput synthesis and screening technologies that result in many hits/leads, efforts are being directed to identify ADME problems at an early stage of the discovery process. It has become common practice to determine cytochrome P450 inhibition, blood levels after intravenous and oral administration, and identification of metabolites at an early stage. Some of this information may be useful in the lead optimisation process so that chemistry can be directed to overcome the problems. Bioavailability studies may be particularly important for evaluating the significance of the *in vivo* biological results, especially, if the results are negative or less convincing. Although ADME studies may be valuable in highlighting the shortcomings of the early hits/leads, these may sometimes result in inappropriate rejection of a lead. In many cases, the physicochemical and toxicological properties of the early hits/leads may be very different to those of the optimised drug candidates.

Examples of Drug Discovery

This section covers the discovery of many of the successful drugs on the market, together with some others which did not make it to the market for various reasons. Although medicinal chemistry along with structural (for example, *x* ray and NMR spectroscopy) and modelling studies has played a major part in all the cases, the starting leads and the final drugs were not always obtained by totally rational design processes. The structure–activity studies in the most relevant *in vitro* and *in vivo* models have played a significant role in converting the initial lead into the final drug that reached the market. Even today, because of the complexities of the drug discovery process, a totally rational approach leading to a marketed drug is not possible. In each of the examples discussed below, chosen to include different design strategies, an attempt has been made to highlight the origins of the starting leads and various rational/semi-rational discovery steps used in the optimisation process. Several interesting points emerge from the examples mentioned below. One of the more interesting and recent developments has been the discovery of non-peptide antagonists and agonists acting at the peptide receptors. Although non-peptide antagonists have been obtained in many cases (for example, ACTH, angiotensin, bradykinin, cholecystokinin, gastrin and LHRH), the agonists have only been obtained in a few cases (for example, angiotensin and bradykinin). These agonist/antagonist discoveries show how small chemical changes can convert an antagonist to an agonist and thus highlight the importance of the screening process.

Receptor Ligands (Agonists and Antagonists)

Early examples

In the past, a number of discoveries have been made in the absence of any knowledge about the receptors or ligands. One of the earliest examples of this kind is morphine which was used for many years as an analgesic (as a constituent of opium, extracted from the poppy plant, *Papaver somniferum*) without any knowledge about its mechanism of action. Only in the last 30 years have various opiate receptor subtypes (for example, μ-, δ-, κ- and σ-receptors) been identified. In addition, endogenous opiate-like peptides, for example enkephalins (Tyr-Gly-Gly-Phe-Met and Tyr-Gly-Gly-Phe-Leu) and endorphins, have been isolated and characterised. Many other opiate-like peptides have been isolated from different species, and enormous number of receptor-selective analogues (agonist and antagonist) have been synthesised in the hope of finding analgesic agents without the side-effects associated with morphine. However, no such compound has yet reached the market. Although there are some reports about peptides acting at the benzodiazepine receptor, the story of morphine and enkephalins is the only example so far where a non-peptide (morphine) acting at a peptide receptor was known before the peptide ligand (enkephalin) was isolated. In all the other examples (described below) the endogenous peptide ligand was isolated first from natural sources and the non-peptide ligands were obtained later by random screening or semi-rational approaches.

Another example of drug discovery without much knowledge of the receptor or the ligand is the discovery of benzodiazepines initially obtained by random (*in vivo*) screening of compounds for anxiolytic activity. The compounds were later found to act as modulators of γ-aminobutyric acid (GABA) at its receptor. Many years later, the discovery and characterisation of benzodiazepine receptors from brain tissue led to the development of *in vitro* receptor binding assays and drugs like diazepam. In a similar manner, histamine had been recognised as a chemical messenger and was shown to stimulate gastic acid secretion many years before the discovery of its receptors. Discovery of antihistamine compounds resulted in the classification of three receptor subtypes (H_1, H_2 and H_3). Histamine acting via H_1 receptors causes contraction in some smooth muscles (for example, in the gut, the uterus and the bronchi) and relaxation in other smooth muscles (for example, in some blood vessels), causing hypotension. Physiologically, histamine plays a role in regulating the secretion of gastric acid by stimulating the parietal cells to produce the acid. This effect is mediated by H_2 receptors. The role of the H_3 receptor is less well defined. Extensive work on antihistamine compounds has resulted in many successful drugs like fexofenadine, cimetidine and ranitidine.

In many cases, including the adrenergic receptors, the nature of the ligand/transmitter (dopamine R1 = R2 = H; epinephrine [adrenaline] R1 = OH, R2 = Me; norepinephrine [noradrenaline] R1 = OH, R2 = H) was known before starting the drug discovery programmes. The availability of many synthetic analogues led to receptor classification (α- and β-adrenergic receptors and other subtypes) and selective ligands. Many of these, for example salbutamol (a β_2-selective agonist used as a bronchodilator for the treatment of asthma), propranolol (a non-selective β-antagonist) and atenolol (a selective β_1-antagonist) both used in the treatment of angina and hypertension, have been successful drugs.

Selective oestrogen receptor modulators (oestrogen antagonists and aromatase inhibitors)

Another example of drug discovery in the absence of any significant knowledge about the receptors has been the discovery of selective oestrogen receptor modulators. Like the above examples, the structures of the ligands were known and were utilised, in some cases, for the discovery of drugs now on the market. The discovery of selective oestrogen receptor modulators (agonists and antagonists) highlights the impact of developing science in any area of drug discovery as new information emerges and new indications become obvious. In the case of oestrogens, over the years it has become clear that oestrogen is important not only in the growth, differentiation and function of tissues of the reproductive system but also plays an important role in maintaining bone density and protecting against osteoporosis. It also has beneficial effects in the cardiovascular (cardioprotective) and central nervous systems (protecting against Alzheimer's disease). In addition, the two isoforms of oestrogen receptor (ERα and ERβ) belonging to a family of nuclear hormone receptors that function as transcription factors on binding to their respective ligands have been identified. Thus tissue-selective oestrogen receptor modulators ranging from full agonist activity to pure antioestrogenic activity may be useful in the treatment and prevention of osteoporosis, treatment of breast cancer, and may reduce the risk of cardiovascular disease and Alzheimer's disease.

Tamoxifen, a non-steroidal anti-oestrogen, demonstrates antiproliferative effects in the breast and is widely used for the treatment of breast cancer. However, it does not show antioestrogenic properties in all tissues. For example, tamoxifen acts as an agonist on bone, liver and the endometrium. This mixed antagonist/agonist profile leads to many advantages in cancer patients. As an antagonist, tamoxifen prevents oestrogen-induced proliferation of breast ductal epithelium and breast cancer, and as an agonist in bone and liver it prevents bone loss in postmenopausal women and reduces cholesterol levels. However, the oestrogenic effects in the endometrium in postmenopausal women can result in an increased risk of endometrial cancer. Many other tamoxifen analogues, for example toremifene and droloxifene, show similar selectivity profiles. An orally active prodrug of the benzopyrene derivative (EM-652) showed a similar agonist/antagonist profile but with more antagonistic effects in the uterus. The activity of raloxifene is also similar to that of tamoxifen, except on the endometrium where it possesses less agonist activity. In comparison with the above mixed agonist/antagonist compounds, the steroidal anti-oestrogen Faslodex (ICI-182780) demonstrates a pure antioestrogenic profile in all tissues.

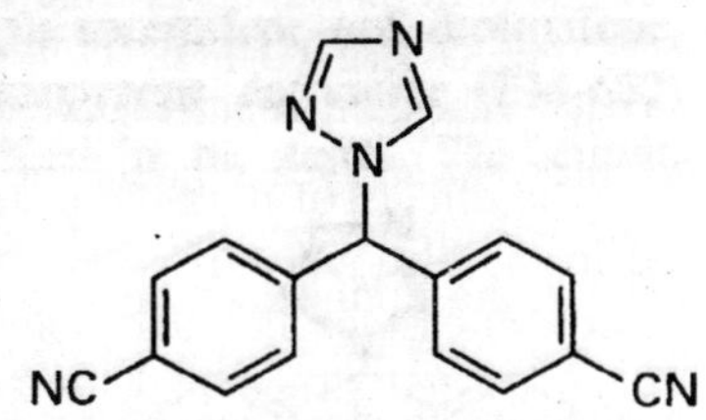

N N N NC CN

Letrozole

As an alternative to blocking the actions of oestrogen with compounds like tamoxifen, similar biological/clinical effects can be obtained by inhibiting aromatase, the enzyme that catalyses the final and rate-limiting step in oestrogen synthesis (conversion of androgens into oestrogens). Steroidal compounds such as formestane and exemestane, that are structurally related to the natural substrate of aromatase, and non-steroidal compounds such as for example anastrozole, letrozole, fadrozole and vorozole have been developed as aromatase inhibitors. Many of these are currently in use for the treatment of breast cancer.

LHRH agonists and antagonists

In more recent times, efforts have been directed towards finding receptor agonists and antagonists acting at the peptidergic receptors. In most of these cases (including LHRH), naturally occurring ligands were first isolated from various animal species, including humans, and crude receptor preparations were then used to screen for other agonist and antagonist ligands. Extensive structure–activity studies are carried out to identify the regions responsible for binding to the receptor and intrinsic activity. In general, SAR studies involve the synthesis of a large number of analogues by carrying out deletion studies (eliminating one or more amino acids from the chain), amino acid replacements with natural and unnatural amino acids, peptide bond replacements, and synthesis of conformationally restricting cyclic peptides. These studies are often followed by conformational studies using various spectroscopy and modelling techniques. Based on the results, further modifications are carried out in a semi-rational manner to obtain compounds with the desired properties.

LHRH [Pyr-His-Trp-Ser-Tyr-Gly-Leu-Arg-Pro-Gly-NH_2] is secreted from the hypothalamus and its action on the pituitary gland leads to the release of luteinising hormone and follicle stimulating hormone. Both of these hormones then act on the ovaries and testes and are responsible for the release of steroidal hormones. Early studies indicated that chronic administration of potent LHRH agonist analogues leads to tachyphylaxis or desensitisation of the pituitary receptors, leading ultimately to a suppression (not stimulation) of oestrogen and testosterone. This finding has led to the use of potent LHRH agonists in the treatment of hormone-dependent tumours. The LHRH antagonists are also expected to be useful for the treatment of these tumours but progress in the antagonist field has been relatively slow. Potent antagonists have been obtained by multiple amino acid substitutions in various positions of the LHRH molecule and a number of the best antagonists have between five and seven amino acid residues replaced by unnatural amino acids. These combinations of multiple substitutions were arrived at in a stepwise manner starting from the first antagonist, [des-His^2]-LHRH. Some antagonists like Abarelix [Ac-D-Nal(2)-D-Phe(p-Cl) -D-Pal(3) -Ser-MeTyr-D-Asn-Leu-Lys (å-isopropyl)-Pro-D-Ala-NH_2] and Ganirelix [Ac-D-Nal(2)-D-Phe (p-Cl)-D-Pal(3)-Ser-Tyr-D-hArg(Et_2)-Leu-hArg(Et_2)-Pro-D-Ala-NH_2] are currently in development for various indications, including as antitumour agents.

For the discovery of potent LHRH agonist and antagonist analogues, a large number of analogues were synthesised by incorporating amino acid changes in single and multiple positions. The most important SAR findings that led to these compounds were:

1. Replacement of the C-terminal glycinamide residue (-$NHCH_2CONH_2$) by a number of alkyl amide (-NH-R) or aza-amino acid amide residues (-NH-N(R)-$CONH_2$), which resulted in a 2–3-fold improvement in potency
2. Substitution of the glycine residue in position 6 by D amino acid residues [for example, D-Ala, D-Leu, D-Arg, D-Phe, D-Trp, D-Ser(Bu^t)], which led to a 2–100-fold improvement in potency
3. A combination of D amino acids in position 6 and an ethylamide or azaglycine amide.

The effects of multiple changes were not always additive. A combination of many of these changes led to the discovery of potent agonists which are currently on the market for the treatment of prostate cancer, breast cancer and some non-malignant conditions such as endometriosis and uterine fibroids. The marketed drugs include Zoladex {[D-Ser(Bu^t)^6, Azgly^{10}]-LHRH} Leuprolide {[D-Leu^6, des-Gly-NH_2^{10}]-LHRH(1-9)NHEt}, Nafarelin {D-Nal(2)^6]-LHRH}, Buserelin {[D-Ser(Bu^t)^6, des-Gly-NH_2^{10}]-LHRH(1-9)NHEt} and Triptorelin { [D-Trp^6]-LHRH}.

The potential of LHRH agonists in human medicine has been greatly enhanced by the development of convenient formulations for the delivery of these peptides. The most successful of these have been the biodegradable poly(d,l-lactide-co-glycolide) depot formulations which release the drug over a period of 1–3 months. A biodegradable poly(d,l-lactide-co-glycolide) sustained-release formulation of Zoladex can deliver 3.6–10.5 mg of the peptide over a period of 1–3 months. The formulation consists of a homogeneous dispersion of the drug (20% w/w) in a rod of the polymer and is administered by subcutaneous injection. Non-peptide antagonists of LHRH were discovered by directed or random screening approaches. A directed screening approach based on the Tyr-Gly-Leu-Arg region of LHRH followed by further medicinal chemistry on a weak lead gave a potent antagonist (T-98475). In binding assays (cloned human receptors and membrane fractions of monkey and rat pituitaries), was as potent as [D-Leu^6, Pro-NHEt] -LHRH. Oral administration of T-98475 (60 mg/kg) to castrated male cynomolgus monkeys resulted in >70% inhibition of plasma LH levels 8 hours after administration of the compound. Medicinal chemistry based on another series of weak non-peptide antagonist leads, discovered by screening the company collection for binding affinity to the rat gonadotrophin releasing hormone (GnRH) receptor, led to a potent compound that demonstrated an IC_{50} of 32 nM in the same binding assay.

Somatostatin agonists and antagonists

The cyclic peptide somatostatin [Ala-Gly-Cys-Lys-Asn-Phe-Phe-Trp-Lys-Thr-Phe-Thr-Ser-Cys, disulphide bridge between Cys^3 and Cys^{14}] and the 28 amino acid precursor containing 14 additional amino acid residues (Ser-Ala-Asn-Ser-Asn-Pro-Ala-Met-Ala-Pro-Arg-Glu-Arg-Lys) at the N-terminus were isolated from extracts of ovine and porcine hypothalamus, respectively. Both peptides are associated with a large number of biological activities, including inhibition of the secretion of growth hormone, insulin, glucagon and gastric acid. Thus, somatostatin may play an important role in many physiological and pharmacological systems. Five human receptor subtypes ($hSSTR_1$–$hSSTR_5$) for somatostatin have been characterised. A large number of analogues have been synthesised in the hope of finding drugs for various diseases. Examples of compounds which have reached the market include octreotide [sandostatin, D-Phe-cyclo(Cys-Phe-D-Trp-Lys-Thr-Cys)-Thr-ol], lanreotide [D-Nal-cyclo(Cys-Tyr-D-Trp-Lys-Val-Cys)-Thr-NH_2 and vapreotide (RC-160) [D-Phe-cyclo(Cys-Tyr-D-Trp-Lys-Val-Cys)-Trp-NH_2]. Daily and slow-release depot formulations of octreotide have been used for the treatment of growth-hormone secreting pituitary tumours, thyrotropin-secreting pituitary adenomas, pancreatic islet cell tumours and carcinoid tumours that express somatostatin receptors. A long-acting formulation of octreotide administered to acromegalic patients for 18 months (once every 4 weeks) suppressed growth hormone and insulin-like growth factor levels in all patients, and signs and symptoms of acromegaly improved during treatment. Reduction of the pituitary tumour was seen in all previously untreated patients.

Progress towards developing small cyclic peptides that are equipotent or more potent than somatostatin was made in several steps. Early SAR established that the Ala^1-Gly^2 residues and the disulphide bridge were not essential for biological activity. Amino acid substitution studies indicated that replacements of Lys^4 by Arg, Phe, Phe(F_5) or Phe(p-NH_2) residues, Asn^5 by Ala or D-Tyr, Phe^7 by Tyr, Trp^8 by D-Trp, D-Trp(5-F), D-Trp (6-F), D-Trp(5-Br), Phe^{11} by Phe(p-I) or Nal(2) and Cys^{14} by D-Cys gave compounds that were either equipotent or more potent than the parent peptide. Amino acid substitutions in other positions gave less potent analogues. For example, most of the analogues obtained by substituting the Phe^6 and Phe^7 residues, except by other aromatic amino acids like Phe (p-Cl), Phe(p-I) and Tyr, were less potent (<10%) than somatostatin. Deletion of the C-terminal carboxyl group or its replacement by an ethylamide group also resulted in compounds equipotent to somatostatin. An equally important finding, useful in designing smaller peptides, emerged by deleting various amino acid residues. Compounds lacking Lys^4 and Asn^5 were found to retain significant biological activity whereas the compounds lacking Phe^6, Trp^8, Lys^9, Thr^{10}, Phe^{11}, Thr^{12} were relatively poor agonists. The deletion and substitution studies led to much smaller peptides like cyclo(Aha-Phe-Phe-D-Trp-Lys-Thr-Phe), cyclo(Pro-Phe-D-Trp-Lys-Thr-Phe) and cyclo(Pro-Phe-D-Trp-Lys-Val-Phe). The most potent analogue, cyclo(MeAla-Tyr-D-Trp-Lys-Val-Phe) was 20–50-fold more potent than somatostatin in inhibiting growth hormone, 70 times more potent in inhibiting insulin and >80 times more potent in inhibiting glucagon. Other more potent cyclic peptides containing disulphide bridges, D-Phe-Cys-Phe-D-Trp-Lys-Thr-Cys-Thr(ol), D-Phe-Cys-Tyr-D-Trp-Lys-Val-Cys-Thr-NH_2, D-Phe-Cys-Tyr-D-Trp-Lys-Val-Cys-Trp-NH_2 and D-Phe-Cys-Tyr-D-Trp-Lys-Val-Cys-Thr-NH_2, were 8 0–200 times more potent than somatostatin. Since the discovery and availability of cloned multiple receptors, additional SAR studies have led to agonist and antagonist analogues that are selective for different receptors. For example, the cyclic peptide Cys-Lys-Phe-Phe-D-Trp-Phe(p-CH_2NH-CH$(CH_3)_2$-Thr-Phe-Thr-Ser-Cys with a disulphide bridge is a potent agonist at human $SSTR_1$ receptors and the N(α-Me)benzylglycine-containing analogue cyclo [(R)-βMeNphe-Phe-D-Trp-Lys-Thr-Phe] is an $hSSTR_2$-selective agonist. The $hSSTR_2$-agonist selectively inhibited the release of growth hormone in rats (equipotent to sandostatin) but had no effect on the inhibition of insulin at the same dose. Cyclo(Phe(N-aminoethyl)-Tyr-D-Trp-Lys-Val-Phe(N-carboxypropyl)-Thr-NH_2 (PTR 3046) a backbone-cyclic somatostatin analogue, and the lanthionine octapeptide displayed high selectivity for the $SSTR_5$ receptor.

In comparison with the agonist analogues, very few antagonists of somatostatin have been obtained by amino acid substitution. Two octapeptide derivatives, 4-NO_2-Phe-c(D-Cys-Tyr-D-Trp-Lys-Thr-Cys)-Tyr-NH_2 and Ac-4-NO_2-Phe-c(D-Cys-Tyr-D-Trp-Lys-Thr-Cys)-D-Tyr-NH_2 (inactive at the SST_1 and SST_4 receptor subtypes; high affinity for the $SSTR_2$ and $SSTR_5$ receptor subtypes) inhibited somatostatin-mediated inhibition of cAMP accumulation in a dose-dependent manner. The more potent antagonist, Ac-4-NO_2-Phe-c(D-Cys-Tyr-D-Trp-Lys-Thr-Cys)-D-Tyr-NH_2], displays a binding affinity to $SSTR_2$ comparable with that observed for the native hormone. H-Nal-c [D-Cys-Pal-D-Trp-Lys-Val-Cys]-Nal-NH_2 was also a more selective $hSSTR_2$ antagonist.

Angiotensin agonists and antagonists (peptides and non-peptides)

Angiotensin II and other members of the angiotensin family are produced by the processing of a protein called α_2-globulin or angiotensinogen, which is synthesised in the liver and found in the blood. The protein is first cleaved by the enzyme renin to generate a decapeptide called angiotensin I (Asp-Arg-Val-Tyr-Ile-His-Pro-Phe-His-Leu), which is further cleaved by ACE to produce the octapeptide angiotensin II [Asp^1-Arg-Val-Tyr-Ile-His-Pro-Phe^8], which is a potent vasoconstrictor. Angiotensin II acts at two receptor subtypes (AT_1 and AT_2). In the case of the agonist analogues, one of the most significant changes has been the replacement of the N-terminal Asp by Sar (N-methylglycine) to give [Sar^1]-angiotensin II, which in a number of *in vitro* tissue preparations was 1.5–2.5 times more potent than the natural ligand. AT_2-receptor selective analogues were obtained by modifications at the N-and C-termini of the peptide. The N-terminally modified compounds, [Me_2Gly^1]-, [Me_3Gly^1] - and [Me_3Ser^1] -angiotensin II, were > 1000-fold more potent at the AT_2 receptor. The analogue modified at positions 1 and 8, [Sar^1, Phe^8] -angiotensin II was 345-fold more potent than angiotensin II at the AT_2 receptor. Modifications of the C-terminal dipeptide (Pro^7-Phe^8) of [Sar^1, Val^5] angiotensin II with constrained aromatic (Tic) and hydrophobic (Oic) amino acids led to analogues with negligible affinity for the AT_1 receptor, but nanomolar affinity for the AT_2 receptor. The most potent and AT_2-selective analogue of the series was Sar-Arg-Val-Tyr-Val-His-Phe-Oic (IC_{50} values of 240 and 0·51 nM, at the AT_1 and AT_2 receptors, respectively).

A conformationally restricted analogue of angiotensin II, [$hCys^3$, $hCys^5$] - angiotensin II, was equipotent to angiotensin II in displacing [^{125}I]-angiotensin II from rat uterus membranes and in inducing contractions in the rabbit aortic rings (pD_2 8·48). Conformational analysis studies indicated that the cyclic peptide-like analogues {for example, c[$hCys^{3,5}$]-angiotensin II} may assume an inverse γ-turn conformation; thus, the amino acid residues 3–5 in angiotensin II were substituted with residues that induce different turns. Most of the analogues were either inactive or much less potent than angiotensin II. However, one of the analogues exhibited AT_1 receptor affinity (K_i 750 nM). A close analogue of containing a nine-membered ring in place of the central ten-membered ring was not active up to a concentration of 10 μM. This example illustrates one of the major difficulties in the synthesis of conformationally restricted analogues: even very small chemical changes lead to relatively large conformational changes and the resulting compounds are usually inactive. Such compounds do not provide much help in the design process. Antagonists of angiotensin II were initially obtained by eliminating the side chain from the C-terminal phenylalanine residue. Antagonists like [Gly^8] -angiotensin II, which competitively blocks the myotropic action of both angiotensin I and angiotensin II in *in vitro* test systems but did not antagonise the pressor response to angiotensin II in anaesthetised cats, were further modified in position 8 to give more potent antagonists, for example [Ile^8] -angiotensin II. A combination of positions 5 and 8 changes along with the N-terminal changes (Sar^1) discovered in the case of agonist series of compounds gave more potent antagonists like [Sar^1, Ala^8]-angiotensin II, [Sar^1, Ile^8] -angiotensin II (pA_2 9.48) and [Sar^1, Pen(SMe)^5, Ile^8]-angiotensin II. [Sar^1, Thr(Me)^5, Ile^8]-, [Sar^1, β-MePhe^5, Ile^8]- and [Sar^1, His^5, Ile^8]-angiotensin II were more potent than [Sar^1, Ile^8]-angiotensin II in the *in vivo* rat blood pressure test. In the cyclic series of antagonists many other cyclic compounds (except [Sar^1, hCys^3, hCys^5, Ile^8]-angiotensin II), for example [Cys^{1,5}, Ile^8] -, [D-Cys^1, Cys^5, Ile^8] -, [Sar^1, Cys^{5,8}]-, [Sar^1, Cys^5, D-Cys^8]- and [Sar^1, hCys^5, D-Cys^8]-angiotensin II, were much less potent.

Non-peptide antagonists of angiotensin II were obtained by random screening approaches. Despite all the progress achieved in discovering potent agonist and antagonist analogues and the information about ligand–receptor interactions derived from the above compounds, it was not possible to design non-peptidic molecules by this rational design procedure. The discovery from a random screening lead of DuP753 (losartan), which is selective for AT_1, opened the way to non-peptide antagonists. The SAR studies indicated that a considerable variation was allowed in the chemical structure of the antagonists. The synthetic medicinal chemistry approaches identified various replacements for the imidazole and the biphenyl tetrazole groups and highlighted chemical changes that led to AT_1- or AT_2-selective or mixed (AT_1 and AT_2) receptor antagonists. Compound (L-162,389) is an example of a mixed antagonist (AT_1 and AT_2 binding affinities of 2–4 nM). In a macrocyclic series of analogues, bound primarily to the AT_1 receptor (AT_1 and AT_2 receptor IC_{50} values 23 nM and 4000 nM, respectively) whereas a very similar analogue bound to both the receptors with similar affinity (IC_{50} 20–30 nM). Another interesting aspect of the non-peptide agonist/antagonist SAR studies has been the identification of both agonists and antagonists in the same series of compounds by minor structural

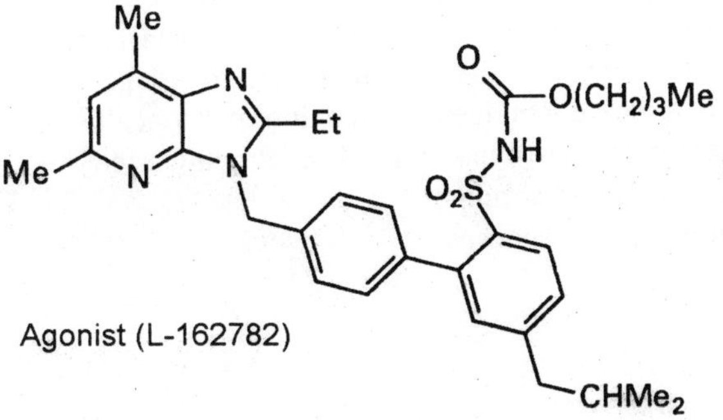

Agonist (L-162782)

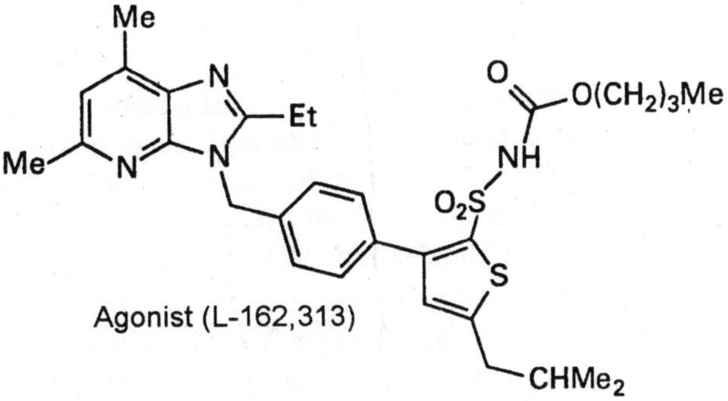

Agonist (L-162,313)

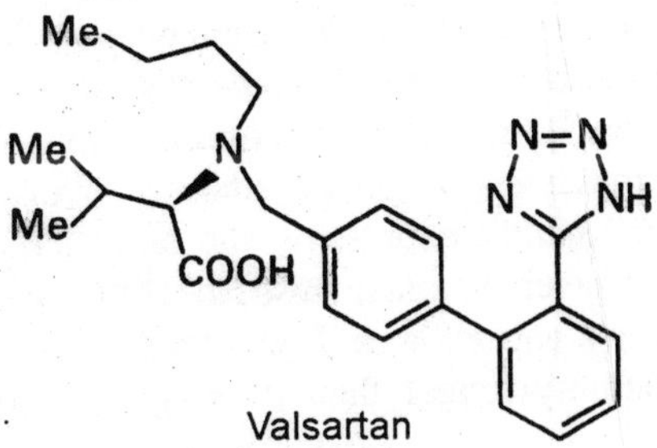

Valsartan

modifications. For example, compound (L-162782) is an agonist whereas a similar analogue that differs chemically by only a single methyl group (L-162,389) is an antagonist. Another close analogue (L-162,313) also displayed agonist activity. At present, it is not possible to predict changes that lead to agonist/antagonist analogues by any rational design approaches. Only by screening the compounds in appropriate tests can selective compounds with the desired biological profile be identified. A large amount of chemical effort in the angiotensin antagonist field has led to the discovery of many successful drugs like losartan, valsartan, candesartan, ibresartan and eprosartan for the treatment of high blood pressure and other cardiovascular complications.

Bombesin/neuromedin agonists and antagonists

Four subtypes of the bombesin receptor have been identified (gastrin-releasing peptide [GRP] receptor, neuromedin B receptor, the orphan receptor bombesin receptor subtype 3 and bombesin receptor subtype 4). The roles of individual receptor subtypes are under investigation and selective ligands for these receptor subtypes are being synthesised. Systematic SAR studies have provided many receptor antagonists. A semi-rational approach was used for the discovery of non-peptide antagonists of neuromedin B. The role of each amino acid side chain was defined by alanine scanning in bombesin(7-14)-octapeptide, Ac-Gln-Trp-Ala-Val-Gly-His-Leu-Met-NH_2 (minimum active fragment), and indicated that Trp^8, Val^{10} and Leu^{13} were most important for the binding affinity to the receptors. A search within the company's compound collection was then initiated for various templates containing Trp, Val/Leu types of side chains. This led to a moderately active lead. Changes at the C-terminus led to more potent (S) α-methyl-Trp derivative. Additional chemical modifications on resulted in a series of "balanced" neuromedin-B preferring (BB_1)/GRP preferring (BB_2) receptor ligands, as exemplified by PD 176252. Compound displays a BB_2 receptor affinity of 1 nM whilst retaining subnanomolar (0·17 nM) BB_1 receptor affinity and is a competitive antagonist at both receptor subtypes.

Bradykinin agonists and antagonists

Peptide SAR studies resulted in potent bradykinin B_2 receptor antagonists like HOE 140 D-Arg-Arg-Pro-Hyp-Gly-Thi-Ser-D-Tic-Oic-Arg. Replacement of some of the amino acids by substituted 1,3,8-triazaspiro[4,5]decan-4-one-3-acetic acids in the B_2 receptor antagonist D-Arg-Arg-Pro-Pro-Gly-Phe-Ser-D-Tic-Oic-Arg gave potent B_2 receptor antagonists like compound (NPC 18521, K_i 0·15 nM) which contains a phenethyl group at position 1 of the spirocyclic mimetic. Another example of a pseudopeptide analogue is compound NPC 18884, which contains three arginine residues. Given intraperitoneally or orally, compound inhibited bradykinin-induced leukocyte influx and exudation. The effects lasted for up to 4 hours and were selective for the bradykinin B_2 receptors. At similar doses compound had no significant effect against the inflammatory responses induced by des-Arg^9-bradykinin, histamine or substance P.

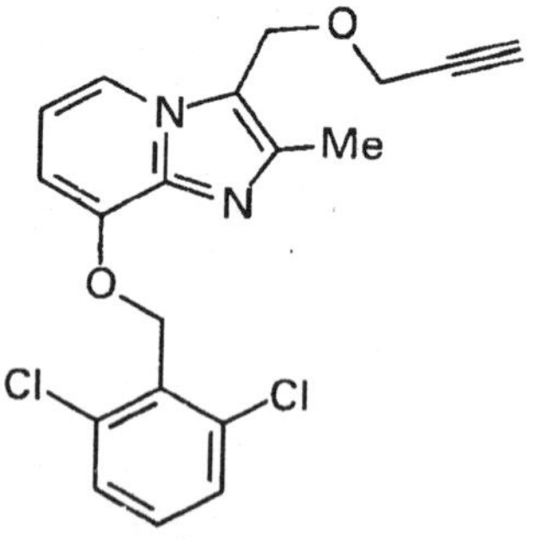

Non-peptide B_2 receptor antagonists and agonists of bradykinin were obtained by random screening approaches. Chemical modifications on a random screening lead led to the non-peptide antagonist, which was active in a number of *in vitro* and *in vivo* test systems (for example, bradykinin-induced bronchoconstriction and carrageenin-induced paw oedema). The non-peptide agonist bound with high affinity to the B_2 receptor (IC_{50} 5·3 nM) but had no binding affinity for the B_1 receptor; at concentrations between 1 nM and 1 μM compound stimulated phosphatidylinositol hydrolysis in Chinese hamster ovary cells permanently expressing the human bradykinin B_2 receptor. The response was antagonised by the B_2 receptor selective antagonist Hoe 140. Intravenous administration of bradykinin or the agonist (both at 10 μg/kg) caused a fall in blood pressure. However, the duration of the hypotensive response was significantly longer than the response to bradykinin.

Lead

Cholecystokinin agonists and antagonists

Peptidomimetic agonist and antagonist analogues of cholecystokinin (CCK) were obtained from the C-terminal tetrapeptide of CCK/gastrin (Boc-Trp-Met-Asp-Phe-NH_2) and analogues like Boc-Trp-MeNle-Asp-Phe-NH_2 and by synthesising conformationally constrained analogues by replacing the Trp-Met/Trp-MeNle dipeptides. The diketopiperazine derivative and the constrained cyclic pseudopeptide CCK_B agonist [(*S*) at the α-carbon of the aminononane moiety (CCK_A/CCK_B = 147)] exhibited full CCK_B receptor agonist properties, and increased gastric acid secretion in anaesthetised rats.

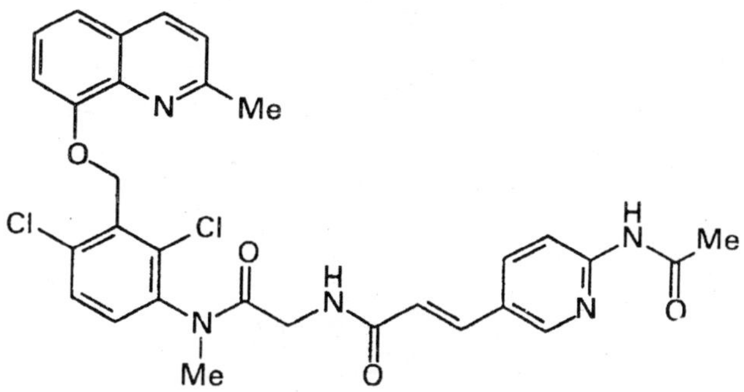

FR173657; antagonist

Non-peptide CCK agonists and antagonists based on a benzodiazepine skeleton were obtained by random screening and lead optimisation. 1,5-Benzodiazepine derivatives were shown to be agonists and antagonists of CCK_A and CCK_B. The substitution pattern at the anilinoacetamide nitrogen played an important role for the activity. While compounds with a hydrogen or methyl substituent were weak antagonists of CCK-8, the ethyl, propyl, *n*-butyl and cyanoethyl derivatives were agonists. Compound displayed 86% CCK-8 functional activity in the guinea-pig gallbladder assay at 30 μM (CCK-8 = 100% at 1 μM) and showed similar affinity for CCK_A and CCK_B receptors. When given orally to rats, the CCK_A agonist (GW5823) reduced food intake to 40% of that in vehicle-control treated animals. When administered orally, the CCK_B/gastrin antagonist YF476 inhibited gastic acid secretion in a pentagastrin-induced acid secretion model and displayed a long duration of action (> 6 hours at a dose of 100 nmol/kg). In addition to the benzodiazepine derivatives, a number of other chemically distinct CCK antagonists have been prepared starting from the random screening leads. The nine-membered ring analogue was a potent CCK_B/gastrin antagonist (rat stomach pK_B 9·08, mouse cortex pIC_{50} 8·3). In comparison, the analogues containing six-, seven- and eight-membered rings were poor CCK_B/gastrin receptor antagonists.

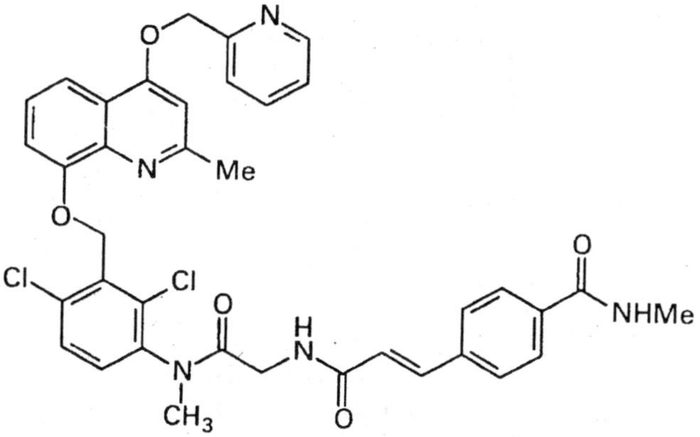

FR190997; agonist

Endothelin antagonists

Endothelin is one of the most potent vasoconstrictor peptides. Antagonists of this peptide are being sought for various cardiovascular disorders. Leads for antagonist design have originated from natural sources, rational design approaches and by random screening. ET_A and ET_B receptor selective antagonists were obtained from cyclic pentapeptides of microbial origin like the ET_A-selective peptide BQ 123 [c(D-Val-Leu-D-Trp-D-Asp-Pro)]. Linear tripeptide derivatives were subsequently developed as ET_A [BQ-485] or ET_B [BQ-788 and BQ-017] receptor selective or non-selective [BQ-928] antagonists. In the BQ-123 series, amino acid replacements converted the ET_A selective antagonist BQ-123 to ET_B selective and non-selective antagonists. For example, c(D-*t*-Leu-Leu-2-chloro-D-Trp-D-Asp-Pro) and

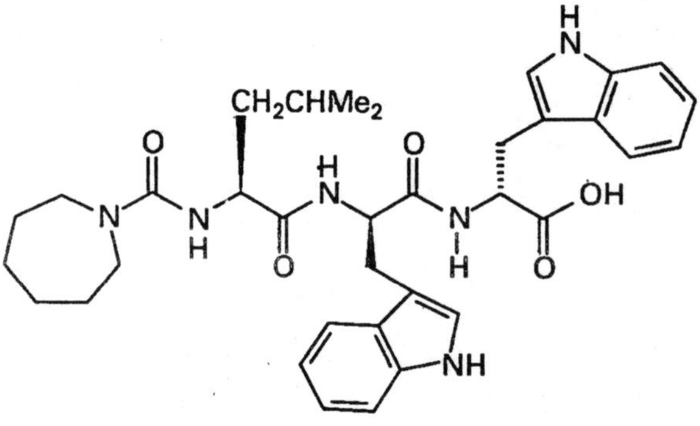

BQ-485

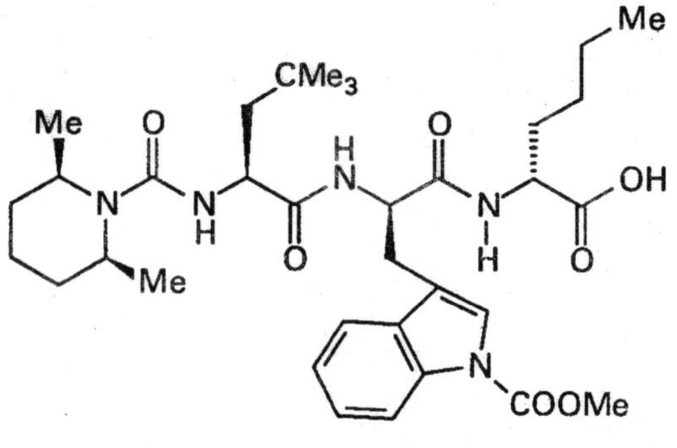

BQ-788

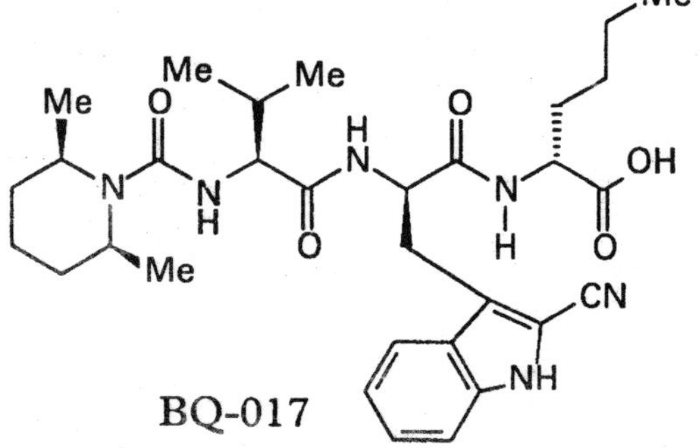

BQ-017

c(D-Pen(Me)-Leu-2- bromo-D-Trp-D-Asp-Pro) were nearly equipotent at both the receptors whereas c(D-Pen(Me)-Leu-2-cyano-D-Trp-D-Asp-Pro) was much more potent at the ET_B receptor. In the *cis*-(2,6-dimethylpiperidino)carbonyl-Leu-D-Trp-D-Nle series of analogues, the 2-bromo-D-Trp, 2-chloro-D-Trp and 2-methyl-D-Trp analogues were potent antagonists at both receptors whereas the 2-cyano-D-Trp and 2-ethyl-D-Trp analogues were more potent at the ET_B receptor.

Antagonists were also discovered using a rational approach starting from the endothelin C-terminal dodecapeptide derivative, succinyl-Glu-Ala-Val-Tyr-Phe-Ala-His-Leu-Asp-Ile-Ile-Trp. Replacing each amino acid in turn with glycine indicated that Phe^{14}, $Ile^{19,20}$ and Trp^{21} were the most important residues. Based on this evidence, a series of compounds with an aromatic moiety attached through a spacer to the amino group of the Trp residue were synthesised. Further work around the initial weak antagonist lead, N-*trans*-2-phenylcyclopropanoyl-Trp, resulted in a 400-fold selective ET_B antagonist. Replacement of the biphenylalanine residue by 2-naphthylalanine, Met, Leu, Ile, Cha, Thr or ethylglycine gave antagonists that were 2–4-fold more potent at the ET_B receptor. The D-Phe-Val derivative displayed similar affinity for ET_A and ET_B receptors (K_i 1–2 nM).

Non-peptide antagonists of endothelin were discovered by random screening approaches. A comparison of compounds demonstrates that it is possible to obtain selective and non-selective compounds in the same series by chemical modifications. Carboxyindoline derivative was about 100-fold more selective antagonist for the ET_A receptor was a non-selective antagonist. Another series of ET_A-selective antagonists included a more selective (> 25000-fold) pyrrolidine carboxylic acid derivative, A-216546. A-216546 was orally available in rat, dog and monkey, and blocked the endothelin-1-induced presser response in the conscious rats. Replacement of the dialkylacetamide side chain in compound resulted in a complete reversal of receptor selectivity, preferring ET_B over ET_A. Compound (A-308165) demonstrated greater than 27000-fold selectivity favouring the ET_B receptor.

Enzyme Inhibitors

Converting Enzyme Inhibitors

Many biologically active peptides are obtained from their precursors by the actions of converting enzymes (zinc metallopeptidases). For example, ACE cleaves a dipeptide from the C-terminus of angiotensin I to generate the pressor peptide angiotensin II. In addition, some of the biologically active peptides (for example, bradykinin, atrial natriuretic peptide (ANP) and enkephalins) are degraded by the converting enzymes into inactive fragments. These enzymes are important in controlling many physiological and pathological processes. In the case of peptides that, in some pathological conditions, produce undesirable effects (for example, vasoconstriction in the case of angiotensin II and endothelin), it is beneficial to prevent the formation of such peptides from their precursors by inhibiting the enzymes involved in the process (for example, ACE and endothelin converting enzyme). On the other hand, in the case of peptides that produce therapeutically beneficial effects (for example, enkephalins and atrial natriuretic factor; ANF), inhibiting the enzymes that inactivate these peptides (for example, enkephalinase and atriopeptidase) is likely to increase the biological half-life of the peptide and thus extend the duration of action. From the point of view of drug discovery, ACE inhibitors, which prevent the formation of a pressor peptide angiotensin II, have been the most successful examples. From the point of view of medicinal chemistry, lessons learned from the ACE story have been very useful in the design of inhibitors of many other metalloproteinases like enkephalinase, atriopeptidase and MMPs.

ACE (peptidyl dipeptidase), known to catalyse the hydrolysis of dipeptides from the C-terminus of polypeptides, belongs to a family of zinc metalloproteinases, which require a zinc atom in the active site. In these enzymes a combination of three His, Glu, Asp or Cys residues creates a zinc binding site. The first major step in the discovery of ACE inhibitors was the isolation of bradykinin-potentiating peptides like $BPP5_a$ (Pyr-Lys-Trp-Ala-Pro) and SQ 20881 (Pyr-Trp-Pro-Arg-Pro-Gln-Ile-Pro-Pro) from the venoms of the Brazilian snake, *Bothrops jaraca* and the Japanese snake, *Agkistrodon halys blomhoffii*. SAR studies on these peptides indicated that a number of pentapeptide analogues of $BPP5_a$, for example Pyr-Lys-Phe-Ala-Pro, were equipotent to the parent peptide in inhibiting ACE. However, smaller di- or tri-peptides, for example Gly-Trp, Val-Trp, Ile-Trp, Phe-Ala-Pro and Lys-Trp-Ala-Pro, were less potent. Although SQ 20881 was studied extensively in the clinic, it could not be used as a drug because of a lack of oral activity. Progress towards the orally active ACE inhibitors was made after the discovery of D-benzylsuccinic acid as an inhibitor of another zinc metalloprotease, carboxypeptidase A. This led to the synthesis of proline derivatives by combining the features present in venom peptides and benzylsuccinic acid. One of the early compounds, succinylproline, was only a weak inhibitor of ACE (approximately 150-fold less potent than SQ 20881). Further modifications in this series led to 2-D-methylsuccinyl-proline and 2-D-methylglutaryl-proline (5- and 10-fold less potent, respectively, than SQ 20881). Replacement of the carboxyl group by a thiol group (a better zinc-ion ligand) resulted in potent ACE inhibitors like captopril (2-D-methyl-3-mercaptopropanoyl-proline), which produced dose-related inhibition of the pressor response to angiotensin I in normotensive male rats and produced marked antihypertensive effects in unanaesthetised Goldblatt two-kidney renal hypertensive rats. Captopril was the first ACE inhibitor to reach the market for the treatment of hypertension.

Since the discovery of captopril, a number of other analogues containing either a different chelating group or a proline replacement have been found to be potent inhibitors of ACE. Some of this work was based on a hypothetical model of the substrate (angiotensin I) binding at the active site of the enzyme. In the case of the ACE inhibitors containing a thiol function (for example, captopril), the thiol group interacts with the zinc ion and the methyl group binds at the S_1' subsite. The proline residue binds at the S_2' subsite and the C-terminal carboxyl group of the proline residue interacts with a positively charged group present in the enzyme. Over the years, medicinal chemistry approaches involving modifications of the chelating group and different groups binding in the S_1' and S_2' subsites have resulted in many potent inhibitors of ACE and many of these, including captopril, enalapril and lisinopril, have become highly successful drugs for the treatment of hypertension and other cardiovascular disorders. The design of phosphorus-containing ACE inhibitors, for example fosinopril, was based on the structure of phosphoramidon [N-α-L-rhamnopyranosyloxy-hydroxyphosphinyl)-Leu-Trp], an inhibitor of another zinc metalloproteinase (thermolysin) isolated from a culture filtrate of *Streptomyces tanashiensis*. In comparison with the effort required for the discovery of ACE inhibitors, progress in identifying potent inhibitors of the enkephalin-degrading dipeptidylcarboxypeptidase (enkephalinase) (used as analgesics) and ANF degrading enzyme (used as antihypertensive agents) was rapid because of the similarities between the enzymes. However, the similarities resulted in problems in achieving selectivity. The differences in the S_1' and S_2' subsites of metalloproteinases were exploited to achieve selectivity. The first potent inhibitor of enkephalinase (thiorphan) was about 30-fold more potent against enkephalinase (K_i approximately 4 nM) than against ACE. Another inhibitor, kelatorphan, was a potent inhibitor of enkephalinase and dipeptidylaminopeptidase and a weak inhibitor of aminopeptidase. Inhibitors like glycoprilat and their orally active prodrugs were potent inhibitors of ACE and enkephalinase; they prevented angiotensin I-induced pressor responses in rats and also increased urinary water and sodium excretion. Similarly, dual metalloproteinase inhibitors like CGS30440 (IC_{50} 19 and 2 nM against ACE and neutral endopeptidase, respectively) inhibited the angiotensin-1 pressor response, elevated the concentration of circulating ANP, and increased the excretion of urine, sodium and cGMP in rats injected with ANP. Candoxatrilat was an inhibitor of atriopeptidase.

It has been much more difficult to achieve complete selectivity in the case of inhibitors of MMPs (for example, collagenases, stromelysins and gelatinases), a family of zinc-containing proteinases involved in extracellular matrix remodelling and degradation. These enzymes have been implicated in diseases like rheumatoid arthritis, osteoarthritis, cancer and multiple sclerosis. The information generated in the case of converting enzyme inhibitors quickly led to inhibitors containing hydroxamate, thiol, N-carboxyalkyl and phosphorous groups for chelating the essential zinc metal and other peptidic and non-peptidic groups for binding to various binding pockets (S_1, S_1' -S_3') in the enzymes. The N-(X = NH) or C-carboxyalkyl (X = CH_2) series of inhibitors also inhibited several of the enzymes (MMP-1, -2 and -3). A proline derivative inhibited MMP-1, -2, -3, -7 and -13; a sulfonamide derivative inhibited MMP-1, -2, -3, -8 and -13, and a conformationally restricted inhibitor like compound (R = H, Ac, Boc or $PhSO_2$) inhibited MMP-1, -3, -8 and -9. Clinical trials on one of the broad-spectrum inhibitors, marimastat, for the treatment of pancreatic, lung, brain and stomach cancers failed to demonstrate efficacy in humans.

Aspartyl protease (renin and HIV protease) inhibitors

Aspartyl proteases are a family of enzymes which, in general, cleave peptide bonds between bulky hydrophobic amino acid residues. The cleavage of the peptide bond is mediated by a "*general acid–general base*" catalysis mechanism using the carboxyl groups of the aspartic acid residues at the active site. Enormous progress has been made in the discovery and optimisation of the pharmacokinetic properties of the inhibitors. Since the antihypertensive market is well served by a number of orally active agents like β-blockers, ACE inhibitors and angiotensin II antagonists, and the condition is chronic, requiring long-term treatment, it is essential to have orally active inhibitors for this indication. Many of the potent and selective renin inhibitors are now approaching the appropriate level of oral bioavailability after more than 25 years of research. In contrast, by using all the chemical information available in the case of renin inhibitors, it has been possible to discover potent orally bioavailable HIV protease inhibitors in a relatively short period of time, and many of these are already highly successful drugs.

Renin inhibitors

A number of chemical approaches have been used in the design of renin inhibitors. In the absence of the purified enzyme, most of the early search for inhibitors was carried out using crude renin preparations. The amino acid sequences of mouse, rat and human renin were obtained later on using either the traditional isolation and sequencing techniques or cDNA methodology. Various three-dimensional models of renin were constructed in the early stages, based on the *x* ray structures of other similar aspartyl proteases, for example endothia-pepsin and penicillopepsin. Later on, the *x* ray crystal structure of recombinant human renin was reported. The inhibitor design process has been based on some of these models.

Initial design of the inhibitors was based on a rational design strategy using the renin substrate as a starting point. Some of the early studies indicated that the octapeptide of horse angiotensinogen (His-Pro-Phe-His-Leu-Leu-Val-Tyr), cleaved slowly by renin between the two leucine residues, was a weak competitive inhibitor of renin. This led to the modifications in the P_1 and P_1' positions (Leu-Leu) of this peptide. The early work indicated that the two leucine residues could be replaced by other natural and unnatural amino acids (for example, Phe, D-Leu). Many of the resulting analogues, like His-Pro-Phe-His-Leu-D-Leu-Val-Tyr, His-Pro-Phe-His-Phe-Phe-Val-Tyr and Pro-His-Pro-Phe-His-Phe-Phe-Val-Tyr-Lys, although more potent than the original substrate-based compounds, were still weak inhibitors of renin. More potent inhibitors were obtained by replacing the peptide bond between the two leucine residues. Many of these peptides, for example Pro-His-Pro-Phe-His-Pheψ (CH_2NH)Phe-Val-Tyr-Lys, His-Pro-Phe-His-Leuψ (CH_2NH)Val-Ile-His and Pro-His-Pro-Phe-His-Leuψ(CH_2NH)Val-Ile-His-Lys (H-142), were potent and selective inhibitors of human renin. The two peptides containing a reduced Leu-Val peptide bond were 800–1000 times more potent inhibitors of human renin (IC_{50} 10–190 nM) than of dog renin (IC_{50} 10–150 mM) and H-12 did not inhibit cathepsin D up to a concentration of approximately 700 mM. One of the smaller peptides, Boc-Phe-His-Chaψ(CH_2NH)Val-NHCH_2CH(Me)-Et, approached the potency of H-142 in inhibiting human renin and lowered blood pressure in salt-depleted cynomolgus monkeys at a dose of 0·1–0·5 mg/kg. Unlike the reduced peptide bond [-ψ(CH_2NH)] analogues, replacement of the scissile peptide bond by -CH_2O-, -COCH_2-, -CH_2S- and -CH_2SO- did not lead to enhanced potency. The reduced peptide bond analogue, H-142, has been studied extensively in various animal and human models. At doses of 1 and 2·5 mg/kg/hr, H-142 produced a dose-related reduction in plasma renin activity and reduced the circulating levels of angiotensin I and II.

Another important step in the discovery of potent inhibitors of renin was the isolation of a naturally occurring aspartyl protease inhibitor pepstatin (Iva-Val-Val-Sta-Ala-Sta [Sta = (3S, 4S)-4-amino-3-hydroxy-6-methylheptanoic acid]), which was a relatively poor inhibitor of human renin but a potent inhibitor of pepsin. Incorporation of the statine residue in the angiotensinogen octapeptide resulted in potent inhibitors of renin. His-Pro-Phe-His-Sta-Val-Ile-His and Iva-His-Pro-Phe-His-Sta-Leu-Phe-NH_2 were equipotent to H-142 as inhibitors of human plasma and kidney renin. Another similar compound, Iva-His-Pro-Phe-His-Sta-Ile-Phe-NH_2, was a five-fold more potent inhibitor of human plasma and kidney renin than was H-142. However, the statine analogue was much less selective. In comparison with H-142, the statine analogue was about 300-fold more potent in inhibiting dog renin. The statine residue [-NH-CH(CH_2CHMe_2)-CH(OH)-CH_2CO-] in the above transition-state analogues was modified in various ways to assess the importance of the side chain isobutyl group, the hydroxyl group and the methylene group. In general, replacement of the isobutyl side chain (occupying the P_1 position) by cyclohexylmethyl or benzyl groups resulted in more potent compounds. The hydroxyl and the methylene groups were not essential for renin inhibition. Several compounds containing difluorostatine, for example difluorostatone, norstatine [(2R, 3S)-3-amino-2-hydroxy-5- methylhexanoic acid], cyclohexylnorstatine [(2R, 3S)-3-amino-4-cyclohexyl-2-hydroxybutyric acid], aminostatine (3,4-diamino-6-methylheptanoic acid) and α, α-difluoro-β-aminodeoxystatine, were potent inhibitors of human renin. Incorporation of the hydroxyethylene, dihydroxyethylene and other statine-like residues in place of the scissile peptide bond in substrate-based analogues, along with other amino acid or non-peptide changes at the N- and C-termini, led to more potent, selective and relatively small molecular weight inhibitors of renin. Examples of such compounds include Ro 42-5892, ICI 219623 and CGP38560. Ro 42-5892 was effective in lowering blood pressure in sodium-depleted marmosets and squirrel monkeys after oral administration (0·1 to 10 mg/kg.). ICI 219623 was effective in lowering blood pressure in anaesthetised sodium-depleted marmosets after intravenous (0·3–3·0 mg/kg) and oral (30 mg/kg) dosing. The indole-2-carbonyl derivative (JTP-3072) caused significant reduction in blood pressure in marmosets at an oral dose of 10 mg/kg for up to 3 hours. Compounds showed some oral absorption. Compound (IC_{50} 1.4 nM) displayed oral activity in a sodium-depleted normotensive cynomolgus monkey at a dose of 3 mg/kg.

In an attempt to design small molecular weight compounds, conformational analysis of the binding mode of CGP 38560 was carried out. This indicated that the S_1 and S_3 pockets constitute a large contiguous, hydrophobic binding site accommodating the P_1 cyclohexyl and the P_3 phenyl groups in close proximity to each other. This led to the synthesis of δ-amino hydroxyethylene dipeptide isosteres lacking the P_4–P_2 peptide backbone. Compound was a moderately potent inhibitor of human renin (IC_{50} 300 nM). Non-peptide inhibitors (R = $-OCH_2COOCH_3$, $-OCH_2CONH_2$ or $-OCH_2SO_2CH_3$) were 15–50- fold more potent inhibitors. Random screening approaches led to non-peptide inhibitors like the tetrahydroquinoline derivative (IC_{50} 0·7 nM [recombinant human renin] and 37 nM [human plasma renin]), which displayed long lasting (20 hour) blood pressure lowering effects after oral administration (1 and 3 mg/kg) to sodium-depleted conscious marmosets. The piperidine derivative also inhibited plasmepsin I and II from *Plasmodium falciparum*.

HIV protease inhibitors

In comparison with the discovery of renin inhibitors, the task of discovering inhibitors of HIV protease has been relatively easy. This is primarily because many of the approaches used successfully in the design of renin inhibitors were also applicable in the design of HIV protease inhibitors. In addition, samples of both HIV-1 and HIV-2 proteases (99 residue peptides), obtained by chemical synthesis and recombinant technology, were available in the early stages of the programme, along with the three-dimensional structure of the HIV-1 protease. Like renin, HIV protease was found to prefer a hydrophobic amino acid (Leu, Ile, Tyr, Phe) in the P_1 position of the substrate and was inhibited by pepstatin. However, unlike renin, incorporation of the statine residue in the P_1 position of the substrate, or the replacement of the scissile peptide bond in the substrate-like peptides with a -CH_2NH-group, did not lead to potent inhibitors. Potent inhibitors of the enzyme were obtained by replacing the scissile peptide bond with a hydroxymethylcarbonyl, hydroxyethylamine, hydroxyethylurea or a hydroxyethylene group. Many such compounds like saquinavir, indinavir, ritonavir, neflinavir and palinavir have reached the market or are in the late stages of clinical trials. In addition, various inhibitors of HIV protease were developed to overcome the problem of viral resistance by modifying the existing inhibitors like ritonavir and amprenavir. Computational studies using HIV-1 protease mutants ($Met^{46}Ile$, $Leu^{63}Pro$, $Val^{82}Thr$, $Ile^{84}Val$, $Met^{46}Ile/Leu^{63}Pro$, $Val^{82}Thr/Ile^{84}Val$ and $Met^{46}Ile/Leu^{63}Pro/Val^{82}Thr/Ile^{84}Val$) and known inhibitors of the enzyme (ABT-538 and VX-478) were used to design inhibitors with better binding affinity towards both mutant and wild-type proteases. ABT-378 inhibited wild-type and mutant HIV protease, blocked the replication of laboratory and clinical strains of HIV type 1, and maintained high potency against mutant HIV selected by ritonavir *in vivo*. Similarly, the allophenylnorstatine-containing dipeptide (JE-2147) (elimination half-life 94 minutes after intravenous administration; oral bioavailability 33–37% in non-fasting and fasting animals) was a potent inhibitor, active against a wide spectrum of HIV-1, HIV-2, SIV, and various clinical HIV-1 strains *in vitro*.

Many other non-peptide inhibitors of HIV protease (dihydropyrone, cyclic urea and sulfamide series of compounds) were obtained by modifications of random screening leads. Examples of these include a cyclic sulfone derivative and PNU-140690, which showed activity against a variety of laboratory strains of HIV-1, clinical isolates and other variants resistant to other protease inhibitors.

Thrombin Inhibitors (Serine Protease)

Thrombin inhibitors like D-Phe-Pro-Arg aldehyde have been known for a long time. However, the compounds lacked oral bioavailability. A semi-rational approach was adopted to modify P_1 to P_3 positions to improve the potency, selectivity and pharmacokinetic properties. Changes in individual positions were followed by multiple changes and synthesis of conformationally restricted analogues. Substitution of the C-terminal arginine aldehyde moiety (P_1 position) by *p*-amidinobenzylamine gave thrombin inhibitors comparable in potency with the transition-state aldehyde analogue but much less potent (130–400,000-fold) against trypsin, plasmin, tissue plasminogen activator and urokinase. Incorporation of a conformationally restricted analogue of arginine in the P_1 position, along with a six- or a seven-membered lactam sulphonamide moiety at P_3 to P_4 positions, gave inhibitors which showed much more selectivity against serine proteases like factor Xa and trypsin. Examples of other conformationally restricted thrombin inhibitors include compounds like (K_i 0·5 nM) which was approximately1 000-fold less potent against trypsin and inactive against plasmin, tissue plasminogen actiator, activated protein C, plasma kallikrein and chymotrypsin. Inhibitor containing conformationally restricting moieties in the P_3–P_2 region showed improved pharmacokinetics in the rat (61% oral bioavailability, elimination half-life 1 hour). A chemically similar inhibitor, inhibited thrombus formation when administered orally (30 mg/kg; bioavailability 55%; 4 hour duration of action) one hour before induction of stasis.

A number of P_3-position-modified thrombin inhibitors exhibited oral bioavailability in rats and dogs, and were efficacious in a rat $FeCl_3$-induced model of arterial thrombosis. Compounds and the corresponding analogues with an unprotected amino group at the N-terminus, showed selectivity (300–1500-fold selectivity for thrombin compared with trypsin) and oral bioavailability (40–76%) in rats or dogs. The arylsulfonylpropargylglycinamide derivative (K_i values 5, 19000, > 30000 nM, > 200000 and > 200000 nM against thrombin, factor Xa, trypsin, plasmin and tissue plasminogen actiator, respectively) also demonstrated oral activity at a dose of 30 mg/kg in rats. Compound containing a Phe(*p*-CH_2NH_2) residue in the P_1 position, was one of the more potent and selective inhibitors of thrombin (K_i values 6·6 and 14 200 nM against thrombin and trypsin respectively) and showed good oral bioavailability in rats (approximately 70%) but low oral bioavailability in dogs (10–15%). Some of the modified D-Phe-Pro-Arg aldehyde analogues like melagatran are undergoing clinical evaluation. Non-peptide inhibitors of thrombin (obtained by random screening procedures) include compounds based around benzothiophene and other ring systems and cyclic and linear oligocarbamate derivatives. The benzothiophene derivative showed antithrombotic efficacy in a rat model of thrombosis after infusion (ED50 2·3 mg/kg/h). The cyclic oligocarbamate tetramer inhibited thrombin with an apparent K_i of 31 nM.

Ras Protein Farnesyltransferase Inhibitors

Cysteine farnesylation of the ras oncogene product Ras is required for its transforming activity and is catalysed by the enzyme protein farnesyltransferase. The enzyme catalyses the transfer of a farnesyl group from farnesyl diphosphate to a cysteine residue of the protein substrate such as Ras. The enzyme recognises a tetrapeptide sequence (Cys-A-A-X, where A is an aliphatic amino acid and X is Met, Ser, Ala, Cys, or Gln) at the C-terminus of the protein. A closely related enzyme, geranylgeranyltransferase, recognises the Cys-A-A-X motif when X is either Leu or Phe, but transfers a geranylgeranyl group from geranylgeranyl diphosphate. Inhibition of farnesyltransferase represents a possible method for preventing association of Ras p21 to the cell membrane, thereby blocking its cell-transforming capabilities. Such inhibitors may have therapeutic potential as anticancer agents.

Semi-rational design approaches for the discovery of farnesyltransferase inhibitors were based on the tetrapeptide Cys-Val-Phe-Met. SAR studies, followed by the synthesis of conformationally restricted analogues, led to inhibitors, which was effective in prolonging the survival time in athymic mice implanted intraperitoneally with H-*ras*-transformed RAT-1 tumour cells. A non-thiol inhibitor (a methyl ester prodrug) showed activity in several *in vivo* tumour models. Examples of other conformationally restricted tetrapeptide analogues incorporating an N-alkyl amino acid residue include compound (HR-11). Further medicinal chemistry approaches on these modified peptides, including the synthesis of a library of secondary benzylic amines, led to orally active methionine derivatives like compound, which attenuated tumour growth in a nude mouse xenograft model of human pancreatic cancer. Compound showed 21–32% oral bioavailability in mice, rats, and dogs. The methyl ester prodrug suppressed the growth of human lung adenocarcinoma A-549 cells in nude mice by 30–90%, in a dose-dependent manner.

Random screening approaches also produced inhibitors of farnesyltransferase. SAR studies on the random screening lead Z-His-Tyr(OBn)-Ser(OBn)-Trp-D-Ala-NH_2 (PD083176) (IC_{50} 20 nM), including the replacement of the N-terminal Z group and the histidine and Trp residues, led to less potent peptides. However, substitution of the Tyr(OBn) and Ser(OBn) residues did not have much effect on the enzyme inhibitory activity. Based on the SAR and truncation studies, potent inhibitors of farnesyltransferase were obtained. The Z-His derivative inhibited isolated farnesyltransferase but was about 4000-fold less potent against geranylgeranyltransferase-1. Compound was also active in athymic mice implanted with H-ras-F cells. When administered intraperitoneally (150 mg/kg/day once daily) for 14 consecutive days after tumour implantation, the tumour growth was inhibited by approximately 90%.

Random screening approaches followed by medicinal chemistry also resulted in chemically distinct farnesyltransferase inhibitors. Compound was orally active in several human tumour xenograft models in the nude mouse, including tumours originating from colon, lung, pancreas, prostate, and urinary bladder. In the piperazine series of inhibitors, compound blocked tumour growth in mice implanted with H-*ras*-transformed cells (approximately 65% inhibition at 1.4 mg/kg/day). The benzodiazepine derivative inhibited anchorage-independent growth of H-*ras*-transformed Rat-1 cells (EC_{50} 160 nM).

Protein Kinase Inhibitors

The protein kinases are a family of proteins (serine/threonine kinases and tyrosine kinases) involved in signal transduction. Signal transduction via these proteins occurs through selective and reversible phosphorylation of the substrates by the transfer of γ-phosphate of ATP (or GTP) to the hydroxyl groups of serine, threonine and tyrosine residues. A large number of protein kinases (>150) have been identified from mammalian sources, and the human genome is expected to provide many more (>2000) in the future. These kinases play a key role in signal transduction pathways involved in many biological processes, such as control of cell growth, metabolism, differentiation and apoptosis. Along with approaches based on monoclonal antibodies, synthetic small molecule inhibitors of kinases are being actively developed for the treatment of various diseases.

A recent example of the antibody-based approach is the discovery of a monoclonal antibody against human epidermal growth factor receptor (HER2), a family of epidermal growth factor receptor tyrosine kinases, including the epidermal growth factor receptor. Many epithelial tumours, including breast cancer, express excess amounts of these proteins, particularly HER2. HER2 is a tyrosine kinase receptor with extracellular, transmembrane and intracellular domains. Initially, several monoclonal antibodies against the extracellular domain of the HER2 protein were found to inhibit the proliferation of human cancer cells that over-expressed HER2. The antigen binding region of one of the more effective antibodies was fused to the framework region of human IgG to generate a "humanised" monoclonal antibody. The antibody (trastuzumab) was investigated alone and in combination with chemotherapy in women with metastatic breast cancer that overexpressed HER2. Compared with chemotherapy alone, treatment with chemotherapy plus trastuzumab was associated with a significantly higher rate of overall positive response and a longer time to treatment failure. Treatment with trastuzumab was associated with some side-effects (chills, fever, infection and cardiac dysfunction).

Examples of compounds in various stages of clinical development include HER2 kinase inhibitors (ZD-1839, CP-358774 and PD-0183805], Bcr-Abl (CGP-57148) and vascular endothelial growth factor receptor kinase inhibitors (SU-5416). Although many of the starting leads were obtained by random screening approaches, further medicinal chemistry was aided by the availability of a number of crystal structures and other modelling approaches.

Protein–Protein Interaction Inhibitors

Many physiological and pathological processes are mediated by protein–protein interactions. The proteins involved in cell adhesion have been most widely studied. The interactions between the integrin family of heterodimeric cell surface receptors and their protein ligands are fundamental for maintaining cell function, for example by tethering cells at a particular location, facilitating cell migration, or providing survival signals to cells from their environment. Ligands recognised by integrins include extracellular matrix proteins (for example, collagen and fibronectin), plasma proteins like fibrinogen, and cell surface molecules like transmembrane proteins of the immunoglobulin family and cell-bound complement. A number of integrins and their ligands have been associated with many processes involved in cardiovascular diseases (for example, thrombosis involving platelet aggregation), inflammation, cancer (for example, metastasis) and bone disorders. The discovery of platelet aggregation inhibitors by blocking the interaction of platelet glycoprotein IIb/IIIa with its natural ligands (fibrinogen and von Willebrand factor) are examples of inhibitors of protein–protein interactions.

Novel inhibitors of glycoprotein IIb/IIIa and fibrinogen/von Willebrand interaction include injectable peptides (for example integrilin), orally active peptidomimetics that act as competitive inhibitors, and a monoclonal antibody c7E3 (abciximab), which irreversibly binds to GP IIb/IIIa. Administered intravenously, circulating abciximab has a plasma half-life of less than 10 minutes. However, the antibody binds tightly to platelets and provides receptor blockade for a period of up to 15 days.

The design of peptide and non-peptide inhibitors of platelet aggregation was based on the early observations that the integrins recognise peptide sequences like Arg-Gly-Asp present in the larger protein ligands like fibronectin and vitronectin. This led to the synthesis of a large number of analogues containing the Arg-Gly-Asp tripeptide or the chemical features of the tripeptide side chains (for example, the guanidino function and the carboxyl group). SAR studies indicated that a basic functional group that mimics the side chain of the arginine and a carboxylic acid group that mimics the Asp side chain are critical to the receptor binding and platelet aggregation activities of these compounds. In addition, a lipophilic group near the carboxylic acid function was found to enhance the potency of the antagonists. These findings led to the synthesis of more stable cyclic peptides like integrelin and many other compounds containing different non-peptide templates to hold the important functional groups in the proper spatial arrangements. All these approaches have resulted in potent injectable or orally active platelet-aggregation inhibitors. Examples of compounds that have reached the market include the antibody abciximab and the injectable peptide integrilin. Many of the orally active compounds like lamifiban, sibrafiban, xemilofiban, orbofiban and tirofiban have been studied extensively in the clinic. However, most of these failed in the late stages of development.

In addition to the well known examples of IIb/IIIa, antagonists of other integrins like $\alpha_v\beta_3$ (vitronectin receptor), $\alpha_v\beta_5$, $\alpha_v\beta_6$, $\alpha_4\beta_1$ and $\alpha_4\beta_7$ have been synthesised. The design of $\alpha_v\beta_3$ receptor antagonists was based on IIb/IIIa antagonists. Therefore some of the compounds, like isoxazoline-containing mimetic, were antagonists of both $\alpha_v\beta_3$ (IC_{50} 0·7 nM) and IIb/IIIa (IC_{50} 0·34 nM). Some other analogues, were more selective against the $\alpha_v\beta_3$ receptor. For example, the diaminopropionic acid derivative was > 500-fold more potent against $\alpha_v\beta_3$ integrin than against $\alpha_v\beta_5$, $\alpha_5\beta_1$ and GPIIb/IIIa integrins. Compound (SC56631) prevents osteoclast-mediated bone particle degradation. The imidazopyridine analogue was active in the $\alpha_v\beta_3$ binding assay (K_i 45 nM) and showed efficacy in an animal model of restenosis.

Further modifications in compounds such as led to non-peptide vitronectin receptor antagonists that had oral activity. For example, compound (K_i 3.5 nM for $\alpha_v\beta_3$ and 28000 nM for $\alpha IIb\beta_3$) showed between 4–14% oral bioavailability in the rat and dog. Another analogue, SB 265123 (K_i 4.1 nM for $\alpha_v\beta_3$, 1.3 nM for $\alpha_v\beta_5$, 18000 nM for $\alpha_5\beta_1$, and 9000 nM for $\alpha IIb\beta_3$), displayed 100% oral bioavailability in rats, and was active *in vivo* in the ovariectomised rat model of osteoporosis.

$\alpha_4\beta_1$ and $\alpha_5\beta_1$ Antagonists

Cyclic peptide inhibitors of VLA-4 and fibronectin/vascular cell adhesion molecule (VCAM)-1 interaction, for example c(Ile-Leu-Asp-Val-NH$(CH_2)_5$CO) were reported. Several of these inhibitors, for example c(Ile-Leu-Asp-Val-NH$(CH_2)_5$CO), c(Ile-Leu-Asp-Val-NH$(CH_2)_4$CO) and c(MePhe-Leu-Asp-Val-D-Arg-D-Arg), blocked VLA-4/VCAM-1 and VLA-4/fibronectin interactions in *in vitro* assays and inhibited oxazolone and ovalbumin-induced contact hypersensitivity responses in mice. The compounds did not affect cell adhesion mediated by two other integrins, VLA-5 ($\alpha_5\beta_1$) and LFA-1 ($\alpha_L\beta_2$). *p*-Aminophenylacetyl-Leu-Asp-Val derivatives containing various non-peptide residues at the N-terminus are reported to be inhibitors of integrin $\alpha_4\beta_1$. Compound (BIO-1211), showed activity in a model of antigen-induced bronchoconstriction and airway hyper-responsiveness in sheep. In various integrin adhesion assays, showed activity against $\alpha_4\beta_7$, $\alpha 1_5\beta_1$, $\alpha_5\beta_1$, $\alpha_6\beta_1$, $\alpha_L\beta_2$ and $\alpha IIb\beta_3$ integrins at much higher concentrations.

Drug discovery has been a continuously changing and evolving field of science over the years. More and more effective and safer treatments have been discovered. Although chemical and biological sciences have always played a major role in the discovery process, new scientific developments and technologies are altering the ways in which these sciences are applied to the discovery process. Advances in rapid DNA sequencing techniques have resulted in the sequencing of the human genome. Finding the disease-related genes, translating the gene sequences into biologically active proteins and evaluating their functions is likely to lead to new drug discovery targets based on new biochemical pathways. The genomic and proteomic studies may also lead to new therapeutic proteins and antibodies. Given the therapeutic success of the interferons, erythropoietin, granulocyte-macrophage colony-stimulating factor, herceptin (trastuzumab), rituximab, and many others, protein drugs are likely to make many additional therapeutic contributions.

Combinatorial library techniques and natural product libraries are providing large numbers of new compounds for screening. Automated high-throughput screening techniques are being developed continuously to test large numbers of available compounds in multiple screens. A combination of these two technologies, along with the discovery of new target proteins (receptors, enzymes, etc.), has the potential to generate leads for various drug discovery programmes. However, before the leads can be taken seriously, it is essential to validate the target appropriately. Otherwise, the optimised leads are likely to fail in the later stages of development. In many cases where some treatments exist along with some knowledge about the causes of the disease, the need for target validation and development of the relevant biological models is less stringent. The discovery of new medicines in these fields becomes a continuous process of identifying medicines that are more efficacious and convenient to administer in a larger number of patients, and display the best possible toxicity profile.

The availability of leads along with advances in multiple parallel solid-phase synthetic and purification techniques would enable the lead optimisation procedure to be carried out in a relatively short period of time. The design strategies for the lead optimisation are likely to be a combination of the types of approaches highlighted in the examples described above. SAR studies, along with structural and modelling studies using cloned proteins (receptors, enzymes, etc.), are likely to make the lead optimisation procedure somewhat more rational. The availability of cloned receptor subtypes and various members of the enzyme classes in the early stages of the programme can be used to build selectivity into the receptor ligands and enzyme inhibitors. Better understanding of the signalling processes will enable the cellular processes to be controlled in a more efficient manner.

2

Clinical Data Management System

This article is intended to be an overview of clinical data management systems and the processes they support. Data management systems are highly dependent on the size and complexity of the organization using them. Systems can range from a set of SAS data sets to a fully integrated, distributed set of applications using a relational database. The entire data management process may employ a variety of technical solutions.

Background

The information presented here is based on experience with processes and technology in a large international pharmaceutical company. Many of these concepts are employed in smaller pharmaceutical companies and contract research organizations (CROs) but on a lesser scale.

Re-engineering

The pharmaceutical industry is under constant pressure to bring drugs to market more quickly and less expensively, without compromising the quality of the products. The desire to achieve a profitable balance between these three objectives—speed, cost, and quality—results in perpetual "*re-engineering*." The investment put into developing and implementing a solid database and streamlining data management tools and processes can contribute greatly to the success of this effort.

How Technology Is Driving Changes in Data Management

The introduction and proliferation of the Internet and web-based applications is having a profound impact on the conduct of clinical trials. The Internet provides us with the ability to communicate easily with CROs and investigators; and them with us, without compromising corporate security. Data sets can easily be placed on a secure web site for being reviewed and updated by a partner. Remote data entry will reach its full potential as a result of the introduction and acceptance of internet technology.

Study Setup

Standardization

To avoid redundancy, many parts of the study and setup processes can be standardized and reused. For example, as case report forms (CRFs) are developed for use across studies, the corresponding components of the study definition (questions, response values), the validation checks, reports, and extract data structures can be reused as well, especially within a drug project. This standardization allows for more efficient use of resources and systems, as well as realization of benefits in CRF design, study definition, validation, analysis, reporting, metrics, and training. Standards for data collection

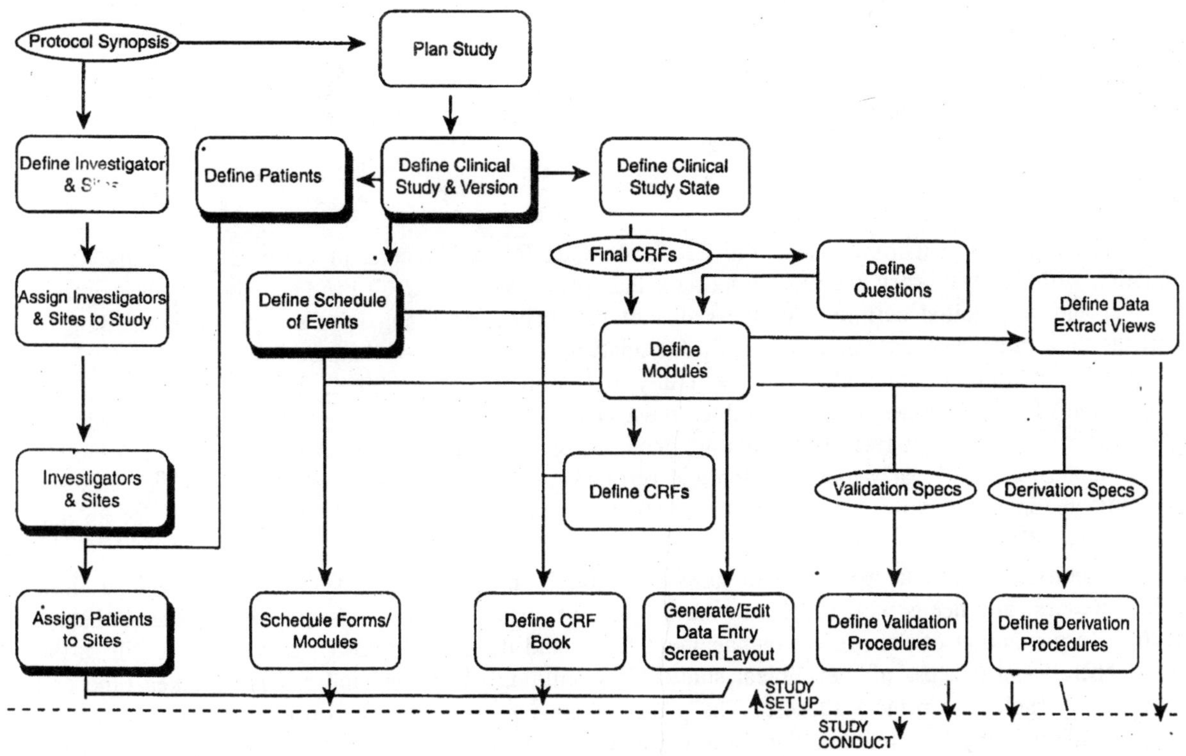

Fig. 2.1. Study setup.

and processing are also necessary to fulfill the reporting requirements for pooled analyses across a project (e.g., safety updates, integrated reports, summaries).

Protocol Development

The protocol must contain a clear statement of the objectives of the investigation (primary and secondary endpoints) and the methods of analysis to be used. The various sections may be written by the appropriate team members and assembled by the clinical representative who is the protocol author. Once the protocol is complete, the CRF is designed. The CRF is the principal document used to collect the study data and guide the study definition in the data management system.

In-House vs. Outsourcing to CROs

Once the project team completes a protocol synopsis, in-house resources should be evaluated. Consideration is given to the type of study required along with the study's priority within the project. The advantages of doing the data management in-house include:

1. All data for project resides on one database
2. Full control over study set-up
3. Re-use of tools already developed
4. Real-time access to data
5. Control over study costs.

If in-house resources are limited and the decision is made to outsource data management activities, the planning process begins by creating a detailed scope of work statement and issuing the request for proposal (RFP). Bids should be solicited from several CROs:

In choosing a CRO, consider the following:

1. Depth of experience in data management
2. Compatibility of computer systems
3. Qualified technical support for data transfer
4. SOPs and policies that meet GCP criteria
5. Interpersonal compatibility
6. Price

Previous sponsor experience with the CRO, the CRO's track record of delivering, and the CRO reputation within the industry are more important than price. When a CRO has been chosen, the contract should include a detailed definition of the scope of work required along with a clear understanding of when the data is considered clean and ready for analysis. A test run of data transfer from the CRO to the sponsor should be done early in the study to identify any problems in data formatting and transmission. The milestones and deliverables must be tracked closely during study conduct in order to ensure that appropriate progress payments are made. The importance of regular communication cannot be overemphasized. The early identification and resolution of technical or process problems is necessary for a smooth database closure and transfer of data. Transfer of data often contains more issues and surprises than anticipated.

The sponsor must take the time to gain a thorough understanding of the CRO's organization, work processes, and needs with respect to the project. In turn, the CRO must understand the sponsor's structure, organization of the project management team, and the rȯle the CRO is expected to fill in the overall operational process of the clinical study. This building of mutual understanding takes time and effort but is crucial for project success. The project team requires reports to track the progress of the study including patient enrollment data, discrepancy counts, outstanding CRF pages, and terminated patients (including dropouts). If the CRO already has adequate tracking systems, the reports should be evaluated and adapted as needed. After study completion, a review of the CRO's performance and a written report of lessons learned will provide information for future planning of projects and outsourcing needs. There are several options for the transfer of CRO-processed data back to the sponsor. Most often, the final data are entered into the CRO's database to produce the final study reports with corresponding datasets. However, with the advances in the Internet and in distributed study conduct, it is possible, and generally desirable from the sponsor's viewpoint, for the CRO to enter data directly into the sponsor's database.

CRF Development

The CRF design process can begin either following or concurrent with the protocol development. Well-designed data collection forms are critical to achieve the objectives of the clinical trial. Consideration should be given to the content, format, and layout of the forms since all these factors contribute to the overall quality and accuracy of the data that will be collected, processed, and reported.

Many disciplines should participate in the CRF design stage. The core team will generally consist of representatives from statistics, data management, forms design, medical and clinical monitoring groups, with other specialists, consulting, as necessary. The primary objective of the team in this process is to optimize and balance the following requirements for the CRF:

1. To facilitate the investigational site in filling out the forms correctly
2. To allow for quick and accurate data entry
3. To ensure that data can be analyzed and that they represent the patient's experience for statistical and clinical reporting

4. To facilitate the pooling of data across a project for safety updates and integrated safety and efficacy reporting
5. Consistency within project or area (e.g., pharmacoeconomics, clinical pharmacology) to allow reuse of tools.

The forms should only collect data that are needed for reporting purposes and avoid collecting unnecessary or redundant data. The standardization of CRFs for use across multiple studies results in significant savings in the design, processing, reporting, and training resources required for a clinical study. Forms can be further broken down into modules (e.g., physical exam, vital signs, demography) or groups of questions. The use of these modules allows for greater flexibility when constructing the forms/pages while retaining the standard use of the question groups. A library of forms can be centrally gathered and maintained that includes "global" forms (those that can be used across projects—e.g., adverse events, demography), project or therapeutic standard forms (used across a project), and study specific forms. There are many applications and systems that can be used to design and generate the CRFs. These range from word processing and desktop publishing packages to customized systems that facilitate the maintenance and use of a library of modules/forms and enforce standards. The CRF may also be in an electronic format rather than on paper, as in the case of remote data entry systems.

Randomization

Randomization is the process by which patients are randomly assigned to a treatment group. It is used to reduce the possibility for investigators and study personnel to bias the results (consciously or unconsciously) in favor of one treatment over another in a study. Randomization also allows for maintaining the blinding of a study when the blind must be broken for an individual patient. In most trials, the randomization data will be kept blinded until data are considered clean and after exclusions are decided to avoid influencing the results of a study. At the end of the trial, it is a requirement to confirm the integrity of the blinding. There must be documentation or an audit trail of all blind breaks and of all data changes post unblinding. The statistician plays an important role in specifying appropriate parameters to be utilized in generating the randomization. The randomization specifications include treatments, centers, block size, study design, blinding requirements, and stratification factors. It is through the usage of stratification or grouping criteria that patient differences can be minimized between treatment groups. Randomization codes are used for packaging and labeling study medications. The systems that are used to generate labels for the treatment bottles may be independent of those that produce the randomization.

Study Definition

A study definition is used to identify to the system characteristics about the data fields stored within, criteria for acceptance of those data, as well as extract formats and file structures. These characteristics may include database variable name, data type (numeric, character, date/time), question name and label, short reference name (e.g., SAS variable name), format (e.g., ddmmyy), field length, acceptable response values (e.g., male/female), coding formats (e.g., 1 = yes, 2 = no), and validation information (e.g., validate against specific thesaurus). Data entry screen layout is also part of the study definition. The ease (or difficulty) of data entry must be balanced with the utility of the data extract file structure, both of which are greatly determined by this process. Therefore, good database design requires the close cooperation and compromise between data management and statistics to ensure quality and efficiency throughout the data processing, management, analysis, and reporting lifecycle.

Many database systems have a catalog of questions or other global library capabilities to facilitate the storage and retrieval of data definition objects. Using these objects as "*building blocks*," standard modules can be established and used across many studies.

This standardization saves considerable resources, not only in the study set-up process but also in training data entry personnel, coding validation checks, producing monitor reports, and for analysis/ reporting. The continued usage of these standards can also allow for constant streamlining and improvement based on experience, with appropriate maintenance and controls. Related to the study definition process, most systems require a schedule of events to be defined to instruct the system when to expect certain forms for tracking purposes and to associate date/visit with the form.

Data Quality Specifications

A data quality plan is a tool to aid in the implementation of data quality. The plan should be developed as soon as the protocol is finalized. Data quality is a shared responsibility across all functions. For example, the monitor assures quality by source document verification (SDV), and the clinician reviews listings of individual patient profiles and study "*outliers.*" New data and corrections to data are usually processed nightly through a batch validation program in the clinical database. The batch validation program will identify new discrepancies that have appeared since the last execution of the validation. The program will also resolve any previously generated discrepancies that are no longer valid because either the data or the associated validation criteria have changed. Batch validation may also be run "on demand" if immediate validation of data is required. With the help of the study team, data management usually prepares the validation procedures document to identify specific variables that must be validated. Edit checks may be defined as part of the data structure and executed during data entry. Programmed checks are user-defined checks executed off-line during batch validation.

These programmed checks include

1. Standard checks developed for all standard CRF pages
2. Project specific checks used within each project
3. Study specific checks used for study specific pages of the CRF.

The completed validation checks should be run against test data to ensure they are written correctly. As the data is received and validated by these procedures, it is important to review the output and add or delete edit checks as appropriate.

Study Conduct

Receipt of Data

Technology is providing a number of options for the transmission of data from the investigator, CRO, or lab, back to the sponsor site. Imaging technology allows for the capture and efficient storage of all CRFs for use in data tracking and electronic submissions. Current and near future imaging technology will allow us to store an electronic copy of signed CRFs as well as easily archive all study-related documents. Images can be read using optical character recognition and bar coding techniques. These technologies, once perfected, will greatly reduce the manpower required to index and enter the data on CRFs into the data management systems. Imaging technology is currently being employed to route documents through the appropriate study conduct workflow.

There have been numerous advances in the area of remote data acquisition. Data can be collected at the site via an electronic CRF or a hand held electronic device. These data can then be transmitted back to the sponsoring company and batch loaded into the sponsor's clinical trial database. Remote data entry technology currently allows for the easy definition and distribution of the electronic CRFs to the investigator site. Some online cleaning can be performed as the data are entered before transmission to the sponsor site, where additional quality checks are applied and transmitted back to the investigator site. This iterative process allows for collection and generally faster cleaning of clinical data. Data can also be transmitted from the CRO, investigator, or lab via electronic data transfer. Laboratory data are most often transmitted this way due to the volume of the data. The data are then batch loaded into the sponsor's clinical trial database. Fax transmissions are often received from the investigator. The fax transmission can be printed out and then data entered, or the fax can go directly to a fax server or be passed through a scanner and an electronic image of the form/document can be created. This image can then be stored, or data entered either by optical character recognition, manual data entry, or a combination of the two. Many studies are still conducted by traditional paper-based methods. CRFs and documents are sent by post (often overnight) to the sponsor site where they are data entered and filed. Today's technology allows for the conduct at multiple sites, with the ability to pool data for interim analyses and integrated safety summaries. The size and complexity of a study should determine which technology should be employed. Most large pharmaceutical companies have a portfolio of study conduct technologies to employ.

Data Entry

In a paper-based data flow, as CRFs are received by the sponsor, the pages or forms can be "logged in" or identified to the system. A document number may be used to uniquely identify a page for further tracking within the database. This document identifier can be scanned from a barcode printed on a form, created using a document number generator, or manually entered. Once the form is recognized as received by the system, a data entry operator can start entry into the database. In the data definition process, screen layouts will have been defined to facilitate the accurate and speedy entry. Some validation or discrepancy checks can be designed to trigger at entry. For example, if a data entry operator attempts to violate the criteria defined to the system for a particular data field (e.g., entering character information into a numerically defined field), a discrepancy can be raised to alert the operator for acceptance or correction to the data. If the entry correctly reflects what is written on the CRF, the value can be accepted and a discrepancy noted for later follow up.

Many systems allow for the option to perform an independent second pass of data entry to ensure that data that is recorded on the CRF matches what is entered into the database. Second pass (double key) should be performed by a different data entry operator than the first pass. In the cases where the first pass and second pass do not match, the data entry operator is prompted and can accept either entry. An audit trail is kept by the system, and reports may be generated to document changes performed during the second-pass process. Data entry conventions are recommended to assist in the consistent handling of the data. These conventions should include guidelines and rules for dealing with expected (and unexpected) issues arising on the forms. Some examples include handling missing data, illegible text or data, investigator comments, acceptable abbreviations, etc.

Not all data are received by the sponsor site on CRFs or paper. For example, data may be entered remotely at the investigator site or generated as an output file from instrumentation and then electronically transferred to the sponsor site via the Web/Internet, other connections, or even diskettes. Alternatives to traditional data entry also include using optical character recognition (OCR) technology. This scanning technique used to populate the database may require the CRFs to be designed with special considerations as to the density of the forms, increased use of coded fields, and legibility of the completed forms.

Discrepancy Management

In addition to the discrepancies generated as a result of study definition (univariate discrepancies), discrepancies may also arise when a batch validation detects data inconsistencies (univariate and multivariate discrepancies). Discrepancies are also identified by a visual review of the data, e.g., monitoring lists, SDV review. Discrepancies may also be created by people responsible for data analysis (e.g., statisticians, pharmacoeconomists, clinical pharmacologists). All discrepancies and data fields requiring verification or clarification are tracked using the clinical database. Quality control for clinical data within data management includes computerized validation of data in the database and second-pass data entry. These activities are performed to ensure that data are complete, accurate, and compliant with the protocol. In addition to discrepancy reports, verification of randomly selected fields may be used to assess the data quality. Discrepancy reports are prepared for investigator review and correction. The sponsor translates the computer output into user-friendly reports. There is direct communication between the investigational site coordinator and the data manager for any error messages that may need clarification. Corrections are made by the site representative directly onto the CRF page and then faxed back to the sponsor. If fax technology is not used, a copy of the corrected CRF page is made and sent to the sponsor by mail or courier. Good clinical practice requires that all corrections must be dated and initialed by the site representative. Once the corrected copies are received, the data manager makes the change in the clinical database. An electronic audit trail is maintained in the clinical database of all data entered and changed. This audit trail tracks the date and time stamp and the identification of the person making the entry correction or change.

Ongoing Monitoring

A number of query tools may be used to track the quality and completeness of CRF and non-CRF data. Many of the tracking reports reside within the data management system, but tracking may also be done using simple ad hoc query tools such as Brio or even SAS. An example of on-going monitoring is the tracking of study enrollment by investigators. Inclusion and exclusion criteria are usually listed on the CRF. The investigator reviews the criteria and either admits or excludes the subject from continuing in the study. This may be reviewed and monitored manually by the monitor reviewing the subjects' medical records to confirm eligibility during source document verification or through reports/ listing of this particular patient data highlighting any irregularities.

Database Closure

At study completion, the data manager is responsible for assuring that the data are clean and then prepares to lock the study/close the database. The purpose of locking the study is to ensure that a full audit trail of any changes exists once the study/patients have been unblinded. Database closure marks the end of the study conduct phase and the beginning of the analysis and reporting phase. The standard definition of clean data is:

1. All outstanding data in-house
2. All outstanding discrepancies resolved
3. SDV completed
4. Clinical review of data complete
5. The allocation of preferred terms to CRF verbatim terms reviewed and complete
6. All non-CRF data revised and processed.

The data management system through a series of reports and internal checks provides the documentation and verification that data have been completely cleaned. When the criteria for clean data are met, a formal sign-off meeting is held for team members and ad hoc functional representatives. With the database closure form signed off, the data manager locks the database. Locking limits the ability to change values for specific privileged users. It also starts a new audit trail of any changes made after locking. The randomization codes may now be entered allowing the statistician to review the data in an unblinded fashion. Any pharmacokinetic data are also loaded at this time. Data management then freezes the database. No changes may be made to the existing database and no new data may be added.

Study Performance Metrics

Performance metrics are used by the study team to track and manage the study. The metrics will aid in the early identification and resolution of problems that may affect data quality and study timelines. For example, metrics involving patient enrollment, visits, forms flow, and discrepancies may be tracked using the clinical database.

Laboratory Data

It is common practice to employ outside laboratories to perform testing for safety and efficacy measures in clinical trials. Along with the results, these laboratories will also provide the units and normal ranges for the tests performed. Since the laboratories are typically utilized by many patients in a study or even across studies, it is practical for the units and ranges to be received and entered once in the system and then linked internally to the patient data to which they apply. This principle of centrally storing values that can be shared across the system is also desirable for maintaining the conversion factors used in deriving lab results into standardized units.

Thesaurus

Medical dictionaries are utilized extensively in clinical trials to assign common terminology to medical events such as adverse events reporting and clinical diagnoses, as well as to link medication trade names to their generic components. Thesaurus management systems facilitate both the ongoing maintenance of base dictionaries (e.g., COSTART, WHOART, MEDDRA) and the linkages to the reported and entered data.

Pharmacokinetic Data

In blinded studies, entering of pharmacokinetic (PK) data on an ongoing basis could jeopardize the blinding of the study. Consequently, the PK data are often entered into a separate database. The data is usually loaded into the data management system only after the study is closed and ready for analysis.

Analysis and Reporting

Extracting Data

A well-designed data management system typically will focus on the primary objective to facilitate the collection and cleaning of clinical data. Although it must also support analysis and reporting, it is not always possible to achieve an equal balance across all these requirements; therefore, data are usually analyzed outside of the clinical database. Data extraction is the process of selecting and copying data fields to an external file. Data extraction procedures generally produce files that are simply a reflection of the database. The data can then be manipulated and/or transposed to achieve an optimal structure for analysis and reporting requirements. Additional fields can be derived, response values standardized or decoded, and variables labeled more clearly. Data may be organized by type of data, such as adverse events, laboratory data, demography, physical exam, etc. Since many of these categories of data exist across clinical trials, standard file structures can be designed and implemented. This standardization allows for the reuse of validated software as well as facilitates the pooling of data across studies for use in project safety summaries and other data reporting across studies.

Derivations

The derivation of data points can be conducted in a number of different ways. Usually they are calculated either in the clinical trials database or as part of the creation of the analysis ready, value added data sets. It is advisable to store derivations for values that are not likely to change, and for which the derivation algorithm is commonly accepted in the clinical trials database. Derivations that are a result of a constantly changing database, or of a complex algorithm particular to a given study, should be conducted outside the clinical trials database and as part of the creation of the analysis ready, value added data sets.

Reporting Tools

Reporting and analysis is usually a continuous process throughout the life of a study. The "final report" is the culmination of the efforts involved in conducting a clinical trial. For ongoing reporting during the life of a study, there are a large number of reporting tools available on the market for the querying of clinical trials data. Each database has a number of tools that are appropriate for creating easy to mildly complex reports against the clinical trials database (i.e., Oracle has several reporting tools). There are also a number of user-friendly query tools that are designed to retrieve data from a number of different databases. Brio can generate query results that join multiple tables and give quite a bit of flexibility over report format and features such as sorting. More complex reports, such as a "missing and overdue forms report," are usually written in third generation language (3gl) such as C++, or taking the data outside the database and using external programming tools. For the final statistical listings and tables, SAS is the industry standard. Where reporting is concerned, the tool that best performs the job should be the one selected.

Electronic Submission of CRFs to Regulatory Agencies

Sponsors may be required to provide selected CRFs as part of the overall package submitted to the regulatory authorities. Recently, regulatory agencies have been encouraging the electronic submission of these CRFs. Given a comprehensive and well-indexed imaging system, it may be possible to subset the requested images and electronically transfer the file with relative ease. For the situations where these files must be manually compiled, a different process may be employed. As CRFs are identified for inclusion, a scanner can be used to produce .pdf files (via Adobe Acrobat Exchangez). An index is required to facilitate the retrieval of the forms, as desired. The collection of indexed images is then transferred onto CD-ROM for the electronic submission.

System Issues

Year 2000

The approach of 2000 A.D. had caused the technology industry to take an in-depth look at all of the automated solutions employed in the industry. Every place where a date was used in an application was examined. Two digit dates were particularly troublesome as we approached the new millennium. The validation effort consumed an enormous amount of resources, both in-house and at the software vendors.

Upgrades

Whether your clinical trials management system was developed in-house or purchased from a vendor, eventually you will have the opportunity to experience an upgrade. At some point you will probably need to upgrade the operating system on the PC or server, the version of the database that your application is built on, or the application software itself. Worst case is when you have to upgrade all of these at once. Ideally your application environment consists of a fully functional and separate test environment. It is in this area that you would test any upgrades. Testing should consist of executing documented test scripts with the goal of proving that existing functionality still works and any advertised new functionality also works. Ideally you would try to avoid upgrading multiple pieces of your environment at the same time, as in the worst case example above. Although multiple rounds of testing is resource intensive, it is much easier to determine the source of any problems and resolve them in a controlled environment. This is a point to be aware of when choosing clinical trial software: Will the vendor support multiple versions of an operating system and database? This will give you the time to test the worst case scenario in a two-phase approach.

Conversion vs. Migration vs. Upgrade

Over time software becomes obsolete, as does hardware. Upgrading to the latest version of the software or hardware is probably the easiest path. But when you find that you must move to a completely new hardware or application environment, there are several things to consider. Often software and hardware vendors can provide the service of migrating or converting your existing data from one system to another. One should carefully investigate what this process would entail. Conversion can be a painful and extremely resource intensive operation. You should realistically look at whether it is feasible to let ongoing trials complete in the legacy system or whether it is feasible to re-enter data into the new system for smaller studies. These strategies are often much more straightforward and less error prone than a conversion would be.

System Validation

Computer systems validation (CSV) is an ongoing process that involves the evaluation and documentation of all components of a system during its life cycle to ensure compliance with approved user requirements and quality standards. A system is defined not only by its hardware and software, but also by the processes surrounding its use. CSV is applicable to a system used to collect, process, capture, or manipulate data that may be included in a submission to a regulatory authority. Validation requires establishing documented evidence that a system meets its predefined specifications and quality attributes. Validation seeks to assure that a system has been developed, tested, and implemented in a controlled manner, performs and will continue to perform accurately and reliably, and is secure from unauthorized or accidental change. In addition to documenting the development and implementation of system components, validation includes documenting hardware and software change control, security management, and training.

Audit Trails and Change Control

It is important to be able to track the reason and source for any changes to data in your clinical trials database. Many applications have built in audit trail capabilities that track the date, time, and ID of the person entering or changing data through the application. Some applications will even prompt for a data change reason. Any changes or deletion of data should be done through the application whenever possible. Sometimes however, the volume of the data to be modified or complexity of the changes requires external intervention. If you plan to modify data in the clinical trials database from outside of the application, the process should be very carefully documented. As in any software development, the program or script that will be run to enter or update data should have a design document, that outlines the modules purpose and expected performance, as well as a set of fully executed test cases. It is common to keep all requests for manual data changes and data change scripts with their respective documents in one directory as backup for a data change log.

3

Clinical Evolution of Drug

The process of developing a new drug, from the identification of a potential drug candidate to postmarketing surveillance, is extremely complex. The drug development process requires input from various members of a multidisciplinary team and the conduct of numerous studies. The time from drug discovery to marketing takes an average of 13 years. Once a chemical is identified as a new drug candidate, extensive preclinical analyses must be completed before the drug can be tested in humans. The pharmacology, toxicology, and preclinical pharmacokinetics must be characterized. The formulations of the drug product that were used in the preclinical studies may be different from the formulation of the final drug product, which may require that additional formulation work and pharmacokinetic analyses be performed. If the characteristics of the new drug candidate arc acceptable for all of the preclinical assessments, it may then be tested in humans. The new drug candidate, at this point, enters the clinical research stage of drug development.

Clinical research represents a vital stage in the development process a stage that is no less daunting than the preclinical research stage. The data obtained from the first-time-in-human, Phase 1 pharmacokinetic studies, and initial safety evaluations in healthy volunteers can make or break the entire developmental program for a drug candidate. The sponsoring company, of course, hopes that the data collected in these initial studies will show minimal safety concerns over an adequate dose range. The pharmacokinetic data can then be used to help design future studies in which efficacy and long-term safety are assessed and additional pharmacokinetic and pharmacodynamic data are collected. Although the basic designs of the initial single and multiple dose-escalating studies are generally straight-forward (but the starting dose is often intensely debated), it is imperative that these studies and future studies be designed to address specific questions. The questions vary depending on numerous specific considerations, including the targeted disease characteristics (e.g., acute or chronic); desired safety, efficacy, and pharmacokinetic evaluations; and assessment of clinical pharmacology (e.g., dosage formulations or dose frequency).

Basic study procedures must also be considered. Thus, the design, conduct, data reporting and analysis, and production of the final study reports can be completed only through the coordinated efforts of a multidisciplinary drug development team. For every clinical study, input is required from multiple personnel with various areas of expertise. Members of a drug development team include physicians, scientists, pharmacists, project managers, statisticians, computer programers, study monitors, regulatory experts, and for some studies, a representative of the formulations group. While some team members may be able to perform multiple tasks, no one team member has the expertise or the time to do everything required to conduct a clinical study. In addition, some members may have overlapping abilities, but other members with particular expertise may be called upon. For example, pharmacokineticists are the experts in pharmacokinetics, but they may also be knowledgeable in pharmaceutics, biostatistics, and clinical care. However, scientists (PhDs) are trained primarily in basic research, while physicians (MDs) are trained in clinical medicine. Since a single drug development program is derived from both of these distinct disciplines, considerable overlap, cooperation, and coordination are necessary to take a drug successfully and efficiently from discovery to market.

Clinical drug development is generally divided into four phases: Phase 1 through Phase 4. For each study conducted within a particular phase, specific information is collected according to the requirements for individual drugs being developed. Collection of safety, efficacy, and pharmacokinetic data is the focus of most clinical trials. Although these topics appear to be distinct disciplines, they are intertwined and represent different ways of evaluating the intrinsic properties of a drug. While the safety, efficacy, and pharmacokinetics of a drug may be assessed in most studies, the team must establish the type and extent of information to be collected, which will vary based upon the specific objectives and designs of the studies. A critical function of the drug development team is the development of the study protocol. The study protocol must clearly describe the study design and methodology that will be used to achieve the study objectives. Input from non-medical and non-scientific members of the team, such as marketing and information technology experts, also is helpful in establishing development strategies and in designing and conducting of clinical studies. Finally, project planning efforts can synchronize team efforts, help contain the soaring costs of pharmaceutical research, and coordinate international development efforts.

The drug development team's primary goal is to gain approval to market the drug, which requires that a marketing application be submitted to a regulatory agency (e.g., a New Drug Application [NDA] is submitted to the Food and Drug Administration [FDA] in the United States and to the Health Products and Food Branch [HPFB] in Canada, while a Marketing Authorization Application [MAA] is submitted to European regulatory agencies). During the conduct of the studies and the compilation and analyses of the data, the team must consider and evaluate many issues, such as how to collect, categorize, and report adverse events. All of these decisions will affect the marketing application that is submitted and may ultimately define how the drug is to be administered. Many of the decisions to be made by the team, and particularly by the investigators, pose ethical dilemmas. Legislation has been enacted to protect human research subjects. Recently, the most pressing ethical dilemma facing the clinical research scientist concerned biotechnology and genetic engineering research. Frequent changes in the regulations and guidelines of various regulatory agencies, differences in interpretations of these rules, and special reporting mechanisms for adverse events represent only a few of the challenges facing a drug development team. Due to continuous advances in scientific information, understanding of disease processes, and gene therapy, change continues to be the rule in modern drug development. However, through the efficient application of sound scientific principles in an ethical manner and with a coordinated team effort, effective new therapies can continue to be developed and marketed.

Roles of the Drug Development Team Members

Physicians

The physician's contribution to drug development and the physician's role on a drug development team have changed over the last few decades. Before the 1960s, medical departments of pharmaceutical companies were primarily composed of physicians who were routinely involved in responding to drug information requests rather than developing new drugs. The Kefauver–Harris Amendment, enacted in 1962, required pharmaceutical companies to demonstrate before marketing that a drug was efficacious, which necessitated that physicians increase their presence on drug development teams. Along with the advent of additional governmental regulations, the increase in complexity of medical knowledge has mandated that physicians become an integral member of any drug development team. In fact, because of the different roles of the physician within an organization, companies may now have various departments (e.g., a clinical research department and a clinical safety department) within the medical department.

Although physicians are trained in patient care, physicians who are typically employed by pharmaceutical companies have more training in scientific methodology than those in the past. The physician on the team is the one qualified to follow the progress of each patient enrolled in a clinical trial and to interpret the results. Some physicians continue to spend time treating patients at a university hospital or a specific clinic where their specialty can be utilized and practiced, which allows these physicians to maintain sharp diagnostic skills. Also, some may perform basic research in academic settings to develop or maintain their knowledge and skills in basic research. However, much of today's clinical research is actually conducted by investigators who are not employed by the company sponsoring the development of the drug. The physician on the drug development team must help in the selection of appropriate investigators to conduct the clinical studies. Pharmaceutical physicians may rely on colleagues who are experts in their respective fields and who have appropriate patient populations and facilities for the targeted research project. The physician is also the expert who deals with emergency situations that may arise during the course of a clinical research project, such as an overdose or severe adverse experience (SAE) that might be experienced with the drug. Similarly, the physician assists investigators who are responsible for evaluating the severity of adverse experiences (AEs) and determining the causal relationship of the AEs to the drug under development.

The physician's involvement in clinical research does not end with the completion of the clinical study. Medical reports, clinical study reports, and sections of NDAs must be written. Interactions with regulatory agencies that require the physician's input may occur frequently. Physicians in clinical research may also be called upon to promote new drugs in a scientific environment by organizing symposia and workshops and by reviewing journal advertisements and promotional material for medical validity and accuracy. The role of the physician in a clinical drug development program has expanded and has been refined in the last 40 years. Physicians increasingly contribute clinical and scientific expertise and administrative skills. Many physicians on drug development teams today spend most of their time designing and implementing studies and interpreting and reporting data rather than being in direct contact with patients. An experienced clinician is an important member of any drug development team.

Scientists

While a drug development team may have only one primary physician, it may have multiple scientists. Pharmacokineticists, pharmacologists, toxicologists, and pharmaceutical scientists are all involved in the clinical development of drugs. The contributions of scientists to a drug development project are derived from their experience in both scientific methodology and basic research.

Although physicians are trained in patient care, scientists are trained in problem-solving skills related to scientific research. To obtain a doctoral degree, a scientist must conduct research and write a dissertation that covers a topic of sufficient scope and depth. During this process, the scientist learns how to solve problems from different perspectives. The scientist also collects extensive data and performs data analyses, thereby gaining valuable insight into the considerations necessary to determine the feasibility of collecting data in a clinical trial. Also, some scientists, such as pharmacokineticists with a pharmacy background, may receive some clinical experience during their training as a scientist.

Scientists help design major portions of study protocols and clinical case report forms (CRFs). The study protocol is the overall plan that the study follows, and it must contain certain types of information, including the following: (1) background data on the targeted disease; (2) the empirical and structural formula of the drug being studied; (3) preliminary pharmacology and toxicology of the drug (specific study objectives and designs); (4) the methods and materials to be used in the study; (5) information regarding drug packaging, labeling, dosage forms, and decoding procedures; (6) overdose management; (7) patient discontinuation procedures; (8) explanation of informed consent and provisions regarding institutional review board approval; and (9) any relevant references and appendices. The CRFs are the forms on which individual patient data are recorded during a clinical trial. From these data, clinical and statistical analyses are performed. All the information that is stipulated in the study protocol must be collected on the CRFs. In conjunction with non-scientific personnel, scientists are responsible for ensuring that the CRFs will capture the appropriate information for each study subject according to the objectives, tests, and evaluations stipulated in the protocol. Careful attention must be given to the administration of special tests or collection of samples so that the timing of the assessments or sample collections do not conflict.

Experience in basic research enables the scientist to function as an important link between the basic research labs within the company and the drug development team. Departments specializing in drug metabolism, microbiology, pharmacology, and toxicology need feedback from early human safety and pharmacokinetic studies so they can continue to plan and conduct appropriate long-term animal studies. Thus, communication between the clinical scientist and the basic scientist is important throughout the progress of the drug development program. Because clinical research has become increasingly more scientific, experts in the methodology of science are necessary for a complete research program. The drug development team's scientists may account for much of the scientific expertise, but the roles of the research team overlap to form a scientifically sound, medically astute cohesive group. In addition to scientific expertise, use of the scientist's administrative talents, such as organizational skills and familiarity with personnel practices, enables effective drug development. Thus, scientists with these skills are often employed in management positions in many organizations.

Pharmacists

The pharmacist's role on the drug development team has greatly expanded the professional opportunities of individuals with backgrounds in pharmacy. Pharmacists can provide valuable therapeutic insight into medical research. Training of pharmacists as clinical scientists with both clinical skills and scientific research skills continues to be an emphasis at many pharmacy schools. Several programs have been devised for the education and development of the pharmacist as clinical scientist. Pharmacists have a broad knowledge in both clinical medicine and pharmaceutics, and therefore are able to bridge the gap between the clinic and the laboratory. Pharmacists' training focuses on drug therapies in disease states, whereas physicians' training focuses on the diagnosis of disease states. Studies regarding drug interaction, positive control, or drug comparison involve drugs that have been studied and marketed. Pharmacists can help in the design of such trials because of their knowledge of marketed drugs. Additional roles of pharmacists appear in the areas of drug information and education and training. Pharmacists have the appropriate expertise in drug therapy to answer inquiries from physicians (and other health professionals) concerning both marketed and investigational drug products. Similarly, the clinic/laboratory bridge that the pharmacist builds makes this team member especially well suited to educate and train new employees in drug development. By offering both general and special skills, the research pharmacist blends clinical medicine with pharmaceutical science and is well qualified as an educator and drug information specialist.

Non-Scientific Personnel

Drug development includes many tasks that may not require the specialized expertise of a physician or a scientist. Administrative skills, creativity, and excellent communication abilities, which are qualities not necessarily emphasized within traditional medical and scientific educational curricula, may be required for many of these tasks. The administrative skills necessary for drug development include incorporating seemingly disparate but vitally linked concepts into a single overall plan. Integration planning may mean organizing study files into a logical sequence or helping to assemble the various parts of an NDA. In the first example, files must be set up in a way that can facilitate internal quality assurance audits and FDA inspections. In the second example, knowledge of the FDA's regulations and good abstracting capabilities are required.

Creativity is a quality that cannot be developed through formal training. Creativity requires bold conjecture and it expresses itself in newer, better ways to accomplish the same goals. An example of creativity in clinical drug research might involve the development of a variable report that could support all of the different research documents that are generated by drug research teams. With such a variable report, common information need not be recreated each time another document is generated. Excellent communication skills may be the most important quality for individuals working in drug development, even for those with strong medical backgrounds. Clinical research requires extensive interactions with personnel within the organization and with outside vendors or clinical sites. The information flow must be both efficient and accurate. For example, marketing departments must communicate frequently with medical departments so that marketing studies, advertising, and package inserts can be planned and evaluated. Individuals who lack strong science backgrounds but who have excellent communication skills often act as liaisons in these situations.

One aspect of clinical research that requires extensive contribution by the drug development team personnel is study monitoring. Study monitors oversee the planning, initiation, conduct, and data processing of clinical studies. While monitoring studies, monitors must communicate frequently with investigators and help ensure the data are being collected properly, FDA regulations are being followed, and any administrative problems are resolved as quickly as possible. Although monitors traditionally have had a non-scientific background, many monitors today have training in the basic sciences, and some even have advanced degrees, which allows them to better understand the scientific aspects of the project. Effective study monitors have a wide range of talents. The many facets of a clinical research program afford individuals with varying types of training, education, and experience, the opportunity to contribute to the drug development process. Although some tasks clearly require the clinical or scientific expertise of a physician or a scientist, other tasks are better suited to those individuals with less specialized and more general capabilities.

Stages in Clinical Drug Development

Before clinical drug development can begin, many years of preclinical development occur, millions of dollars are spent, and countless decisions are made. Basic research teams consisting of chemists, pharmacologists, biologists, and biochemists first identify promising therapeutic categories and classes of compounds. One or more compounds are selected for secondary pharmacology evaluations and for both acute and subchronic toxicology testing in animal models. A compound that is pharmacologically active and safe in at least two non-human species may then be selected for study in humans. Before the drug can be tested in humans, an Investigational New Drug (IND) application, which contains supporting preclinical information and the proposed clinical study designs, must be filed with an appropriate regulatory agency.

Clinical drug development follows a sequential process. By convention, development of a new drug in humans is divided into four phases: preapproval segments (Phases 1 through 3) and a postapproval segment (Phase 4). The definitions of the three preapproval phases have relatively clear separations. However, the different phases refer to different types of studies rather than a specific time course of studies. For example, bioequivalence studies and drug–drug interaction studies are both Phase 1 studies, but they may be conducted after Phase 3 studies have been initiated. The generalized sequence of studies may be tailored to each new drug during development.

Phase 1

After the appropriate regulatory agency has approved a potential drug for testing in humans, Phase 1 of the clinical program begins. The primary goal of Phase 1 studies is to demonstrate safety in humans and to collect sufficient pharmacokinetic and pharmacological information to permit the determination of the dose strength and regimen for Phase 2 studies. Phase 1 studies are closely monitored, are typically conducted in healthy adult subjects, and are designed to meet the primary goal (i.e., to obtain information on the safety, pharmacokinetics, and pharmacologic effects of the drug). In addition, the metabolic profile, adverse events associated with increasing dosages, and evidence of efficacy may be obtained. Because most compounds are available for initial studies as an oral formulation, the initial pharmacokinetic profile usually includes information about absorption. Additional studies, such as drug-drug interactions, assessment of bioequivalence of various formulations, or other studies that involve normal subjects, are included in Phase 1.

Generally, the first study in humans is a rising, single-dose tolerance study. The initial dose may be based on animal pharmacology or toxicology data, such as 10% of the no-effect dose. Doses are increased gradually according to a predetermined scheme, often some modification of the Fibonacci dose escalation scheme, until an adverse event is observed that satisfies the predetermined criteria of a maximum tolerated dose (MTD). Although the primary objective is the determination of acute safety in humans, the studies are designed to collect meaningful pharmacokinetic information. Efficacy information or surrogate efficacy measurements also may be collected. However, because a multitude of clinical measurements and tests must be performed to assess safety, measurements of efficacy parameters must not compromise the collection of safety and pharmacokinetic data. Appropriate biological samples for pharmacokinetic assessment, typically blood and urine, should be collected at discrete time intervals based upon extrapolations from the pharmacokinetics of the drug in animals. Depending on the assay sensitivity, the half- life and other pharmacokinetic parameters in healthy volunteers should be able to be evaluated, particularly at the higher doses. The degree of exposure of the drug is an important factor in understanding the toxicologic results of the study. Pharmacokinetic linearity (dose linearity) or non-linearity will be an important factor in the design of future studies.

Once the initial dose has been determined, a placebo-controlled, double-blind, escalating single-dose study is initiated. Generally, healthy male volunteers are recruited, although patients sometimes are used (e.g., when testing a potential anticancer drug that may be too toxic to administer to healthy volunteers). These studies may include two or three cohorts, with six or eight subjects receiving the active drug and two subjects receiving placebo. The groups may receive alternating dose levels, which allow assessment of dose linearity, intrasubject variability of pharmacokinetics, and dose- response (i.e., adverse events) relationship within individual subjects. Participants in the first study are usually hospitalized or enrolled in a clinic so that clinical measurements can be performed under controlled conditions and any medical emergency can be handled in the most expeditious manner. This study is usually placebo-controlled and double-blinded so that the drug effects, such as drug-induced ataxia, can be distinguished from the non-drug effects, such as ataxia secondary to viral infection. The first study in humans is usually not considered successfully completed until an MTD has been reached. An MTD must be reached because the relationship between a clinical event (e.g., emesis) and a particular dose level observed under controlled conditions can provide information that will be extremely useful when designing future trials. Also, the dose range and route of administration should be established during Phase 1 studies.

A multiple-dose safety study typically is initiated once the first study in humans is completed. The primary goal of the second study is to define an MTD with multiple dosing before to initiating well-controlled efficacy testing. The study design of the multiple-dose safety study should simulate actual clinical conditions in as many ways as possible; however, scientific and statistical validity must be maintained. The inclusion of a placebo group is essential to allow the determination of drug-related versus non-drug-related events. The dosing schedule, which includes dosages, frequency, dose escalations, and dose tapering, should simulate the regimen to be followed in efficacy testing. Typically, dosing in the second study lasts for 2 weeks. The length of the study may be increased depending on the pharmacokinetics of the drug so that both drug and metabolite concentrations reach steady state. Also, if the drug is to be used to treat a chronic condition, a 4-week study duration may be appropriate. To obtain information for six dose levels with six subjects receiving active drug and two receiving placebo for each of two cohorts, a minimum enrollment of 24 subjects should be anticipated. Similar to the first study in humans, these subjects would be hospitalized for the duration of the study.

Also similar to the first study, pharmacokinetic data must be obtained. These data will be used to help determine dosage in future efficacy trials. The new pharmacokinetic information that can be gathered includes the following: (1) determination regarding whether the pharmacokinetic parameters obtained in the previous acute safety study accurately predicted the multiple dose pharmacokinetic behavior of the drug; (2) verification of pharmacokinetic linearity (i.e., dose proportionality of C_{max} and AUC) observed in the acute study; (3) determination regarding whether the drug is subject to autoinduction of clearance upon multidosing; and (4) determination of the existence and accumulation of metabolites that could not be detected in the previous single-dose study. A number of experimental approaches can be used to gather this information, and all require frequent collection of blood and urine samples. The challenge to the clinical pharmacokineticist is to design an appropriate blood sample collection schedule that will maximize the pharmacokinetic information, yet can be gathered without biasing the primary objective—determination of clinical safety parameters.

Phase 2

After the initial introduction of a new drug into humans, Phase 2 studies are conducted. The focus of these Phase 2 studies is on efficacy, while the pharmacokinetic information obtained in Phase 1 studies is used to optimize the dosage regimen. Phase 2 studies are not as closely monitored as Phase 1 studies and are conducted in patients. These studies are designed to obtain information on the efficacy and pharmacologic effects of the drug, in addition to the pharmacokinetics. Additional pharmacokinetic and pharmacologic information collected in Phase 2 studies may help to optimize the dose strength and regimen and may provide additional information on the drug's safety profile (e.g., determine potential drug-drug interactions). Efficacy trials should not to be initiated until the MTD has been defined. In addition, the availability of pharmacokinetic information in healthy volunteers is key to the design of successful efficacy trials. The clinical pharmacokineticist assists in the design and execution of these trials and analyzes the plasma drug concentration data upon completion of the efficacy studies.

During the planning stage of an efficacy trial, the focus is on the dosage regimen and its relationship to efficacy measurements. Plasma drug concentrations for various dosages can be simulated based upon the data collected in the first two studies in humans. The disease or physiological states of the test patients (e.g., organ dysfunction as a function of age), concurrent medications (e.g., enzyme inducers or inhibitors), and the safety data obtained earlier must be considered when choosing an optimal dosage regimen for the study. In addition, if the targeted site of the drug is in a tissue compartment, theoretical drug levels in this compartment can be simulated, which may help scientists determine the appropriate times for efficacy measurements.

On completion of the efficacy trial, a therapeutic window for plasma drug concentrations can be defined by reviewing the correlation between plasma drug concentrations and key safety and efficacy parameters. The goal is to improve efficacy and safety of the drug by individualizing the dosage based upon previous plasma drug concentration profiles in the same patient.

Phase 3

If the earlier clinical studies establish a drug's therapeutic, clinical pharmacologic, and toxicologic properties and if it is still considered to be a promising drug—Phase 3 clinical trials will be initiated. Phase 3 studies enroll many more patients and may be conducted both in a hospital or controlled setting and in general practice settings. The goals of Phase 3 studies are to confirm the therapeutic effect, establish dosage range and interval, and assess long-term safety and toxicity. Less common side effects and AEs that develop latently may be identified. In addition, studies targeted to evaluate and quantify specific effects of the drug, such as drowsiness or impaired coordination, are conducted during this phase. Phase 3 studies are also used to identify the most appropriate population or subpopulation for the study drug and to establish a place for the drug in its therapeutic class. A drug may be developed in a therapeutic class that already has effective alternatives, but the investigative compound may have a better safety profile than its established competitors. A Phase 3 clinical study can be designed to assess relative safety profiles.

Closer inspection of drug interactions is warranted in Phase 3 clinical trials. In many disease states, the use of polytherapy is quite common, and the risk of drug–drug interactions is high, both from pharmacokinetic and pharmacodynamic perspectives. The likelihood of drug interactions and semiquantitative estimates of magnitude may be predicted from in vitro data. The potential for interactions needs to be evaluated from two perspectives: the potential that the new drug may affect the pharmacokinetics of other drugs, and the potential that other drugs may affect the pharmacokinetics of the new drug. The former generally depends on the ability of the new drug to affect various enzyme and carrier-mediated clearance processes. Most notably, this concerns the cytochrome P450 (CYP) isoforms but could also involve conjugative enzymes and transporters, such as p-glycoprotein. Drugs may be an effective inhibitor without being a substrate of a CYP isoform, as is the case for quinidine's inhibition of CYP2D6.

The potential for significant drug–drug interactions caused by other drugs requires knowledge of the components of clearance for the new drug and the likelihood that known inhibitors will be coadministered. For drugs with multiple pathways and a broad therapeutic index, the need for formal interaction studies may be limited. Population pharmacokinetic analyses of data obtained from Phase 3 studies may be used to help discover and quantify drug interactions due to classes of drugs often associated with inhibition (e.g., macrolides, systemic antifungals, calcium channel antagonists, fluoxetine, paroxetine) or induction (e.g., anticonvulsants, rifampin). Most early clinical trials are conducted at university medical centers with physicians who specialize in a certain area of medicine. When study drugs are eventually marketed, however, general practitioners will be prescribing them as well. Therefore, it is important that family physicians are exposed to study drugs during this phase because they represent the segment of clinicians who will be writing most of the prescriptions. Similarly, to maximize the commercial return on drug development, a multi-indication strategy may be pursued (sometimes designated as Phase 5 if conducted postapproval). In addition, testing of the drug in foreign countries is appropriate during Phase 3; however, other countries may operate under different regulatory obligations than in the United States.

Phase 4

Whereas Phase 1, 2, and 3 studies are conducted prospectively using subjects or patients whose entrance into the study depends on strict inclusion and exclusion criteria, Phase 4 studies employ mainly observational, rather than exclusionary, study designs. Post-marketing surveillance and any additional studies requested by the regulatory agency as conditional approval of the NDA are conducted during Phase 4. Data collection in premarketing clinical trials is an extensive, scientific exercise. Detailed blood work, special laboratory tests, and careful physiologic monitoring are typical in these studies.

Postmarketing studies, however, are often targeted for much larger patient populations (5000–10,000 or more), which limits extensive data collection from each patient and emphasizes collection of safety information. These studies are complemented by reports of AEs from patients not enrolled in a study. The large numbers of patients in Phase 4 studies make it easier for researchers to determine rare AEs and can help identify patient populations that are at particular risk for certain AEs. For example, demographic trends toward side effects involving geographic locus, gender, or race may be determined from postmarketing surveillance data.

Protocol Considerations

The task of designing a clinical study cannot be undertaken until the study objective of that trial has been rigorously defined. The objective should explicitly state what is being investigated and vague language should be avoided. Once an unbiased and specific objective has been developed, scientists can build the study design around it and then develop and write the protocol. One of the main considerations when designing an investigational study concerns the type and number of comparative groups that will be involved. A control group of subjects may be evaluated in addition to the group taking the investigational drug. Sometimes more than one control group is used in a study. The control groups take either placebo or active medication and are compared with the group taking the investigational drug. This design is used to rule out the possibility of a placebo effect or to assess the efficacy and safety of the investigational drug relative to other drugs currently marketed.

Regulatory agencies frequently require the pivotal Phase 3 studies, which will be used to support an NDA, to be placebo-controlled studies. Placebo medication should be as similar as possible to the drug being investigated (e.g., same color, taste, and shape). No statistically significant difference in response between this group and the subjects taking the investigational drug is evidence against that drug having any real effectiveness. Similar to the placebo considerations, active medication taken by the control group also should be as similar as possible to the drug being investigated (e.g., same color, taste, and shape). If the formulations cannot be made with similar appearances (e.g., tablet, suspension, etc.), a placebo of each formulation could be made so subjects would take one active formulation and the placebo of the other formulation to maintain the blind. No statistically significant difference in response in this group relative to the subjects taking the investigational drug is evidence that active medication has no advantage therapeutically over the existing therapy. However, a higher incidence of AEs in the control group and an equal rate of efficacy relative to the subjects taking the investigational drug are evidence of the new drug's advantage over the existing therapy.

In addition to determining the types and number of control groups that should be included in a study, the drug development team must decide between a parallel and a crossover design. For example, in a placebo- controlled clinical trial, a parallel design is one in which each study group takes the same medication (i.e., either placebo or active drug) throughout the study. With a crossover design, each study group eventually receives both placebo and active drug (e.g., one group may take placebo for a 6-week period and then cross over to receive active drug for the following 6-week period).

An advantage of the crossover design is that it allows each group to be its own control, thereby allowing a demonstration of efficacy to occur during the treatment with the drug. A disadvantage of the crossover design is that residual effects from one treatment period may carry over into the other treatment period. Absolute determination of efficacy and safety of the different treatments is difficult and sometimes impossible. One way to avoid the problem of residual effects on crossover studies is to have washout periods between the different treatment phases. During the washout period, the patient is either given a placebo or no treatment for several days or weeks so that any possible metabolite or effect of the drug is "washed out" of the patient before the next treatment phase begins. An advantage of the parallel design is that it avoids the problems associated with possible residual effects of one treatment period influencing the other treatment period(s) because each treatment group is only exposed to one drug. Compared with a crossover study, more patients may be required for a parallel study so that statistical significance can be established between the study groups. In a parallel study, recruiting the required larger numbers of patients who fit the study criteria takes longer, but the duration of that study is usually shorter than the duration of a crossover study. Crossover designs span greater periods of time because each group must sequentially take an active and a control medication over a period that is long enough to allow a treatment effect to emerge. When washout periods are added, the time required to conduct these studies becomes longer still, and more study subjects may drop out. These difficulties are often outweighed by the fact that statistical significance can be achieved with fewer patients in crossover studies.

Once the study design has been chosen, there are many other issues to consider when developing and writing clinical protocols. Among the topics to be considered are criteria for patient eligibility, efficacy and safety parameters, timing of the events, packaging and dispensing of the clinical trial material, and the informed consent form. Also, to be determined is how the study will be blinded. For most well- controlled studies, subjects are assigned to the various groups by using a randomization process so that biased selection is eliminated, the overall collection of the subjects' variables is comparable in each group, and statistical power is guaranteed. In these double- blind studies, neither the subject nor the investigating scientists know to which group the subject has been assigned. Thus, extensive input from the drug development team is required when designing studies and writing protocols.

Drug Development Considerations

Most drugs are tested in humans to treat a specific disease entity or some adverse clinical condition. Because the pathogenesis of diseases and the exact mechanisms of action of drugs are often poorly understood, the process of evaluating a drug's efficacy can be complicated. Upon treatment, a patient's adverse clinical condition may improve; however, for many diseases this occurrence can only be evaluated indirectly by clinical assessments (e.g., via blood pressure measurements in the treatment of hypertension). However, a drug's characteristics can also be measured directly. For example, measurement of blood concentrations of the drug enabling calculation of pharmacokinetic parameters is a direct evaluation of the drug.

Similar to efficacy assessments, evaluation of the safety of a drug may also involve indirect measurements. One of the primary methods of obtaining safety information in a clinical trial is through a patient's reporting of AEs. Although the exact biochemical mechanisms responsible for many AEs cannot be evaluated directly, the indirect evaluation of the drug's adverse effect can be seen clinically. Because clinical assessments are indirect measures, AE reporting leads to several complex questions. The degree of drug- relatedness or causality, the effect of concomitant medication, the severity of the AE, the complications of the disease state, and the effects of other clinical conditions or diseases are usually difficult to determine, particularly early in the drug development program. Also, all reports of AEs in a clinical drug research program are recorded, tabulated, and cross- referenced to form a safety database, regardless of whether the AE is determined to be drug related. The information contained in this database is used to generate the package insert.

Although the clinical effect of a drug is perhaps the primary concern of drug development, an understanding of the drug's biochemical and physicochemical properties and mechanism of action is also desired. These direct measures are of equal concern in drug development as are the indirect evaluations of a drug's clinical effects. The primary tool used to study the intrinsic physicochemical properties of a drug is pharmacokinetics, which is a branch of biopharmaceutics. Pharmacokinetics describes the relationship between the processes of drug absorption, distribution, metabolism (biotransformation), and excretion (collectively abbreviated ADME) and the time course of therapeutic or adverse effects of drugs. Efficacy is determined by the drug concentration at the site of action, which generally is correlated with the drug concentration in the blood. The ultimate goal of pharmacokinetics is to characterize the sources of variability in the concentration time profile, which may be correlated with variability in efficacy and adverse events.

Pharmacokinetics can be used to guide dosage regimen selection and thereby optimize pharmacologic effects and minimize toxicologic effects when a drug is administered to an individual patient. Thus, although the basic pharmacokinetic properties of a drug are identified during the earliest stage of clinical drug development, the many factors affecting the pharmacokinetics in the patient population must be identified throughout the drug development process to enable proper dose selection for individuals. Thus, both indirect and direct measures are used to evaluate a drug.

Marketing Input

A successful pharmaceutical company has an appropriate blend of both research and marketing to enable a symbiotic, rather than antagonistic, relationship. Because an effective scientific and clinical research team often designs and executes experiments and clinical trials that involve costly overhead expenses, it is essential for marketing decisions to be geared toward company profitability being made allow the company profitable so these expenses can be met. Therefore, both medical and marketing input are necessary if a pharmaceutical company is to be successful.

By gathering data on all facets of the needs in the marketplace from clinicians and by maintaining a profile awareness of new products under development by competitors, marketing personnel are in an excellent position to advise their colleagues in the research arena who are responsible for the drug development program. Also, a marketing expert can help identify the problems other companies are having in selling their product and thereby avoid the same difficulties. For instance, sales problems may be related to ineffective advertising or faulty packaging; therefore, they do not concern clinical research. However, problems in sales can also be related to a drug's undesirable effects. An effective drug that does not lead to the AEs associated with an already approved drug would have a marketing advantage. Someone in marketing research may suggest conducting clinical studies that would evaluate the relative incidence of the AE with the hope that the data could be used to support effective advertising.

Thus, research and marketing are mutually benefical in a successful pharmaceutical company. Marketing groups help clinical research teams by supplying them with information about competing products, the needs of the marketplace, and suggestions for new formulations. Clinical research teams provide the data to support therapeutic and marketing claims and act as chief advisors to marketing personnel concerning drug research studies and promotional claims.

Effective Global Planning

Because drugs are frequently marketed worldwide and the clinical development of drugs may involve studies that are conducted internationally effective global planning can present its own difficulties. Obviously, medical practice, regulatory guidelines, and the cultural environment may be different in various countries, but also the manner in which research is conceived can differ vastly between countries. Medical researchers in some countries may be more conservative than researchers in other countries, which could potentially lead to the underdosing of drugs. These differences in research approaches actually stem from differences in ethical standards. Another reason that international planning may be difficult in drug research concerns the way in which various countries view early clinical trials and drug safety. Some countries view volunteer subjects and patients differently from a regulatory perspective, making it easier to recruit and enroll subjects for Phase 1 studies than it is to recruit and enroll patients for Phase 2 or Phase 3 studies. In the United States, both patients and volunteers are viewed in the same way, and studies with patients and volunteers cannot be initiated until the FDA has authorized an IND. In addition to regulatory guidelines, the regulatory process is still another aspect of clinical drug development that can differ widely between countries. In England, sponsoring research firms do not interact very much with the British drug regulatory agency the Committee on Safety of Medicines. This lack of direct interaction stems from the desire to keep commercial influence away from the objective evaluation of a pharmaceutical company's study data. This lack of communication results in British companies treating government guidelines for conducting clinical research as a routine checklist rather than an aid in forming the most appropriate development strategy.

In the United States, federal guidelines (Code of Federal Regulations, CFR) have been established by the FDA to help sponsoring research firms conduct good, consistent clinical studies. However, some of the items in these guidelines may not be appropriate for all clinical studies, and some items that may be appropriate to include in a clinical study may not have been incorporated into the federal guidelines. These variations occur because each drug and disease state is unique, and complete guidelines cannot be established for all cases. For these reasons, several meetings are held between clinical research teams and the FDA before an NDA submission to ensure that all appropriate methodology and experimentation is being incorporated into the overall drug development project.

Beginning in the early 1990s, the FDA participated in a collaborative effort to harmonize the technical procedures for development and regulatory approval of human pharmaceuticals internationally. Forces that led the agency in this direction included increased trade, the multinational nature of the pharmaceutical industry, trade agreements such as the North American Free Trade Agreement and the General Agreement on Tariffs and Trade by the World Trade Organization, European activism, and pressures on the industry to control costs. These pressures included intense competition and health care reimbursement controls. This harmonization effort is the work of the International Conference on Harmonisation (ICH) of Technical Requirements for Registration of Pharmaceuticals for Human Use. ICH has focused on achieving harmonization of technical requirements in three major regions of the world: the United States, the European Union, and Japan. Some of the earliest ICH guidelines addressed the format and content of the Investigator's Brochure, stability testing, and genotoxicity testing. The FDA also works with the World Health Organization and other international organizations to set standards for health care products. Clinical drug research is a complicated, multidisciplinary task that may be conducted internationally. In fact, many pharmaceutical companies are multinational, with locations in several countries. Planning and coordination become even more complex for such global drug development programs. Despite the differences among countries in medical practice, regulation, and culture, international drug development and marketing are vital parts of many organizations. The successful multinational pharmaceutical company will plan its clinical research strategy according to any differences among nations before to implementing its international development plans.

Ethical Considerations

No topic in clinical drug development is more controversial and emotionally charged than the myriad ethical dilemmas that face physicians and scientists involved in clinical research. Given that clinical research has generally proved to have moral consequences through its direct and indirect influence on alleviating suffering, steps must be taken to ensure that abuses do not occur during the course of drug development. Therefore, guidelines for the protection of human subjects have been developed, proposed, and accepted worldwide. Because of the atrocities committed by Nazi medical researchers in the 1930s, the Nuremberg Code was written, and highlighted the importance of obtaining all research subjects' voluntary consent to their participation in clinical studies. The Declaration of Helsinki, which was published by the World Medical Association in 1964 and has been updated several times since, takes the informed consent issue one step further by giving only qualified medical scientists and physicians the right to conduct clinical research. However, similar concerns go back at least to the 1830s, when

Dr. William Beaumont developed a contract with a patient, and in the late 1800s, when a leprosy worker experimented on a patient without her consent.

Legislation that ensures the protection of human research subjects in the United States includes the 1979 publication of the Belmont Report on the Ethical Principles and Guidelines for the Protection of Human Subjects of Research. This report concerns the fine line between biomedical research and the routine practice of medicine and explores the criteria that determine the risk-benefit ratio in the consideration of conducting clinical research. It also addresses basic guidelines for the proper selection of human research subjects and further defines the elements of informed consent.

Other important legislation in the United States includes the FDA's Guidance for Institutional Review Boards (IRBs) for further guarantees of protection for human research subjects. IRBs are independent committees that review proposed clinical research projects before the commencement of the research. These committees decide whether the risk to research subjects outweighs the potential benefit of the research; they can suggest modifications in the research proposal or disapprove the project altogether. IRBs must consist of both men and women of varying professions. At least one member must have his or her primary concern in a non-scientific area (e.g., a lawyer or clergyperson), and at least one member must not be affiliated with the institution at which the research will be conducted. Closely related to the rights of human research subjects are the rights of routine patients involved in non-research medical matters. In 1973, the American Hospital Association published the Patient's Bill of Rights, which requires that the acting physician give his patients complete information concerning their diagnosis, treatment, and prognosis; that the patient be given respectful care; that the patient be given the opportunity to refuse treatment; and that the patient's records, condition, and medical care be treated confidentially.

Another ethical issue facing clinical research scientists concerns study design, in particular, the placebo-controlled clinical trial. The reason placebo-controlled clinical trials are conducted is quite compelling from a scientific standpoint: to ensure that the evidence supporting the efficacy of an experimental drug is actually due to the properties of the drug and not to the psychologic properties of the study subjects. In other words, if a placebo effect from the experimental drug occurs rather than a true therapeutic effect, then a comparison of the drug group with the placebo group will show statistically similar response rates. It is a way to help separate actual drug responses from placebo responses, especially in studies investigating psychiatric compounds, but also in other therapeutic areas with a clearer "*physiologic*" or "*biochemical*" basis.

One defense for conducting placebo-controlled clinical trials is that the subjects chosen for the placebo group are randomly chosen, so that no malicious withholding occurs. Also, many study protocols have provisions of study extension that guarantee subjects in placebo groups have the opportunity to take the drug as an extension of the study after they complete the original part, or they are offered the chance to receive alternative therapy. Study subjects may be given monetary compensation for their participation in studies, in addition to free, thorough physical exams, lab work, and physician visits.

Interestingly, experimental drugs have unknown side effects that can cause serious biochemical and physiologic problems, whereas placebo medication does not. This fact makes possible the contrary argument and objection, on purely ethical grounds, to giving study subjects experimental and hence unproven drugs. Of course, informed consent and careful monitoring by trained medical personnel help to alleviate the ethical problems associated with giving subjects an active, investigational drug. The most important aspect of all studies is that the patient be completely informed of all study procedures and agree to willingly participate in the study. The most recent pressing ethical dilemma facing the clinical research scientist surrounds the increasing amount of research that is being conducted in biotechnical and genetic engineering. Ethical issues will continue to play important parts in the medical and legal worlds. Whereas pure science is value-neutral, its application is always open to debate. Undesirable extremes are likely to exist at both ends of the spectrum.

Future Prospectives

To conduct a clinical study for the evaluation of a new drug, a vast array of personnel is required. Physicians are largely used because of their knowledge of clinical medicine and patient care, whereas scientists are used because of their knowledge of the methodology and the science. Pharmacists serve a bridging function due to their unique training in therapeutics and the pharmaceutical sciences. Non-scientific personnel are indispensable because of their ability to coordinate the many facets of a drug development project. The clinical evaluation of drugs involves many different levels of scrutiny before a drug product can be marketed. These levels include Phase 1 for safety testing, Phase 2 for evaluating efficacy and determining the correct therapeutic dose, Phase 3 for large-scale studies and determination of drug interactions, and Phase 4 for postmarketing surveillance. Phase 1 studies are typically conducted in healthy volunteers, and Phase 2 through 4 studies are conducted in patients. Study design plays a critical role in the clinical evaluation of drugs. A clinical study cannot be conducted without specifically outlined objectives and a definitive plan, which are vital components around which the study protocol is constructed. The use of placebo or active drug control groups in the study, and whether the design should be open, parallel, or crossover, must be determined. In most studies, patients are assigned to study groups randomly.

The developmental objectives facing the clinical research team include indirect evaluations of a drug's safety and efficacy, such as effects on vital signs or behavior, and direct evaluations of a drug's intrinsic properties, such as its pharmacokinetics and mode of action. Also, the marketing medical liaison is important if research is to support future sales plans and advertising is to reflect study results. Finally, effective global planning is necessary because drugs are more frequently developed and marketed worldwide, and therefore involve differing patient populations and different government regulations. ICH guidelines have helped to standardize regulations worldwide. The ethical dilemmas facing clinical research scientists affect much of the legislation that currently regulates the conduct of clinical trials. The goal of drug development research is to develop effective pharmacotherapy for mankind's ailments, and regulatory agencies have enacted legislation to prevent unethical research. Although traditional medicines continue to be discovered and developed, the fields of biotechnology and gene therapy continue to advance. In addition, new methods to collect and evaluate clinical data on a real-time basis will help to speed the development process.

4

Clinical Perspectives

The eventual clinical implications of the large efforts in pharmacogenomic research throughout the world described in other chapters may be profound and widespread, but the actual utility of pharmacogenetic knowledge in clinical practice to date remains limited and largely untested. Changes in clinical practice represented by changes in dose or in the drug administered that result in real changes in health outcomes would be important measures of progress toward the "*personalized medicine*" or "*precision prescriptions*" so frequently predicted. Such outcomes might include the avoidance of a specific toxicity or the achievement of a specific therapeutic effect, but, as with all measures of success in medicine, must also include real clinical outcomes. It seems inevitable that significant improvements will continue to be made in the proportion of patients that are treated well, as is heralded by the recent reports of the effectiveness of a generally *ineffective* drug, gefitinib (Iressa) in lung cancer in patients who carry sensitizing mutations of the tyrosin kinase domain of the epidermal growth factor receptor (EGFR). We would not be surprised at this progress, if we recognized that such improvements are actually part of a continuum of improvement in the quality and individualization of patient care.

Individualization of therapy to an individual patient is not a new concept in medicine, but one central to its practice since the beginning. The writings of Hippocrates, Garrod, Jenner, and Osler all emphasize the centrality of treating the patient as an individual. There are multiple recent successes in targeting therapy to individual patients, supported by outcomes data and in wide clinical use already. To take the field of breast cancer as an example, such advances would include the evolution from the simple individualization of dose of chemotherapy by weight and body surface area to the use of estrogen and progesterone receptor status to target endocrine therapy by specific estrogen receptor modulators or aromatase inhibitors, to the use of the Gail index to identify patients most worth of preventive treatment, and to the use of BRCA1 mutations and HER2 status to target trastuzumab (Herceptin) therapy. We should not delude ourselves either by thinking that pharmacogenetic testing will usher in a new revolution in therapy or that the need for it represents an insult to our collective ability to individualize treatments in the past. "*Personalized medicine*" is nothing new. We have been doing it all along. That said we have to admit that we have been doing it when we had time and when it was possible in busy clinical practice environments and that the pressures to adopt a "*one dose fits all*" approach are real. Quality has always mattered in health care, but now the quality of our performance as effective prescribers is being measured by hospitals, by health care systems and by government agencies.

Pharmacogenomics should be seen as a stimulus to quality prescribing, a salve to the impersonalization of mass health care, and an invitation to advance the quality of our care beyond what is possible when we have time to do it and less medication to choose from. It should be designed as a "*tool for quality improvement*" along with the legions of administrators monitoring the number of new and return patients we see, the multiple digital assistants marketed to us, and the digitizing of our medical records. A large number of potential pharmacogenetic tests have been proposed, and so it is necessary to have some simple means of separating, which tests are likely to be most valuable.

In guiding drug therapy, pharmacogenetic tests should help to prevent serious adverse reactions, reduce hospitalizations and mortality, and should thereby reduce health care costs, but also avoid the prescribing of drugs to patients who are likely not to respond. In fact, preventing ineffective treatment possibly is as effective in reducing costs of health care as adjusting doses to minimize adverse effects and improve efficacy. While tests that are robust, reliable and cheap to perform will inevitably have an edge over those that are not, it is also important that a test provides added value above what is currently available. If we can measure LDL-cholesterol as a metric to follow statin efficacy, or if the physician of a patient with hypertension can tell at the next weekly visit whether a diuretic or an *angiotensin converting enzyme* (ACE) inhibitor is working, it makes less sense to develop a pharmacogenetic test to predict the effects of statins and anti-hypertensive drugs, than to search for one that predicts the response to an antidepressant or cancer treatment, where our current predictive powers are more limited. However, we constantly learn and better understand the reasons for variability in drug response. For instance, the somewhat smaller reduction in total cholesterol and LDL cholesterol in some patients treated with pravastatin recently was explained by a common variant of the HMG-CoA reductase gene.

We should not be naïve to the fact that our scientific forbearers have developed numerous useful predictors of treatment response. To return to the example of breast cancer treatment: no pharmacogenetic test is likely to have value unless it can improve on the currently widely used and useful predictive clinical parameters: the number of lymph nodes, grade of tumor, etc. An excellent example of a rigorous approach has been provided by the group at the Netherlands Cancer Institute, who showed that a customized tumor gene expression array was a more powerful predictor of the outcome of disease in young patients with breast cancer than standard systems based on clinical and histologic criteria. Last, but NOT least, a pharmacogenetic test, as any other diagnostic procedure, must be economically viable for companies that make test kits and for laboratories that do the testing. With these criteria in mind we have reviewed the approximately 45 pharmacogenetic situations or genes that have been associated with drug response in more than one clinical study. Monogenic traits were considered in regard to their possible clinical impact or the potential that they may consistently affect the choice and/or dose of a drug treatment. Of the seven genes and situations, the role of CYP2D6 in the use of neuroleptics and antidepressants is discussed in other chapters, and the testing for the presence of HER2 in breast cancer or for variants of HCV is well established.

N-Acetyltransferase (NAT2) and Isoniazid

One of the first pharmacogenetic traits to be recognized more than 50 years ago was the slow acetylation of the antituberculosis drug isoniazid now known as the polymorphism of N-acetyltransferase 2 (NAT2) and inherited as an autosomal recessive trait. Isoniazid is the treatment of choice for latent tuberculosis infection and is included in most first-line therapy regimens in combination with rifampicin, ethambutol and pyrazinamide. However, acute or chronic hepatitis frequently develops in patients receiving these drugs, with an incidence of 1–36%, depending on different regimens and how one defines hepatic injury, from transient elevations of liver function tests to serious injury or even death. Of the various drugs used in the combination therapy, isoniazid appears to be the main drug to induce hepatotoxicity. Additional risk factors are alcohol consumption, advanced age and pre-existing chronic liver disease. In numerous studies, slow acetylators treated with isoniazid and rifampicin had a higher risk of hepatotoxicity than rapid acetylators and among patients with hepatotoxicity, slow acetylators had significantly higher serum aminotransferase levels. Additional genetic risk factors were a homozygous "wild-type" genotype for CYP2E1 (CYP2E1 c1/c1) conferring high activity to this enzyme. In other studies, the acetylator genotype was a good predictor of isoniazid plasma levels and isoniazid-induced hepatotoxicity. These data suggest that genotype-derived dosage regimens, e.g., 400, 300, and 200 mg per day for slow (homozygous for two defective alleles), intermediate (heterozygous) or rapid (homozygous for two active alleles) acetylators, should be considered in future prospective studies.

The resurgence of tuberculosis in many countries as a serious threat because of a growing prevalence of drug resistance and its association with high risk patients such as HIV-seropositive individuals, convicts, homeless, or drug users has reemphasized the role of genetic risk factors for the hepatotoxicity associated with antituberculous regimens. The incidence of NAT2 slow acetylators can vary from 5% to 95%, depending on the geographic/ethnic origin of the population studied. In addition to isoniazid, the NAT2 polymorphism affects the pharmacokinetics of a wide variety of arylamine and hydrazine drugs and chemical carcinogens. They include sulfonamides such as salazosulfapyridine, the anti arrhythmic procainamide and the anticancer drug amonafide, for all of which dose adjustments according to the acetylator genotype or phenotype have been recommended, but are not part of common practice.

CYP2C9 and Warfarin

Warfarin is a commonly used anticoagulant that requires careful clinical management to balance the potentially lethal risks of over-anticoagulation and bleeding with the equally daunting risks of under anticoagulation and clotting. It is a legitimate target for a pharmacogenetic test because the surrogate for clinical effect, the international normalized ratio (INR) of the prothrombin time takes several days to reach its steady state, and improvements in both adverse outcomes and efficacy would be obtained if a pharmacogenetic test could more accurately predict dose. The CYP2C9 is known to be the primary catalyst of the human metabolism of the S-enantiomer of warfarin, and the scientific association is sufficiently strong that warfarin was the substrate chosen for the crystallization of a human cytochrome

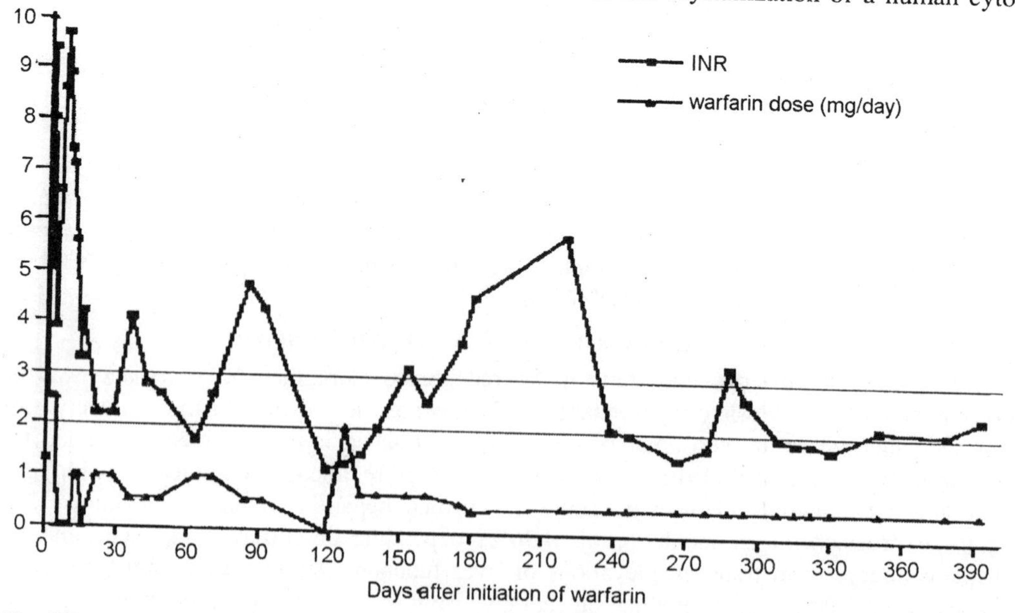

*Fig. 4.1. The INR values and warfarin doses of a patient with CYP2C9*3 allele variant requiring over 1 year to maintain a therapeutic INR.*

CYP2C9 with its bound substrate. Multiple retrospective studies from investigators all over the world have shown that variant alleles of the CYP2C9 gene encoding the *2 [Arg144Cys] and *3 [Ile359Leu] alleles increase the anticoagulant effect of warfarin and decrease the mean daily dose required to maintain the INR of the prothrombin time within the target therapeutic range. It is clear that the cost of caring for such a patient would likely outweigh the cost of a pharmacogenetic test. This anecdotal observation is supported by other case reports, and by a number of trials.

The more persuasive of these are studies that take into account the other clinically available predictive factors, including specifically Vitamin K intake. Aithal et al., the first group to report a clinical association between CYP2C9 genotype and warfarin dose went on to study the contribution of CYP2C9 genotype, age, body size, and vitamin K and lipid status to warfarin dose requirements. The multiple linear regression models for warfarin dose indicated significant contributions from age ($r = 0.41$, $p < 0.001$), genotype ($r = 0.24$, $p < 0.005$), and age and genotype together ($r = 0.45$, $p < 0.005$). The CYP2C9 genotype had a significant effect on S-warfarin clearance ($r = 0.34$, $p < 0.0001$) but none on R-warfarin clearance. In addition, Khan et al. studied the influence of dietary Vitamin K on dosage requirements and showed that, while dietary vitamin K had no effect, CYP2C9 genotype ($p = 2\%$) and age ($p < 1\%$) significantly contributed to inter-patient variability in warfarin dose requirements.

While data have been available for some time in relation to maintenance dose, the effect of CYP2C9 polymorphisms on dose requirements during the induction phase, when the danger of bleeding complications likely is greatest, has also been studied: patients with 2C9*2 or 2C9*3 variant alleles more frequently had INR values above the upper limit of the target range (3.0) (65% for 2C9*2/- and 66% for 2C9*3/- Vs. 33% for 2Cp*1/1; p = 0.006 and .012, respectively). In elderly patients, a genetic influence on response to warfarin does exist as in younger patients. In work carried out by Siguret et al. The CYP2C9 genotype was performed in 126 patients, with a mean age 87 ± 6 years. The mean daily dose of warfarin was 3.0 ± 1.4 mg, with 3.1 mg in patients with the wild type *1/*1 genotype ($n = 80$), 2.7 mg in *1/*2 heterozygotes ($n = 20$), 2.9 mg in *1/*3 heterozygotes ($n = 18$), 1.2 mg in *2/*2 homozygotes ($n = 2$), 2.3 mg in compound heterozygotes *2/*3 ($n = 6$).

Most importantly, the aggregated data prompted Higashi et al. to design a trial to test whether CYP2C9 genotyping could predict outcomes of patients on warfarin therapy. In this retrospective cohort study, 200 patients receiving long-term warfarin therapy for various indications underwent CYP2C9 genotyping and were evaluated by outcome measures, including anticoagulation status, measured by time to therapeutic INRs, rate of above-range INRs, and time to stable warfarin dosing or to serious or life-threatening bleeding events. They found that the mean maintenance dose varied significantly among the six-genotype groups (*1/*1 [$n = 127$], *1/*2 [$n = 28$], *1/*3 [$n = 18$], *2/*2 [$n = 4$], *2/*3 [$n = 3$], and *3/*3 [$n = 5$]) (by the Kruskall–Wallis test, $\chi^2 = 37.348$; $p < 0.001$). Compared with patients with the wild-type genotype, patients with at least one variant allele had an increased risk of above-range INRs of 1.40 (95% CI, 1.03–1.90). The variant group also required more time to achieve stable dosing (HR, 0.65; 95% CI, 0.45–0.94), with a median difference of 95 days ($p = 0.004$). In addition, patients with a variant genotype had a significantly increased risk of a serious or life-threatening bleeding event (HR, 2.39; 95% CI, 1.18–4.86).

More prospective studies are needed to test the feasibility and cost effectiveness of using algorithms based on these parameters for adjusting initial warfarin dose to meet individual needs, but the data at present make a strong case for the use of CYP2C9 genotyping testing prior to warfarin treatment, especially in the elderly. The main alternatives to warfarin, the coumarin derivatives acenocoumerol and phenoprocoumon, are widely or exclusively used instead of warfarin in certain European countries. Again the S-enantiomers of these closely related chemicals are substrates of CYP2C9. The presence of even one copy of CYP2C9*3 profoundly decreases the metabolic clearance of S-acenocoumarol. S-acenocoumarol, which normally is clinically inactive will now exert the main anticoagulant activity. The CYP2C9*3 allele therefore is related to low-dose requirements of racemic acenocoumerol, a higher frequency of over anticoagulation and an unstable anticoagulant response. Phenoprocoumon not significantly affected in its kinetics by the CYP2C9 polymorphism and appears to be a clinically useful alternative to warfarin in patients carrying CYP2C9*2 and *3 alleles.

Thiopurine S-Methyltransferase and Mercaptopurin

The therapy of cancer almost always involves multiple drugs with considerable toxicity. Pharmacogenomic approaches to cancer therapy have already briefly been discussed at the beginning of this chapter in regard to breast cancer. In general, these strategies include variations in germline DNA (e.g., genetic polymorphisms), acquired somatic mutations in tumor cells (e.g., sensitizing mutations in the tyrosine kinase domain of the EGFR gene that is the target of genitifib) or variations in RNA expression. Perhaps one of the best studied examples for the application of pharmacogenomic strategies to prevent adverse drug reactions is the polymorphism of the thiopurine S-methyltransferase (TPMT) gene, which has been extensively reviewed. The TPMT catalyses the S-methylation of thiopurine drugs such as mercaptopurine and its prodrug azathioprine. These drugs are successfully used to treat *acute lymphoblastic leukemia* (ALL) of childhood. Moreover, gastroenterologists prescribe thiopurine drugs as second-line (off-label) therapy for Crohn's disease and ulcerative colitis. Because methylation by TPMT is the pre-dominant pathway for inactivation of thiopurines, patients with TPMT deficiency accumulate active thioguanine nucleotides and this can lead to severe and life-threatening hematological toxicity. The TPMT activity in erythrocytes is trimodally distributed among Europeans, European-Americans, and African-Americans, which corresponds well to the genotypes or the respective presence of 2, 1, or 0 functional TPMT alleles.

In fact, the concordance rate between TPMT genotype and phenotype is >98%. Twenty mutant alleles of TPMT have been associated with low TPMT activity and three of these variants (TPMT*2, TPMT*3A, and TPMT*3C) account for approximately ~95% of low TPMT activity phenotypes. Approximately 1 in 150–300 individuals is homozygous for inactive TPMT alleles, approximately 10% of patients are heterozygous and have intermediate activity and ~90% are normal or high methylators in a Northern European Caucasian population. Interestingly, a subpopulation of ultrarapid TPMT metabolizers also was identified in these population studies. Because of the genotype–phenotype concordance and the severe toxicity associated with high concentrations of thioguanine nucleotides, several cancer centers routinely genotype patients for TPMT mutant alleles and use genotype-derived algorithms for dosing. Intermediate metabolizers receive ~65% and poor metabolizers 5–10% of standard doses of mercaptopurine. Dose reductions in patients with variant TPMT alleles lead to similar or superior survival compared to patients with wild-type alleles. Expectedly, there is considerable variability in the frequency of TPMT alleles in populations of different ethnic origins.

Despite the obvious robustness and cost-effectiveness of TPMT genotyping, additional factors and "*resistance of physicians to change*" so far have limited genotyping to specialized cancer centers. The arguments that full TPMT activity does not preclude possible myelotoxicity with multi-drug regimens and that partial TPMT activity does not always mandate reduced doses appear not very convincing. The information from genotyping obviously is only one type of information to be used in making decisions on drug and dosage regimens in following a patient with ALL, but it has an important function of telling the physician which patients have to be monitored more closely. Of major concern is a report of an increased incidence of secondary brain tumors after radiotherapy in children with decreased TPMT activity phenotypes and/or high concentrations of thioguanine nucleotides in blood cells. The implications for therapeutic decisions regarding prophylactic radiotherapy in ALL therefore must be further investigated.

UDP-Glucuronosyltransferase (UGT) 1A1 and Irinotecan

Results from several recently published trials suggest that patients who are homozygous for a UGT gene variant known as UGT1A1*28 (the "7/7" genotype) are at greater risk for irinotecan-induced severe diarrhea or neutropenia. Irinotecan is a camptothecin analog and inhibits topoisomerase I as an antineoplastic principle. It is used to treat several solid tumors. The disposition of irinotecan is quite complex and involves numerous metabolic enzymes and transport proteins. The SN-38 is the active metabolite of irinotecan and is eliminated via UGT1A1 conversion to SN-38G, an inactive glucuronide cleared via biliary excretion.

Reduced activity of UGT1A1 is linked to an approximately fourfold increased risk of severe toxicity, including dose-limiting diarrhea and neutropenia. Significant correlations between patients carrying one or two copies of the UGT1A1*28 allele and reduced UGT1A1 expression and reduced SW38 glucuronidation have been well documented. More than 50 mutations in UGT1A1 have been reported by Tukey and Strassburg, 2002 many of which are found in patients with Gilbert's syndrome, a form of mild non-hemolytic unconjugated hyperbilirubinemia. The most common mutant gene is UGT1A1*28, it contains seven dinucleotide repeats in the TATA box of the promoter [A(TA)$_7$TAA] instead of the normally six repeats, which leads to approximately 70% reduction of transcriptional activity. Many rare mutations also lead to Gilbert's syndrome, and individuals with this syndrome are pre-disposed to SN-38 initiated toxicity. Although, as always, a number of additional factors influence the toxicity of SN-38 in the intestine and bone narrow, assessment of the presence of the UGT1A1*28 allele in patients prior to irinotecan treatment will allow to start with lower dose or change to alternative therapies.

CYP2D6 and Codeine

It involves a large number of drugs, including many antidepressants and neuroleptics, antiarrhythmics, and many others commonly used drugs. In fact, recent recommendation for adjusting the doses for a number of antidepressant and neuroleptic drugs in the four genotypes/phenotypes poor metabolizers, extensive metabolizers, intermediate metabolizers, and ultrarapid metabolizers have been proposed. Prospective studies are planned to evaluate these recommendations, as genotyping tests for the multiple mutations of CYP2D6 are available. Here we discuss the striking differences in the responses to opioids that are associated with the CYP2D6 polymorphism. Dextromethorphan, codeine, hydrocodone, oxycodone, ethylmorphine, and dihydrocodeine all are dealkylated by polymorphic CYP2D6. The polymorphic O-demethylation of codeine is of clinical importance when this drug is given as an analgesic. About 5% of codeine is O-demethylated to morphine, and this pathway is deficient in poor metabolizers. Poor metabolizers therefore experience little analgesic benefit from treatment with codeine. Similarly, respiratory, psychomotor, and pupillary effects of codeine are decreased in poor metabolizers compared with extensive metabolizers.

Codeine is frequenctly recommended as a drug of first choice for treatment of chronic severe pain. Physicians must appreciate that no analgesic effect is to be expected in the 5–10% of Caucasians who are of the poor metaboliser phenotype, or who are extensive metabolizers receiving concomitant treatment with a potent inhibitor of CYP2D6. No morphine or morphine metabolites were detected in plasma when codeine was coadministered with quinidine. Although codeine may seem on the surface a poor candidate for a pharmacogenetic test, since the patient knows whether the medicine has worked or not, in fact there are many situations where analgesia is imperfect and even in situations where a patient can tell that codeine is having no analgesic benefit, his or her physician may not be aware, and self-reporting about pain is a notoriously variable and subjective phenomenon. It follows that the test may be valuable as a means of indicating which patients should not receive codeine as an analgesic, and who would most likely benefit.

Therapeutic Lessons

Pharmacogenetics has provided a number of therapeutic lessons that make us understand clinical drug response and it has influenced the drug development process. Among the therapeutic lessions are that most drug effects vary considerably from person to person and that all drug effects are influenced by genes. But it has also been realized that the most drug responses and toxicities are influenced by many genes interacting with environmental and behavioral factors. Genetic polymorphisms of single genes, including mutations in coding sequences, gene duplications, gene deletions, and regulatory mutations affect numerous drug-metabolizing enzymes. Several cytochrome-P450 enzymes, *N*-acetyltransferases 2 (NAT2), TPMT, and a UDP-glucuronosyltransferases (UDP-GT) are the examples discussed here. Individuals who possess these polymorphisms are at risk of experiencing more adverse drug reactions or inefficacy of drugs at usual doses.

Genetic polymorphisms of drug targets and drug transporters also are increasingly recognized (receptors, ion channels, and growth factors) as causing variation in drug responses, but they have not been studied enough in regard to their clinical importance that would advocate genotype-based dose adjustments. Several targets of cancer therapy, for example, the epidermal-growth-factor receptor, respond to treatment only in subgroups of patients who carry sensitizing mutations of these targets. Finally, the frequency of variation of drug effects, whether multifactorial, or genetic, varies considerably in populations of different ethnic origins.

Future Perspectives

One of the major challenges in the future is the interpretation of multigenic and multifactorial influences on drug responses. Indeed, as already mentioned, most drug effects and treatment outcomes, or the individual risk for drug inefficacy or toxicity are due to complex interactions between genes and the environment. Environmental variables include nutritional factors, concomitantly administered drugs, disease, and many other factors including lifestyle influences such as smoking and alcohol consumption. These factors act in concert with several individual genes that code for pharmacokinetic and pharmacodynamic determinants of drug effects such as receptors, ion channels, drug-metabolizing enzymes, and drug-transporters. The challenge will be to define polygenic determinants of drug effects and to use a combination of genotyping and phenotyping tests to assess environmental influences.

The increasing use of the term pharmacogenomics reflects the evolution of pharmacogenetics into the study of the entire spectrum of genes that determine drug response, including the assessment of the diversity of the human genome sequence and its clinical consequences. Rapid sequencing and genotyping of SNPs will have a major role in associating sequence variations with heritable clinical phenotypes of drug or xenobiotic response. The SNPs occur approximately once every 300–3000 bp if one compares the genomes of two unrelated individuals and represent 90–95% of all variant DNA sites. Any two individuals thus differ at approximately 3 to 10 million base pairs.

How can we use this information to predict drug responses particularly with the view that in a few years technologies will be available to sequence an entire human genome in a few hours and at a reasonable prize? Once a large number of SNPs and their frequencies in different populations are known, they can be used to correlate an individual's genetic "*fingerprint*" with the probable individual drug response.

It has been proposed that high density maps of SNPs or the so-called haplotype blocks in the human genome might allow the use of these SNPs as markers of xenobiotic responses even if the target remains unknown, providing a "*drug-response profile*" that is associated with contributions from multiple genes to a response phenotype. A recent "*proof of concept*" was provided by Xu et al. 2004 for tranilast-induced hyperbilirubinemia. Whole genome screening for regions of linkage disequilibrium associated with this adverse effect was used to identify three SNPs of UGT1A1 gene to be responsible for this drug-induced adverse reaction. In practice, and because of the complexities of defining disease phenotypes and clinical outcomes, the validity of this concept is limited.

Genomic technologies also include methods to study the expression of large groups of genes and indeed the entire complement of products (mRNAs) of a genome. Most drug actions produce changes in gene expression in individual cells or organs. This provides a new perspective for the way in which drugs interact with the organism and also provides a measure of the drug's biological effects.

For instance, numerous drugs induce their own metabolism and the metabolism of other drugs by interacting with nuclear receptors such as arylhydrocarbon receptor (AhR), peroxisome proliferator activated receptor (PPAR), pregnane × receptor (P × R), and constitutive androstane receptor (CAR). These receptors act as "*xenosensors*" and transcription factors that activate a response that includes increased biotransformation of drugs. The phenomenon of induction has major clinical consequences such as altered kinetics, drug–drug interaction or changes in hormone and carcinogen metabolism. Genomics is providing the technology to better analyze these complex multifactorial situations and to obtain individual genotypic and gene expression information to assess the relative contributions of environmental and genetic factors to variations in drug response.

Clinical Potential of Pharmacogenetics

Why is pharmacogenetics so rarely applied in clinical practice, in spite of well-established genetic polymorphisms and available genotyping methods? Numerous reasons for the slow acceptance of pharmacogenetic principles have been brought forward. The lack of large prospective studies to evaluate the impact of genetic variation on drug therapy is one reason for the slow acceptance of these principles. On the other hand, pharmacogenetic information is only reluctantly included in product information or drug data sheets alerting the physician to dosing problems.

A recent search for pharmacogenetic information in the prescribing information available to physicians provided the following bleak results. Seventy-six drug package inserts (PIs) from the Physician's Desk Reference (PDR) contained pharmacogenomic data. The gene usually was either a drug-metabolizing enzyme or the information was related to the variability in viral genomes as predictors of response to antiviral therapy or drug resistance. Information to guide treatment decisions was found in only 25 PIs, representing 22 drugs. Of these four were ranked in the top 200 prescribed drugs (celexocib, fluoxetine, pantoprazole, and divalproex sodium). Advice for treatment decisions based on specific genetic conditions were found in four PIs, namely that prolastin (α1-proteinase inhibitor) is not indicated in patients with certain α1-antitrypsin deficiency phenotypes, trastuzumab indicated only in patients with overexpression of the HER2 protein, tretinoin, and imatinib are to be given only in patients with either a specific subtype of acute myelogenous leukemia or Philadelphia chromosome-positive chronic myeloid leukemia, respectively.

Surprisingly, information on increased risk for potentially life- threatening adverse effects or treatment failures with conditional recommendations for genetic evaluation were found for only four drugs, namely recombinant factor X, somatotropin, divalproex sodium, and valproic acid. Only for one drug, thioridazine, did the PI contain a contraindication for a genetic subgroup, namely CYP2D6 poor metabolizers, which may develop QTc (prolonged heart-rate-corrected QT interval) interval prolongation in the electrocardiogram and develop ventricular arrhythmia.

Clearly, PIs at present do not contain useful information for gene-guided dose adjustments or therapeutic decisions. In particular, there are no explicit recommendations for drug dosing in TPMT deficient patients in the PIs for mercaptopurine or azathioprine or in the PI for warfarin for patients with low activity alleles of CYP2C9. Similarly, the PI for irinotecan does not contain information on the risk of patients with UGT1A1 deficiency. A major effort is underway at the Food and Drug

Administration to correct these obvious deficiencies in alerting physicians to potential problems, and this has included the first approval of a pharmacogenetic test: an oligonucleotide microarray test for CYP2D6 and CYP2C19 genotypes in December of 2004. In the future, not performing a pharmacogenetic test may have legal consequences.

Pharmacogenomics offers the potential to provide better health care through improved rational prescribing. We believe that is gradual acceptance in clinical practice will contribute to the education of health care professionals as prescribers. In addition, we must recognize an increasingly important source of pressure to improve pharmacotherapy: increasingly educated patients will come to expect the application of genomics and other technologies to drug selection and dosage when possible. The personalized medicine that many view as a new goal is actually what physicians always intended, and is becoming what patients, and the regulatory bodies that protect them, expect.

5

MOLECULAR DIAGNOSTICS

Pharmacogenomics is a rapidly evolving area driven by the new genetic information and new molecular technologies arising from the mapping and sequencing of the human genome. The field of pharmacogenomics has a parallel with the more traditional area of molecular diagnostics, in which molecular techniques are used for identification of a disease mutation in a particular patient population with a genetic disorder. Both fields have been impacted greatly by new genetic information and technologies, and have certain similar challenges to overcome. This chapter will focus on describing technologies and general issues in molecular diagnostics, and similarities to pharmacogenomic molecular applications.

Molecular diagnostics is an integration of molecular genetic knowledge and technology and conventional laboratory medicine for patient diagnostics. Due to the cost of performing testing, molecular diagnosis has historically been restricted to testing of a limited number of individuals at high risk, typically people who are suspected of being affected or carriers of a particular monogenic inherited disorder. This scenario is beginning to change as diagnostics expands into higher-volume testing of larger patient groups and at-risk populations. For example, widespread population carrier screening for cystic fibrosis carriers using molecular diagnostic methods has recently been implemented in the United States, with the goal of identifying carrier couples prior to the birth of an affected child. The increased volume of testing produced by these new applications has required the development of higher-throughput and lower cost molecular diagnostic assays to detect nucleotide changes. Large-scale molecular diagnostic applications parallel molecular pharmacogenomic testing requirements for high throughput and cost-effective molecular diagnostic tests suitable for screening a large number of individuals for multiple genetic changes. An important issue in a discussion of typical molecular diagnostics and pharmacogenomics is the difference in the interpretation of testing for mutations in a single gene disorder vs. testing for mutations in one or more genes involved in multifactorial disorders.

The majority of current molecular diagnostic assays are used to test for mutations in monogenic disorders. For example, cystic fibrosis is a relatively common single gene disorder caused by mutations in the cystic fibrosis transmembrane conductance regulator (CFTR) gene. Many diagnostic laboratories routinely test for 25–30 of the most common CFTR mutations, which account for the majority of cystic fibrosis mutations in most populations. The finding of a mutation is diagnostic in that a prediction of disease can be made on the basis of finding two mutations in the CFTR gene carried by an individual. In contrast, multifactorial diseases such as hypertension and obesity are more complex as disease onset is likely to be dependent on changes in several genetic regions, each with a different influence on disease progression, plus environmental factors. Individuals with a family history of hypertension may carry mutations in several genetic regions that lead to an increased susceptibility for hypertension. However, due to environmental differences only a portion of the individuals who carry these mutations will develop hypertension. The interpretation of molecular testing in multifactorial diseases is complex, as it requires interpretation of the results of testing several genetic regions and involves gene–environment interactions that are difficult to predict. Many individual drug responses are likely to be multifactorial traits, and these same issues will complicate prediction of drug response outcome based on molecular testing results.

Types of Genetic Variations

Genetic diseases can be divided into two main groups based on whether they are caused by relatively few common mutations or by many unique mutations. Tay-Sachs disease, a fatal neurodegenerative disorder caused by a deficiency of hexosaminidase A, is common in the Ashkenazi Jewish population. Three hexosaminidase mutations account for ~96% of the disease in the Ashkenazi Jewish population. In contrast most patients with Fabry disease, a metabolic disorder caused by deficiency of the enzyme galactosidase A, have unique mutations in the galactosidase A gene. This distinction is significant, as the detection of a small number of known mutations in a gene requires quite different technologies than the analysis of a complete gene to search for unknown mutations. Other types of genetic variation known to cause genetic disorders include deletions and duplications that can range in size from a single base to large regions encompassing whole exons or entire genes.

Deletions and duplications are of particular significance in molecular diagnosis, as they require special assays for detection, such as quantitative PCR to determine gene copy number. Genetic mutations can also alter function at levels other than the DNA coding sequence, such as mutations at conserved splice site sequences, which alter RNA splicing. The methods of detection of these different types of genetic changes vary depending on the type of mutation to be detected. Methods of mutation detection include specific assays designed to identify a certain nucleotide change at a particular base pair in a sequence, or the use of direct sequencing to detect many unique mutations. Direct sequencing may be preceded by the scanning methods to highlight particular exons of a gene that may contain a mutation. If a genetic disease is caused by a few recurrent mutations that account for the majority of disease, it is often more appropriate to test for these few mutations by a specific assay rather than by sequencing. In contrast, diseases caused by a large number of mutations in a single gene are more appropriately tested by direct sequencing methods. Therefore, it is critical that a molecular diagnostic test be appropriately matched to the types of mutations to be detected for a particular gene.

Methods to Detect Known Mutations

There is a vast array of techniques that are currently being used to look for mutations for clinical molecular diagnostic use. The following overview of methods describes some of the most common techniques to detect recurrent mutations used in many diagnostic laboratories.

PCR-Restriction Enzyme Assays

Certain genetic changes alter a restriction enzyme recognition site, either by creating a new site or destroying an existing site. In these cases, a molecular diagnostic assay can be designed in which a region containing the potential mutation site is amplified via PCR and digested with the appropriate restriction enzyme to determine if the restriction digest pattern is altered due to the presence of the mutation. In some cases, designing a PCR primer containing a mismatch that anneals near a mutation site can artificially produce a restriction enzyme site. When combined with the mutant genetic sequence, the mismatched PCR primer sequence and the mutation alters a restriction enzyme site and so produces altered restriction enzyme patterns. Quality control for this type of assay requires that appropriate positive and negative control samples must be present in each assay in order to confirm that the enzyme is properly active. An example of a PCR-restriction enzyme assay to detect variation for a pharmacogenomic application is the original detection of mutations in the gene for the cytochrome isozyme P250D6 (CYP2D6), which cause the "*poor metabolizer*" of debrisoquine phenotype. Since this paper was published, many assays using different methods have been designed to detect mutant alleles in the P250D6 gene, highlighting the complexity in choosing a method for molecular analysis of mutations in a particular gene. The main advantage for molecular diagnostics using a PCR-restriction enzyme assay is that it is simple to develop and perform, likely accounting for its continued use in many diagnostic laboratories. The major disadvantage is that the assay is time consuming, as each mutation must be individually analyzed. Although this assay is effective for testing a small number of samples in specific cases, it is not suited for testing samples for multiple mutations or for screening large numbers of samples.

Allele-Specific Oligonucleotide Assay

The basis of the *allele-specific oligonucleotide* (ASO) assay is that DNA duplexes which contain a mismatch are destabilized and have a lower melting temperature than correctly paired duplexes. To test for mutations using ASO, two probes, one containing the normal sequence and one containing the mutant sequence, are produced and hybridized to the patient's DNA. For each normal and mutant probe, conditions can be found where the probe will hybridize to only its perfectly matched duplex. If the patient sample contains only normal sequence, only the normal probe will hybridize. In a heterozygous sample, both the mutant and normal probes will hybridize, and in a homozygous mutant sample only the mutant probe will hybridize. An advantage of the ASO method is that it can be used to simultaneously test samples for several different mutations by the use of multiple probes bound to a solid matrix.

In practice, the success of this method relies on precisely establishing conditions for optimal oligonucleotide hybridization in order to ensure specific probe hybridization, and so multiplex ASO assays can be difficult to develop. Molecular diagnostic kits for use in genetic disorders based on ASO methods are available. There have been improvements to the ASO assay, specifically by development of a multiplex allele-specific diagnostic assay (MASDA) in which the ASO technique is adapted to a solid support and multiple regions are probed simultaneously. This has been achieved by altering probe hybridization conditions, so that hybridization of multiple probes at a single temperature is feasible. Using these improvements, it has been possible to analyze >500 samples simultaneously for >100 known mutations in multiple genes.

Allele-Specific Amplification Assay

The *allele-specific amplification assay* (ASA) assay is based on the fact that Taq polymerase will not initiate amplification from a primer that has a mismatch at the 3' ends. Two primers are designed so that the 3' base of the primer corresponds to the site of the genetic mutation to be tested, with either the normal or the mutant sequence at the 3' base positions. An unknown sample can then be tested for the presence of the mutation by using both the normal and the mutant primers in PCR with a common reverse primer. If the sample contains only normal sequence, a PCR product will only be produced when the normal primer is used, and similarly when the sample contains mutant sequence a product will only result from use of the mutant primer. Like the PCR-restriction enzyme method discussed, the ASA approach has also been applied to the detection of mutations in the CYP2D6 gene.

In the original ASA protocols, the mutant and normal PCR primers were separated into two reactions, so that lack of amplification could occur in one PCR reaction depending on the sequence present in a test sample. This is not ideal for a diagnostic test due to the possible misinterpretation of a false negative result, and the ASA protocol is usually modified to be a multiplex reaction that includes a positive internal control in each PCR reaction. For example, an ASA assay has been developed, which detects 12 common CFTR mutations simultaneously. However in this assay, two reactions must still be run in parallel for every sample to be analyzed, since the mutant and normal products produced are the same size and so must be physically separated in order to be distinguished.

The ASA can be improved by the use of fluorescent-dye labeled primers, which avoids the need for two separate reactions by using flourochromes to distinguish normal and mutant sequences. We have developed molecular diagnostic ASA assays to detect mutations causing Tay-Sachs and Canavan disease using fluorescent-dye labeled PCR primers. The mutant and normal primers are labeled with different color dyes, so that the PCR products resulting from either the normal or the mutant allele-specific primer will be a different dye color, allowing discrimination of normal and mutant sequence. The use of fluorescent dyes thus simplifies the assay, and allows one sample to be tested for multiple mutations in a single reaction. The advantage of the ASA method is that multiplex reactions to detect several mutations simultaneously can be developed. Multiplex reactions reduce the labor and costs and so are ideal for detection of a larger number of mutations. The main disadvantage of the ASA method is that achieving specific product amplification can be problematic.

Oligonucleotide Ligation Assay

The *oligonucleotide ligation assay* (OLA) is similar to allele-specific amplification in that specific interrogation of a mutation site is achieved by two oligonucleotides that contain the normal or mutant base at the 3' end of the primer. However, in the OLA assay, the normal or mutant primer anneals directly downstream and adjacent to a common primer. The two primers are directly adjacent to one another, and thermostable ligase is able to join the annealed primers. In the case of a normal DNA sequence, only the normal and common primers will anneal and so be ligated, while a mutant DNA sequence will produce ligation of only the mutant and common primers. This method has also been applied to the detection of CYP2D6 alleles.

A recent improvement in the OLA assay is the use of sequence-coded separation (SCS), in which non-nucleic mobility altering compounds are attached to the specific primers. The mobility altering compounds are designed so that the products from each primer are a different size, and so will allow discrimination between primer pairs for different mutations. This technology is used in a diagnostic assay for cystic fibrosis in which 32 mutations in the CFTR gene can be detected simultaneously. This novel method of size separation may expand the utility of the OLA assay, as it will allow multiplex assays for a large number of mutations. The main advantage of the OLA technique is the ability to multiplex several mutations; while the disadvantage is that without SCS the assay is of somewhat limited application. Many diagnostic laboratories currently use the commercially available OLA assay for mutations causing cystic fibrosis.

Primer Extension/Minisequencing Assay

The primer extension assay is similar to the dideoxy method commonly used in sequence analysis. In the primer extension assay, a region containing the mutation to be assayed is amplified in a first PCR reaction. A specific primer, which is designed to anneal directly upstream of the base which is the site of a known mutation, is then used in a second reaction. Radioactively labeled dideoxy nucleotides corresponding to either the normal or the mutant base at the potential mutation site are added in separate tubes. During the reaction, the labeled nucleotide added to the 3' end of the primer will depend on the sequence at the potential mutation site. If the normal sequence is present at the potential mutation site, only the reaction containing the normal labeled dideoxy nucleotide will produce a labeled primer. Conversely, if the mutant sequence is present at the mutation site, only the reaction containing the mutant nucleotide will produce a labeled primer. Individuals who are heterozygous for the mutation will produce labeled primers in both dideoxy tubes, due to the presence of both sequences at the potential mutation site. Primer extension assays are very sensitive for mutation detection and may be advantageous for large-scale testing with some modifications to the basic protocol. Primer extension assays have been designed to use fluorescent dye labeled nucleotides to eliminate the need for radioactivity and may also be adaptable to use on solid supports. For molecular diagnostics purposes, there are also commercially available kits and protocols for diagnostic applications.

Technical Advances in Molecular Diagnostic Techniques

In recent years, there have been major technical advances in genetic analysis methods due primarily to use of new technologies developed for genomic applications. This is leading to an increased emphasis on faster, more efficient methods of detecting genetic mutations facilitated by the use of novel methods and equipment, with increased automation to reduce labor intensive steps in genetic analysis. Major technological advances will be essential as routine molecular diagnosis of genetic disorders adjusts to increasing volumes and large-scale population screening. Most current molecular diagnostics assays are not highly automated, and are generally labor-intensive and expensive. For large-scale molecular diagnostic testing, more automation with reduced personnel involvement is essential in order to reduce the cost of testing. Other requirements of large-scale testing will be improved software programs capable of dealing with large amount of data.

Capillary Electrophoresis

A significant advance in common molecular diagnostic applications is capillary electrophoresis, in which traditional slab electrophoresis gels are replaced by capillaries. The electrophoresis of samples is carried out in a thin capillary tube filled with a matrix, and the movement of DNA molecules through the tube is detected and recorded. Capillary electrophoresis is amenable to automation as samples can be automatically loaded from reaction plates. Capillary electrophoresis can be readily applied to many genetic tests that traditionally would be analyzed on a slab gel, including methods for recurrent mutation detection, fragment analysis and direct sequencing. Capillary electrophoresis with equipment containing 96–384 capillaries has greatly reduced the labor required for certain molecular diagnostics tests, particularly direct sequencing for mutation detection.

DNA Chip Technology

The DNA chips are high-density arrays, in which many nucleic acid sequences are anchored on glass supports similar in size to microscope slides. The DNA chips can be designed in certain formats depending on the application of the chip. The current applications of DNA chip technology of relevance to diagnostics include use in determining sequence of an unknown fragment by hybridization, detection of SNPs or gene expression profiling in various tissues. The major benefit of the use of DNA chips for these applications is that information on thousands of genetic regions can be obtained from a single chip experiment. For example, chips that are used to determine expression profiles from various genes can analyze thousands of RNA fragments on a single chip. This has been used for cancer applications, in which gene expression profiles from tumor tissues are compared to normal tissues to determine, which genes are differentially regulated in the cancer tissues. Currently, DNA chips for use in gene expression studies work well. However, sequencing and SNP chips are still not accurate enough for routine use in identifying genetic changes in a clinical molecular diagnostic laboratory. In addition, there are ethical considerations regarding provision of molecular diagnostic testing of a large number of genes or mutations on DNA chip, which need to be addressed.

Denaturing High Pressure Liquid Chromatography Analysis

New applications for Denaturing High Pressure Liquid Chromatography (HPLC) may also have important future applications for testing for genetic variation. The HPLC has been adapted to DNA fragment analysis for separation of fragments under partially denaturing conditions. Fragments to be analyzed for the presence of a mutation are amplified by PCR and then run on a denaturing HPLC column. The DNA heteroduplexes containing a mismatched base due to the presence of a mutation have a different mobility through the HPLC column from normal matched homoduplexes, due to the altered melting temperature of the heteroduplex. The mobility difference between the normal and the mutant sample allows for screening of fragments for genetic changes.

The main application of DHPLC technology for diagnostics is likely to be its use as a screening tool for genetic variation prior to sequencing, which is similar in principle to traditional methods of scanning such as single-strand conformational polymorphism (SSCP) and denaturing gradient gel electrophoresis (DGGE) assays. However, DHPLC also has the potential to be a method to screen samples for previously known mutations. The advantages of DHPLC are its automated nature, the simplicity of preparing fragments for analysis and the short run times required for fragment analysis.

MALDI-TOF Mass Spectrometry

Mass spectrometry is also being applied to genetic analysis by the use of matrix-assisted laser desorption/ionization time-of-flight (MALDI-TOF) mass spectrometry. The principle of this application is that sequence differences can be determined by analyzing the inherent mass differences of the four-nucleotide bases. For molecular diagnostic applications, the most obvious application of MALDI-TOF is the use of modified primer-extension assays, in which the base extended is at the nucleotide site of a known sequence change. MALDI-TOF is promising for high throughput applications, as more than one genetic region or mutation can be simultaneously analyzed and the assays. An example of the use of MALDI-TOF in diagnostics is in detection of mutations in CFTR causing cystic fibrosis.

Real-Time PCR

Additional developments in PCR technologies are also impacting on molecular diagnostics. One of the most important has been the development of PCR machines that have the capability of detecting product formation during the PCR reaction, known as real-time PCR. Assays can be designed in which the binding of a sequence-specific probe to its homologous PCR product results in an increase in fluorescence during the PCR reaction, allowing for real-time detection of the PCR product. This has been achieved using various probe designs that maintain a fluorescent reporter dye in close proximity to a quencher dye. Upon hybridization to its specific sequence the quencher is separated from the reporter thus generating a fluorescent signal from the reporter dye. This technology has been applied to detection of mutations causing genetic disease as well as for pharmacogenomic research. The advantage of real-time PCR techniques is that they do not require any post-PCR analysis such as gel electrophoresis, since the amplification and detection of the specific product are completed within the PCR reaction.

Robotics

A common objective of all of the new technologies discussed is to reduce the labor and expense required for large-scale testing. High-throughput detection machines require high sample input rates, which are not feasible without the use of robotics. Robotics will be required to automate the isolation of DNA, to prepare reactions for PCR, and to load detection machines after PCR. For example, the labor associated with manually preparing DNA samples for analysis on a 384-sample capillary electrophoresis machine would negate the benefit of using the advanced equipment. Robotics instruments are now available that can perform various functions, including nucleic acid extraction and preparation of PCR reactions. Robotics is likely to become more flexible in future, with robots specifically designed to interact with specialized equipment for specific applications. An important aspect of increased robotic use will be the development of software programs able to perform data analysis on the high volume of data generated. The increasing use of robotics will allow genetic diagnostic laboratories to increase the number of tests it is able to perform, without continually increasing laboratory staff, due to the ability to perform more tasks in less time. The methods listed above are some of the major areas of interest in the development of biotechnology-based molecular diagnostic procedures. Some private companies are currently offering genetic testing based on new biotechnology-based large-scale molecular diagnostic methods. An overview of some companies involved in developing diagnostic strategies for large-scale genetic testing for pharmacogenomics is provided in Persidis. The need to develop high-throughput, sensitive and cost-effective molecular testing for genetic variation remains a significant challenge in molecular diagnostics, which is shared with pharmacogenomic applications.

Since many individuals will require testing, and many genetic changes may need to be tested, the diagnostic methods will need to be robust, cost-effective and specific. Some of the new advances in genetic analysis, such as real-time PCR and MALDI-TOF, hold promise for meeting these demands. In addition, as the throughput of molecular diagnostic testing improves, testing is likely to still be limited by uncertain significance of new sequence changes detected. This is also an issue in common with pharmacogenetics, as the application of routine pharmacogenomics still requires a more thorough understanding of the genetic causes underlying drug response variations. The genetic variations may be simple changes, or they may be complex alterations that are also influenced by environmental factors. Significant research on the effect of genetic variation on enzyme activity and the resultant effect on drug response will be required. New technologies for DNA analysis and mutation detection, and improved understanding of the interpretation of mutations, will make it possible to meet the demands of both future molecular diagnostic and pharmacogenomic applications.

6

Clinical Pharmacology Overview

Clinical pharmacology is the branch of pharmacology that focuses on the study of drugs in humans. A comprehensive understanding of the principles of clinical pharmacology facilitates the clinician prescribing optimal therapy to an individual patient. Over the last 30 yr the clinical pharmacology of many drugs has been elucidated with advances in sophisticated, accurate, and precise analytical tools to determine plasma drug and/or metabolite concentrations in biological fluids. This has permitted a better understanding of the relationship between the pharmacokinetics (derived from the Greek *pharmakon* [drug] and *kinisis* [movement] and meaning drug concentration over time) and the pharmacodynamics (derived from the Greek *pharmakon* and *dynameostis* [power], meaning drug action or power) for many drugs. Oncology has, only somewhat belatedly, generated adequate data on these pharmacological properties of many widely used cytotoxic drugs. This is to some extent unfortunate, because cytotoxic drug therapy demands close attention to pharmacological principles as the therapeutic index of many anticancer agents is narrow, that is, $TD_{50}/ED_{50} \leq 2$. To achieve the primary therapeutic endpoint (tumor

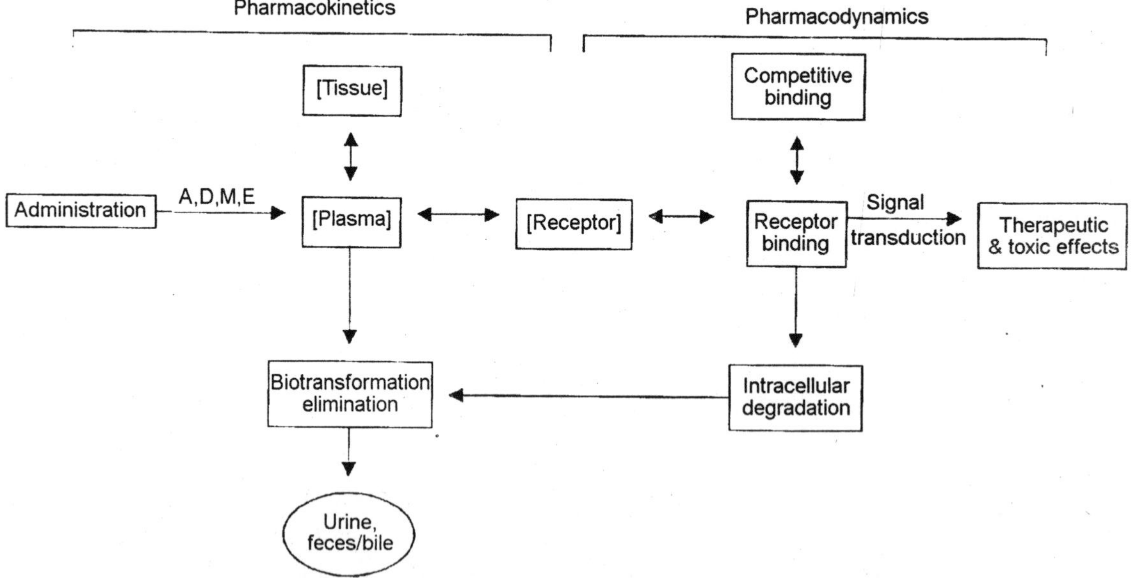

Fig. 6.1. Schematic representation of the physiologic processes determining drug disposition in the human body and the relationship of pharmacokinetics and pharmacodynamics to these processes.

cell death leading to tumor shrinkage), the limits of tolerable drug toxicity to normal tissues are often encroached. Importantly, adverse events, both anticipated and unexpected, must be integrated into therapeutic decisions to optimize patient outcome; thus ongoing assessment and reassessment of the cytotoxic drug effects on tumor and normal tissues are required. Drug–drug, drug–herb/food and drug–comorbid disease interactions, if not considered and anticipated, can have dire consequences for cancer patients. Furthermore, the rapidly increasing numbers of genetic polymorphisms in proteins involved either in the primary mechanism of a drug action and/or the processes that determine drug pharmacokinetics (absorption, distribution, metabolism, and excretion) further increase the complexity of optimal drug prescribing. This chapter focuses on the principles of clinical pharmacology applied to cytotoxic chemotherapy, and forms a basis as to why these principles assist the oncologist in optimizing the efficacy/toxicity ratio for cancer chemotherapeutic agents in individual patients.

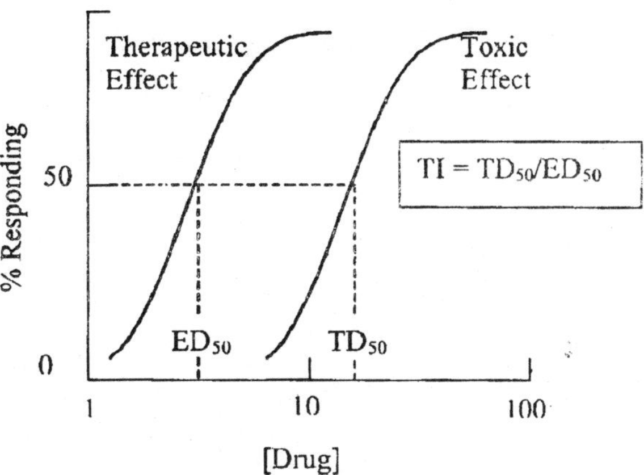

Fig. 6.2. Therapeutic index (TI): the ratio of the TD_{50} to the ED_{50} is an indicator of a drug's selectivity for producing the desired therapeutic effect in relation to its toxic effects.

Mechanisms of Drug Action (Pharmacodynamics)

The study of the effects of drugs on biologic and physiologic processes is termed pharmacodynamics. Most drug effects result from interactions with specific macromolecules or *targets* that induce a biochemical or physiologic change. The target of the drug may be an enzyme found in the plasma or sited intracellularly; a cell-membrane-located protein; an ion channel protein or a structural protein; or DNA, RNA, or other macromolecules (e.g., microtubules). The site of action of many drugs is a *receptor* which normally binds an endogenous regulatory ligand (e.g., hormones, growth factors, neurotransmitters); the receptor function is modified on drug binding. Drugs that bind to receptors and mimic the endogenous ligand are termed *agonists* (e.g., recombinant human erythropoietin [rhEPO], granulocyte colony stimulating factor [G-CSF], opioids). When a drug binds to a receptor and blocks the effects of the endogenous ligand, the drug is termed an *antagonist* (e.g., flutamide, an androgen receptor antagonist; ondansetron, a 5-hydroxytryptamine type 3 [5-HT3] antagonist, trastuzumab [Herceptin] monoclonal antibody against HER-2 /neu). Certain agents have both agonist and antagonist properties at receptors and are termed partial agonists (e.g., tamoxifen-mixed estrogen receptor agonist/ antagonist, nalbuphine-mixed $\mu/\kappa/\delta$ opiate receptor agonist/antagonist). Many established and novel anticancer agents inhibit the function of endogenous enzymes by binding directly to an enzyme and are thus termed *enzyme inhibitors* (e.g., dihydrofolate reductase inhibitors—methotrexate; topisomerase I inhibitors, such as members of the camptothecin family; epidermal growth factor receptor [EGFR]-associated tyrosine kinase I inhibitors—OSI-774 [Tarceva] and ZD 1839 [Iressa]; and the farnesyl transferase inhibitor trifarnib).

Drug Action

The binding of a drug to its target is often highly specific and dictated by the three- dimensional structure of both the ligand and target as well as electrostatic, dipole–dipole, ionic, van der Waals, hydrophobic, and hydrogen bond forces. The greater the net sum of these forces, the higher the binding affinity of the drug to its target. Occasionally, a drug will form irreversible covalent bonds with its target, for example, alkylation of the 7-nitrogen and 6-oxygen atom in the guanine ring by ifosforamide

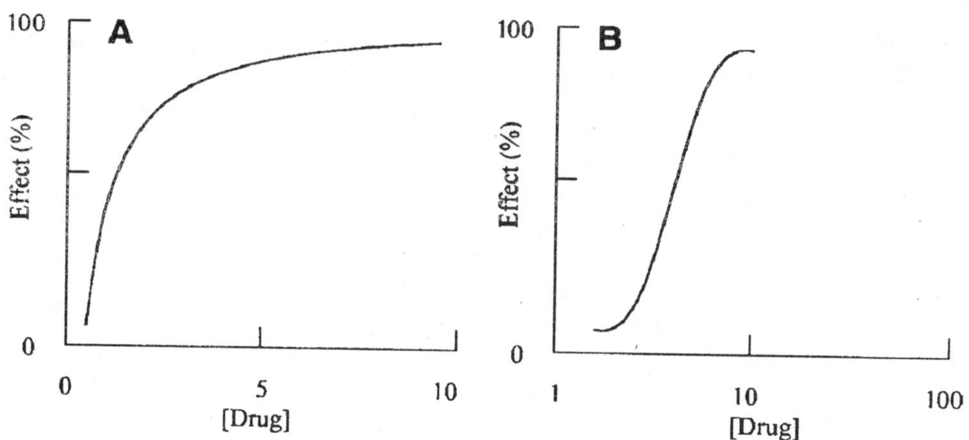

Fig. 6.3. Dose-response curves plotted (A) arithmetically and (B) semilogarithmically.

mustard, the active metabolite of the ifosfamide. The pharmacologic effects of any drug most often occur in a graded, effect site concentration-dependent manner. In many cases the plasma drug concentration is linearly related to the dose of the drug administered; the graphical representation of drug effect is thus often referred to as a *dose–response curve*. Agonist drugs produce a graded dose response up to a maximum value (E_{max}), above which increasing the drug concentration no longer produces a significant increase in effect. Antagonists produce no response and partial agonists have a reduced effect and reduced maximal effect–response. Each drug has a specific shape to its dose (concentration)–response curve at its target site. In clinical therapy its importance underpins the need for dose titration of a drug to optimize the desired response.

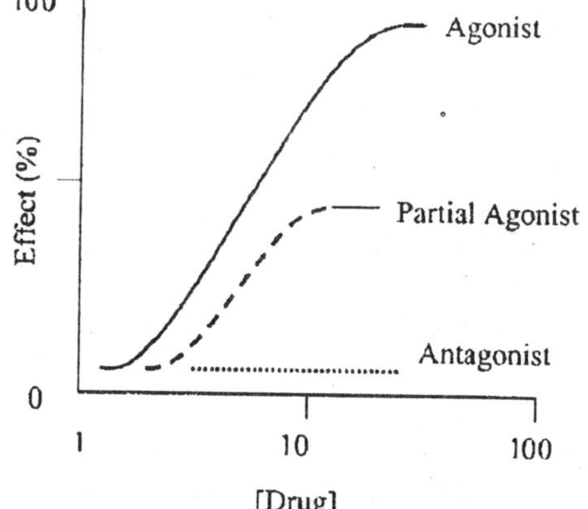

Fig. 6.4. Semilogarithmic plot of percent maximal effect vs drug concentration for an agonist, partial agonist, and antagonist.

Receptor Pharmacology and Function

Molecular cloning techniques, along with advanced biochemical methods, have greatly enhanced our ability to discover and characterize physiological receptors, signal transduction pathways, and effector proteins. Receptors for endogenous ligands are classified into four "*superfamilies*" with distinct functional properties. Three families are localized to the cell membrane: ligand gated ion channel receptors (e.g., glutamate, nicotinic acetylcholine, and γ-aminobutyric acid receptors); G-protein coupled receptors (e.g., opiate receptors), and receptors with enzymatic activity (e.g., EGFR and platelet derived growth factor receptor [PDGFr]). A fourth family of receptors is located within the cell and is known as nuclear transcription factor receptors (e.g., steroid hormone receptors, retinoic acid [RA] receptors, and retinoid X receptors [RXR]). Agonist binding to any one of these receptors, regardless of family, activates a signal transduction pathway, for example, activation of a specific enzyme or cascade of enzymes, release of a second messenger(s), or transcription of a particular gene, and it is this intracellular physiologic change that mediates the effect of a ligand stimulating the receptor.

Agonists

Agonists (e.g. morphine, bromocriptine, lutenizing hormone-releasing hormone agonist, [leuprolide]) produce an effect by interacting with and activating specific receptors for endogenous ligands. The particular signal transduction pathway linked to a receptor determines the process of receptor activation. Drugs that bind directly to and inhibit the activity of enzymes or proteins are not considered agonists because they do not first interact with an endogenous receptor. A useful parameter to compare drugs with equal maximal effect is EC_{50}, the concentration of drug at which a 50% maximal response is observed. Agonist properties can be quantified in terms of potency and magnitude of effect. Potency depends on four factors: receptor density, efficiency of receptor signal transduction, drug affinity for the receptor, and the degree of signal transduction induced by the drug binding to the receptor (*efficacy*). The latter two are properties of the drug itself and can be quantitated by plotting the percentage maximal effect vs log drug concentration for two comparison drugs, which will give relative potency or relative efficacy.

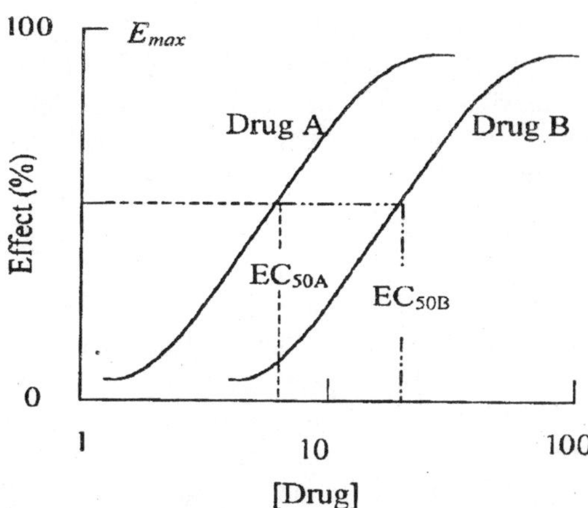

Fig. 6.5. Relative potency: semilogarithmic plot of percent maximal effect vs drug concentration for two drug (A and B) with equal maximum pharmacologic effect (E_{max}).

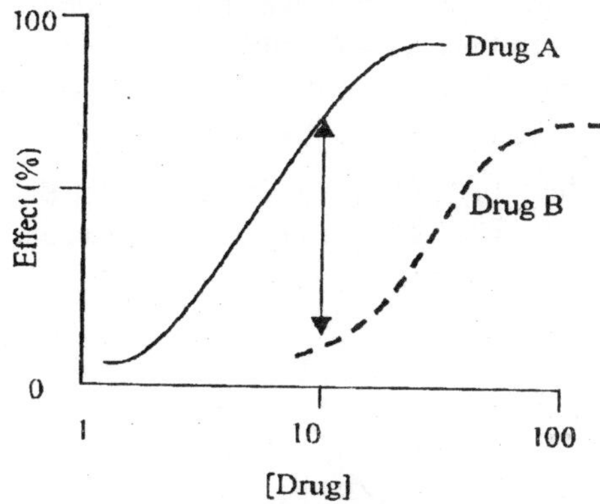

Fig. 6.6. Relative efficacy: semilogarithmic plot of percent maximal effect vs drug concentration for two drugs (A and B) with differing maximal effects.

Competitive antagonists

Competitive antagonists (e.g., trastuzumab, alemtuzumab, rituximab) bind the same endogenous receptors as agonists, but they fail to induce a response (i.e., there is no receptor-mediated downstream signal transduction). Agonists in the presence of competitive antagonists simultaneously compete for the same receptors. The drug concentration in the effect compartment and receptor affinity determine the degree of receptor occupancy of each agent at any given moment in time. The effects of a competitive antagonist can be overcome by increasing the concentration of the agonist. Noncompetitive antagonists, on the other hand, in effect decrease the number of "*effective*" receptors and attenuate the maximal response to an agonist. The effects of a noncompetitive antagonist cannot be overcome by increasing the agonist concentration.

Enzyme inhibition

Similar concepts can be applied to drugs that are enzyme inhibitors (e.g., methotrexate, camptothecins, EGFR tyrosine kinase inhibitors). Thus the drug and the endogenous substrate compete for the same binding site on the enzyme. When the drug is bound, the enzyme can no longer bind substrate and the rate of the enzymatic reaction is reduced. One of the most successful molecularly targeted agents that possesses such a mechanism is imatinib mesylate (STI571/Gleeve), which inhibits ATP binding to the tyrosine kinases activity of the protooncogene *KIT*, PDGFr, and BCR–ABL, inhibiting protein phosphorylation and signaling. Alternatively, some drugs (e.g., chloradenosine as its anabolite chlorodeoxy ATP and the non-nucleoside reverse transcriptase inhibitors [NNRTI] of HIV-

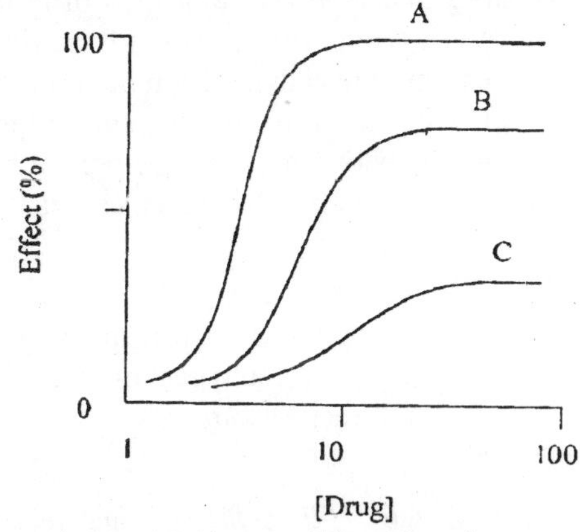

Fig. 6.7. Noncompetitive antagonism.

1, nevirapine, and efavirenz) bind to enzymes at sites other than the endogenous substrate-binding site and induce a conformational change in the enzyme structure. This structural change modifies the three-dimensional shape of the endogenous substrate binding site so that the endogenous substrate is no longer recognized and is unable to bind. These drugs are termed allosteric or noncompetitive enzyme inhibitors.

Partial agonists

Partial agonists (e.g., tamoxifen [a partial agonist at the estrogen receptor], bryostatin [a partial agonist of protein kinase C], certain opioids [nalbuphine, buprenorphine]) stimulate endogenous receptors, but to a lesser degree than full agonists because of their intrinsically low efficacy. When an agonist is administered in the presence of a partial agonist, the maximal effect of the agonist is diminished because some receptors are occupied by the less effective partial agonist, which implies that partial agonists are also partial antagonists. The partial agonist properties of a drug can be overcome by increasing the concentration of the pure agonist.

Non-Receptor-Mediated Drug Action

Some drugs exert their effects based solely on the physical or chemical nature of the drug. In cancer therapy, examples of drugs that work via this mechanism are purine analogs (e.g., 6-mercaptopurine and thioguanine) and certain pyrimidine analogs (e.g., fludaribine), which do not target specific endogenous receptors. They are incorporated into nucleic acids causing the impairment of DNA or RNA synthesis. This mechanism has been termed "*counterfeit incorporation.*"

Pharmacodynamic Models

Pharmacodynamic models quantify the pharmacologic effect of a drug as it relates to the concentration of drug at its site of action (effect compartment concentration). These models are dependent on the assumptions of receptor *occupancy theory*. This theory states that the intensity of the drug effect is proportional to the number of receptors bound by drug and that the maximum effect occurs when all receptors are occupied by the drug. The assumptions of the receptor occupancy theory are as follows: (1) drug--receptor association/dissociation is rapid and at equilibrium, (2) each receptor binds only one drug molecule at a time, (3) drug-receptor binding is reversible. The clinically most pertinent pharmacodynamic model is the E_{max} model, which is based on the hyperbolic relationship between pharmacologic effect and drug concentration. The effect (E) can be quantitated by the following equation:

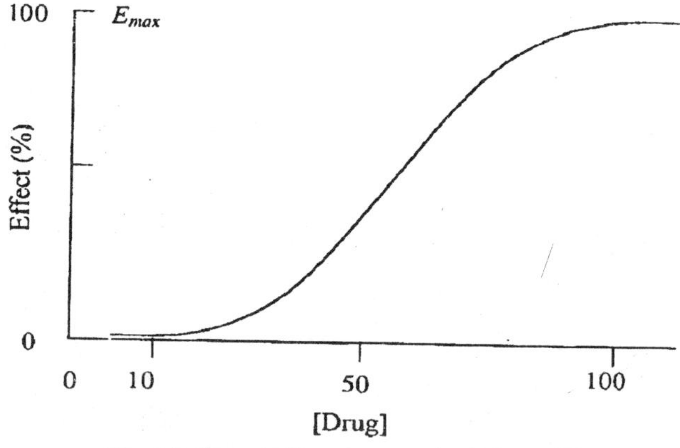

Fig. 6.8. Sigmoid E_{max} pharmacodynamic model.

$$E = (E_{max} \times C)/(EC_{50} + C)$$

where E_{max} is the maximal effect, C is the plasma drug concentration, and EC_{50} is the concentration of drug at which 50% maximal response is observed. If a receptor can bind more than one drug molecule simultaneously (e.g., oxygen binding to hemoglobin), then the sigmoid E_{max} model is used and the equation for effect becomes:

$$E = (E_{max} \times C^{\gamma}) / (EC_{50}^{\gamma} + C^{\gamma})$$

where γ is the "*Hill coefficient*" and relates to the number of drug binding sites per receptor; it determines the slope of the curvilinear relationship.

PHARMACOKINETICS

The study of the time course of drug absorption, distribution, metabolism, and elimination by the human body is termed *pharmacokinetics*. An adequate understanding of the basic principles of pharmacokinetics combined with the specific pharmacokinetic parameters for an individual drug enable the prescriber to choose the most appropriate route of administration, dose, and dosing frequency to obtain an optimal pharmacologic response while minimizing toxicity.

Absorption

Most drugs must enter the systemic circulation to reach specific sites of action (usually intracellular targets for cancer drugs), which are often distant from the site of administration. Drug absorption is a highly variable process dependent on the physicochemical properties of the drug such as molecular size and shape, lipid solubility, degree of ionization, and protein and tissue binding characteristics. Passive diffusion is by far the most important process by which drugs move across cell membranes. The thickness of the cell membrane and the presence or absence of drug efflux pumps (e.g., ATP binding cassette [ABC] transporters, e.g., ABCB1—also known as MDR-1 and P-glycoprotein) also determine the rate and extent of drug absorption. Oral (enteral) drug administration is the most common route of drug delivery because it is convenient, safe, and economical. The majority of cancer drugs, however, are either poorly absorbed from the gastrointestinal tract or undergo significant metabolism or excretion by the gastrointestinal mucosa and/or liver prior to entering the systemic circulation. This process is known as the *first-pass effect*. Drugs with a high first pass effect have low *bioavailability* (F), a term used to describe the fractional extent to which a dose of drug reaches the systemic circulation.

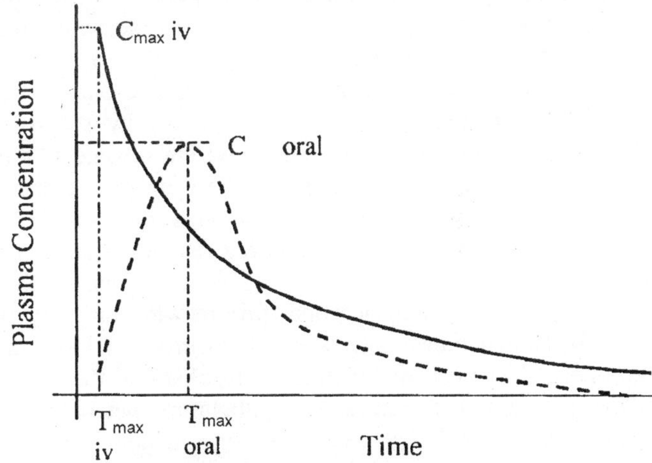

Fig. 6.9. Plasma drug concentration time curves following intravenous (solid line) and oral (dashed line) administration.

Examples of drugs with low oral bioavailability include morphine, many cytotoxics (e.g., paclitaxel, docetaxel, daunorubicin), and monoclonal antibodies (which are proteins and therefore degraded by acid in the stomach). Intravenous administration of drugs used in cancer chemotherapy circumvents the factors related to absorption and the first-pass effect, and by definition provides 100% bioavailability. Other routes of drug administration (e.g., subcutaneous, intramuscular, intra-arterial, intrathecal, and topical) are important in cancer therapeutics.

Distribution

Once a drug enters the systemic circulation, it begins to equilibrate (distribute) throughout the body. Many factors contribute to drug distribution including cardiac output, regional blood flow and blood flow within a tumor, pH of the local environment, presence of drug efflux pumps (especially ABCB1 [MDR-1/P-glycoprotein] and other ABC transporters that are present in many tumors), and the physicochemical properties of the drug, especially its lipid solubility. Binding to plasma proteins (mainly albumin for acidic drugs and α_1 acid glycoprotein for basic drugs) can limit the degree of drug distribution because only unbound (free) drug can passively diffuse through cell membranes. Some drugs accumulate in certain tissues preferentially, usually because they are highly lipophilic or secondary to tissue-specific binding (e.g., paclitaxel to beta-tubulin). Many chemotherapeutic agents have to enter tumor cells to produce a cytotoxic effect. Distribution into tumor cells can be facilitated by transport proteins (carriers) and may be energy dependent (i.e., active transport). Active transport moves drugs against electrochemical and concentration gradients, which can significantly increase drug concentration in tumor cells. Examples of drugs that are actively transported into cells in addition to their transmembrane flux by passive diffusion include fludarabine, gemcitabine, and methotrexate.

Metabolism (Biotransformation)

Many drugs undergo enzymatic modification (metabolism), which most commonly reduces their pharmacological activity and enhances the body's ability to excrete the drug. In some instances, the metabolite is more pharmacologically active than the parent drug (e.g., conversion of ifosfamide to ifosforamide mustard; CPT-11 to SN-38) or an active metabolite may be cleared more slowly than the parent compound (e.g., CPT-11 metabolite SN 38, morphine metabolite, morphine-6-glucuronide). Drug metabolism can be categorized into two phases: phase 1 reactions, which involve metabolic modifications of the drug (often oxidation, reduction, or hydrolysis), and phase 2 reactions, which are synthetic conjugation reactions involving the covalent linkage of a highly polar molecule (glucuronic acid, sulfate, amino acid, glutathione, acetate) to the drug or its metabolite. The products of phase 2 reactions have increased water solubility and are readily excreted in the urine (or bile). The primary site of drug metabolism (both phase 1 and phase 2 reactions) is the liver, although the gastrointestinal tract, kidney, and lungs play important roles for some drugs. Within the liver, the cytochrome P450 (CYP450) monooxygenase system accounts for the vast majority of phase 1 drug metabolism. There are more than 50 known functionally active cytochrome P450's in humans, with only eight isoforms accounting for more than 90% of all drug metabolism. CYP 3A4 and CYP 3A5 (nearly identical isoforms and also expressed in the intestinal epithelium) metabolize approx 50% of all drugs; CYP 2D6 (20% of drugs) and CYP2C9/19 account for the metabolism of another 20–25% of drugs; all the other active isoforms (CYP1A1/2, CYP2B6, CYP2A6, CYP2E1) accounting for the remaining CYP450 metabolic activity. Many drugs are substrates for (and thus metabolized by) more than a single member of the CYP450 enzyme family, having differing affinities for binding to the different CYP450s. Drugs can be both substrates for the CYP450 enzymes and inducers or inhibitors of these enzymes.

Concurrent use of drugs that interfere with the metabolism of another drug may result in significant toxicity or therapeutic failure. The recent identification of multiple genetic polymorphisms for many of the CYP450 enzymes has in part allowed us further insight into the interindividual variability in drug metabolism. The best example of this is the four different CYP2D6 phenotypes; which yield poor, intermediate, extensive, and ultrarapid metabolism of drugs that are substrates for this enzyme.

Phase 2 conjugation reactions also take place in the liver, the most important of which is glucuronidation. This involves the addition of a glucuronide group to the drug by uridine diphosphate glucuronosyltransferase (UGT). More than 15 isoforms of UGTs have been identified, and as with the CYP450 system, functional polymorphisms have been identified (UGT1A1 catalyzes the glucuronidation of SN-38 to SN-38 glucuronide). The same holds true for *N*-acetyltransferase (NAT) and accounts for the "slow and fast acetylator" phenotypes, which affects the metabolism of amonafide to *N*-acetylamonafide (NAT2) and its toxicity profile (fast acetylators experience greater myelosuppression). Intracellular metabolism is another important mechanism of drug biotransformation. Many antimetabolite drugs are dependent on intracellular anabolism/metabolism to yield pharmacologically active entities (e.g., 5-fluorouracil, gemcitabine, 6-mercaptopurine).

Excretion (Elimination)

Drugs can be eliminated from the body either in an unchanged form or as metabolites. Lipid-soluble drugs generally are metabolized to more polar compounds to facilitate their elimination from the body via the kidney. The kidneys are primarily responsible for the excretion of drugs and their metabolites while biliary excretion plays an important role for certain drugs (e.g., taxanes, SN-38 glucuronide). Elimination of drugs via the urine is dependent on three processes: glomerular filtration, active tubular secretion, and passive tubular reabsorption. The glomerular filtration rate is reduced in the elderly and many disease states and is dependent on cardiac output and intravascular volume. Drug molecules that are not protein bound ("free drug") can be filtered. Other physicochemical properties of drugs and metabolites that facilitate renal excretion include small molecular size (mol wt < 500 Da) and being unionized at physiological pH, which depends on the pK_a of the compound.

Pharmacokinetic Parameters

A simple plot of plasma drug concentration vs time offers the prescriber useful pharmacokinetic data. C_{max} is defined as the maximal plasma concentration following a specific dose and t_{max} is the time at which C_{max} is observed. The area under the plasma drug concentration vs time curve (AUC) is a useful measure of the body's total drug exposure.

Volume of distribution

The concept of volume of distribution can be demonstrated by the theoretical administration of a drug as a rapid intravenous bolus injection with sampling and measurement of plasma concentrations at specified time intervals. The resultant log plasma drug concentration vs time graph for a drug that rapidly distributes and equilibrates throughout the body (i.e., the one-compartment, well-stirred model with first-order elimination) will appear similar to the plot representing drug A. Extrapolation of the line back to time zero gives a theoretical plasma drug concentration (C_0) that would have occurred if drug equilibration were instantaneous. This theoretical concentration results from the dilution of a known amount of drug (usually milligrams) into an unknown volume of the human body, which is known as the *apparent volume of distribution* or V_d. Dividing the dose (D) by C_0 gives the value for V_d (usually expressed in liters): $V_d = D/C_0$. Factors affecting the volume of distribution include the physicochemical properties of the drug and many patient-dependent factors such as body size, fat composition, water content, and plasma protein concentration. The V_d is often referred to as the "apparent" volume of distribution because it does not represent a true physiologic single space or compartment within the human body, but rather a theoretical composite value for all the compartments to which the drug distributes. The one-compartment model is a convenient mathematical representation of drug distribution and elimination for many, but not all drugs. More complex models are required for drugs that have protracted distribution times (e.g., paclitaxel, daunorubicin). In the two-compartment model represented for drug B (e.g., docetaxel), the body is divided into two theoretical spaces, a smaller central compartment (blood volume plus the extracellular space of highly perfused tissues; heart, lung, liver, kidneys) and a larger peripheral compartment, which represents all other tissues. A semilogarithmic plot of plasma drug B concentration vs time reveals a biphasic decline in plasma drug concentration over time. The first phase, known as the alpha phase, represents redistribution of drug B out of the

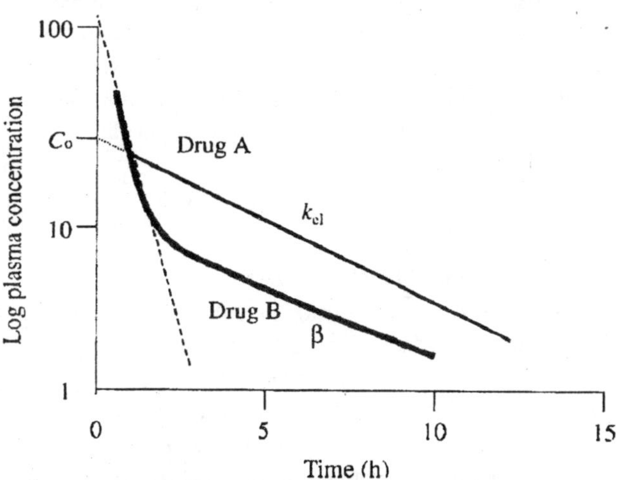

Fig. 6.10. Plasma drug concentration time curves following intravenous (solid line) and oral (dashed line) administration.

central (sampling) compartment and into the peripheral tissues. The beta phase, also known as the terminal elimination phase, occurs after drug B has equilibrated between the two compartments and primarily represents drug elimination. Three-compartment models are necessary to describe some drugs (e.g., paclitaxel, many anthracyclines) that have two distribution phases preceding the terminal elimination phase. The volume of distribution for drugs following a multicompartment model is conceptually the same as for one-compartment modeling, but calculated in a slightly different way.

Clearance

Clearance represents the rate at which a drug is eliminated from the body and is expressed in terms of volume per unit time for first-order elimination. The volume term represents the theoretical volume of blood (or more often plasma) totally cleared of drug during a given time interval, which remains constant and independent of plasma drug concentration. The amount or mass of drug removed from the body per unit time, however, is constantly changing (depending on plasma drug concentration) during first-order elimination and is therefore not a convenient means to express clearance. When clearance mechanisms are saturated (i.e., operating at full capacity), zero-order elimination kinetics is followed and a constant mass (milligrams) of drug is cleared from the body per unit time regardless of the plasma drug concentration.

Most drug pharmacokinetics fit a one-compartment, first-order elimination kinetics model with an elimination rate constant (k_e) equal to the slope of the line for the log plasma drug concentration vs time plot. The total body clearance, Cl_T (which is a summation of all clearance mechanisms; renal, hepatic, and other) of a drug is directly proportional to k_e and V_d: $Cl_T = k_e \times V_d$. Another useful equation to calculate Cl_T for first order elimination is:

$$Cl_T = F \times \text{dose/AUC}$$

where F is the bioavailability and AUC is the area under the log plasma drug concentration time curve.

Elimination half-life ($t_{1/2}$)

The amount of time it takes for the plasma drug concentration to decline by 50% is defined as the half-life ($t_{1/2}$). Half-life is also related to the ke: $t_{1/2} = 0.693/k_e$. Substitution of Cl_T/V_d for k_e yields the equation: $t_{1/2} = 0.693 \times V_d/Cl_T$.

$$t_{1/2} = 0.693 \times V_d/Cl_T$$

Thus, $t_{1/2}$ changes as a function of both Vd and Cl_T (under steady-state conditions). The half-life of a drug is useful in determining the dosing interval for many drugs that are dosed to a steady state and the time required to reach steady-state plasma concentrations (i.e., four half-lives to reach 94% of steady state) as well as being useful for estimating the time for a specific percentage of administered drug to be removed from the body (i.e., on cessation of drug therapy, the plasma drug concentration will decrease by 50% for each $t_{1/2}$ time interval).

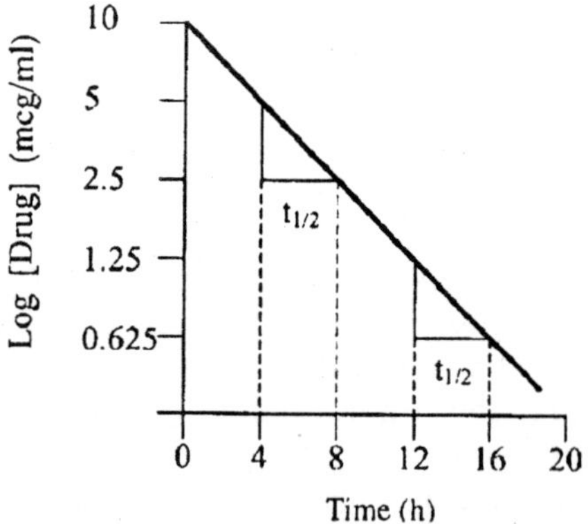

Fig. 6.11. Half-life: log plasma drug concentration vs time plot for a drug following first-order elimination kinetics and a half-life of 4 h.

Noncompartmental modeling

Noncompartmental modeling uses statistical moment theory to derive the same pharmacokinetic parameters and provides the additional parameters of AUMC or area under the first-moment curve (analogous to AUC) and the mean residence time (MRT). The primary advantage of noncompartmental modeling is the requirement for fewer model specific assumptions.

Nonlinear "dose-dependent" pharmacokinetics

Clearance, for most drugs, remains constant (proportional to plasma drug concentration) over the therapeutic dose range and as a result, first-order kinetics are obeyed. Occasionally, clearance mechanisms become overwhelmed (i.e., saturated) and there is no longer an exponential decline in plasma drug concentration over time (i.e., zero-order kinetics are followed). Under such circumstances in which clearance mechanisms are saturated (e.g., enzyme saturation, Michaelis–Menton kinetics apply), small increases in dose can dramatically increase plasma drug concentration or AUC. In such cases (e.g. paclitaxel at doses > 135 mg/m^2 administered over 3 h), the pharmacokinetics are considered "*dose dependent*" or "*capacity-limited.*" This is also termed Michaelis–Menton pharmacokinetics as the nonlinear relationship of concentration and dose can be fitted to the classical enzyme kinetic model. The processes of drug absorption (e.g., oral methotrexate, melphalan), distribution, and excretion can also become saturated, which in turn leads to a drug exhibiting nonlinear pharmacokinetics.

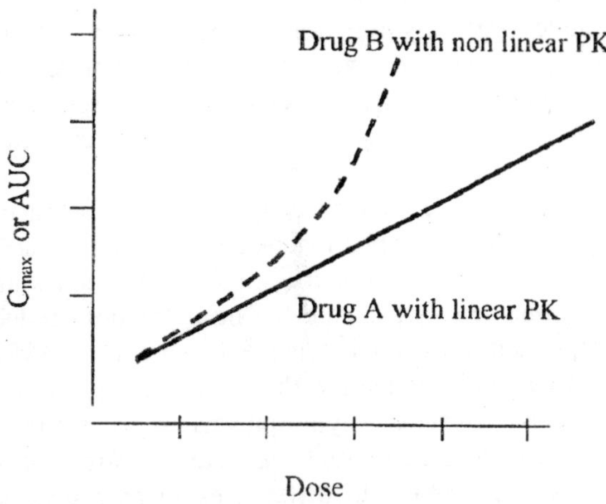

Fig. 6.12. Drug A has linear pharmacokinetics with dose proportional increases in C_{max} and AUC.

Population Pharmacokinetics

Pharmacokinetic parameters can vary widely from one patient to the next, which may lead to significant toxicity in some patients and therapeutic failure in others. Population pharmacokinetic modeling of pharmacokinetic data from many different patients can help quantify some of this variability. This can be especially useful when the target population for the drug is heterogeneous or when the therapeutic window is narrow (i.e., effective plasma drug concentrations approach toxic concentrations). These models can simultaneously quantitate the effects of identifiable patient demographic variables (e.g., age, sex, weight, etc.), pathophysiological variables (e.g., renal or liver function, congestive heart failure, etc.), and therapeutic variables such as concomitant drug therapy on drug disposition. Another advantage is that the residual variability (the variability not accounted for by the other specified covariates) is quantitated, which includes intraindividual variability, model misspecification, and measurement error.

Pharmacokinetic-Pharmacodynamic Relationship

Pharmacokinetic modeling describes the change of plasma drug concentration over time and pharmacodynamic modeling relates drug concentration to pharmacologic effect (without regard to time). Pharmacokinetic–pharmacodynamic (PK–PD) modeling relates pharmacologic effect to the change of plasma drug concentration over time. The goal is to predict not only the magnitude but also the duration of pharmacologic effect based on the pharmacokinetic parameters of a particular drug. PK–PD models are predicated on the assumption that the concentration of drug in the plasma (accessible compartment) is proportional to the drug concentration at the receptor site (effect compartment). There are some drugs for which there is no correlation between plasma concentration and pharmacologic effect; however, toxicity may be correlated to plasma concentration in some cases (e.g., methotrexate). Such models have perhaps been best used in oncology to predict drug toxicity rather than antitumor effect.

Interpatient Variability

The pharmacokinetic parameters and the pharmacologic response from a specific dose of a drug may vary widely from patient to patient. There are multiple reasons for the observed interpatient variability in drug response that involves both pharmacokinetic and pharmacodynamic processes. These include organ dysfunction, disease state, concurrent medications, receptor and metabolic enzyme phenotype, age, sex, and other demographic characteristics. Drug bioavailability may vary from patient to patient secondary to increased or decreased expression or activity of intestinal enzymes that metabolize drugs or varying expression of drug efflux pumps (i.e., ABCB1-MDR-1 or P-glycoprotein). ABCB1 (P-glycoprotein) also pumps drugs out of cells, thus lowering the intracellular drug concentration, its overexpression in tumor cells is a well-documented mechanism of tumor cell resistance. One of the primary causes of pharmacokinetic variability is interpatient differences in the rate of drug clearance. In the case of drugs (or drugs with active metabolites) that are primarily cleared by the kidney, decreased renal function will dictate the need for dose reduction to avoid excessive toxicity (e.g., methotrexate). Drugs that undergo extensive hepatic biotransformation and/or biliary excretion may require dose modification in patients with severely compromised hepatic function (e.g., taxanes, anthracyclines, vinca alkaloids). Genetic polymorphisms in the CYP450 enzyme and other phase 2 enzyme systems (e.g., *N*-acetylation transferase-2, glutathione-*S*-transferase, and uridine diphosphate glucuronosyltransferase) will also contribute to differences in an individual's ability to metabolize anti-cancer drugs. Another major reason for altered CYP450 activity is the use of concurrent medications that either inhibit or induce one or more isoforms, which may result in significant changes in the rate of drug clearance.

Variability in the volume of distribution of a drug can also account for some of the observed interpatient variability. Age is particularly important for volume of distribution because infants have approx 70–80% total body water compared to 60% for adults. Elderly patients have relatively more adipose tissue and less water content as well as decreased muscle mass. Disease-related alterations in plasma protein concentrations in cancer patients can affect the volume of distribution of drugs that are highly protein bound (e.g., α_1-acid glycoprotein which binds docetaxel and UCN-01) influencing free drug concentrations and drug clearance. Pharmacodynamic variability is produced not only by differences between patients in the concentration of drug at the effect site as a result of pharmacokinetic variation but also by receptor/target polymorphisms. Examples of these polymorphisms include cases in which a receptor is more or less responsive to a certain drug concentration, as is the case for opioid receptors, or where paclitaxel resistance is linked to variants in the β-tubulin.

7

PROMISE OF PERSONALIZED MEDICINE

The concept of individualized drug therapy has been a central focus in clinical pharmacology and medicine for many decades. In practice, there are two key elements concerning customized therapies: choice of the dosing regimen and/or the drug itself. Both of these factors contribute to personalized medicine. Despite its apparent simplicity, individualization of treatment is a daunting challenge due to molecular heterogeneity in human diseases and marked patient-to-patient and between-population differences in drug effects as well as therapeutic dose requirements.

Therapeutics as a science relies on the degree of predictability of drug effects and the mechanisms governing their predictability. A clear understanding of the factors that influence dose–response and time-course of drug action allows rational choice of drugs and their dosages. There are also degrees of personalized medicine. The resolution of customization may vary, on the one hand, from drugs that are targeted for a very small group of individuals, to those that are intended for use in most members of the population without regard to individual characteristics of the patients. The latter group is also known as blockbuster drugs and represents majority of the medications that are currently in clinical use. Thus, the notion of personalized medicine reflects a fundamental conceptual departure from the traditional lore of pharmacotherapy that asserts the use of pharmaceuticals uniformly in broad patient populations, rather than smaller subpopulations wherein drugs may exhibit enhanced efficacy and optimal safety.

Interest in personalized medicine and rational choice of therapies can be traced back to the first formal comparative trial in the 18th century. James Lind, a naval surgeon, demonstrated in 1747 that citrus juice, and not the other leading remedies recommended by physicians of the day, cured scurvy. At the turn of the 20th century the British physician, Archibald Garrod wrote presciently on the topic of chemical individuality. More recently in the second half of the 20th century, the impetus for customized pharmacotherapy was fueled by adverse drug reactions (ADRs). The early reports of aplastic anemia in patients exposed to chloramphenicol, followed by the thalidomide disaster in 1961 led to recognition of at risk populations, or conditions (e.g., renal failure) and drug–drug interactions that may predispose to drug toxicity. These developments and the ensuing scientific scrutiny culminated in the publication, for the first time, of formal principles pertaining to individualization of drug treatment based on disease, genetic, or environmental chemical influences.

Why is there a strong emphasis on personalized medicine now? Interindividual variability in drug effects and the lack of reliable predictors of this variability are increasingly recognized as important barriers to science-based therapeutics. Moreover, the public health consequences of uncertainty in drug efficacy and safety have been increasingly documented by recent pharmacovigilance studies. A number of policy initiatives, particularly those on ADRs, further added to the momentum for personalized therapies in health care. Notably, present genetics-based efforts to individualize drug therapy have a more *mechanistic* focus in contrast to the previous empirical initiatives on personalized medicine using less precise demographic and descriptive clinical characteristics of the patients or the attendant disease. Hence, a common thread that runs through current pharmacogenomic strategies aimed at personalized medicine is the intent to relate the descriptive results of pharmaceutical interventions or patient characteristics to molecular and mechanistic underpinnings of drug response that, by extension, may allow more precise and rational predictions on clinical outcomes.

The advances made by completion of the Human Genome Project (HGP) 4 years ago and the high throughput genomic technologies that spun off from this effort now make it entirely feasible to apply this vast knowledge-base in the clinical practice and diagnosis of human diseases as well as drug efficacy and safety in each individual patient. The HGP presents unique research opportunities to identify novel drug targets for common complex diseases. This offers the promise in the near future for improvements not only in drug safety but also therapeutic efficacy by selective prescriptions in subpopulations identified by genetic testing of drug targets. The individualization of drug therapy is thus evolving from traditional dose titration methods to more radical approaches concerning prescription decisions and the choice of drugs based on individuals' genetic make-up. These changes, understandably, are attracting much attention from all stakeholders including patients, physicians, academic investigators, pharmaceutical industry, insurers and experts in regulatory science. Collectively, these recent developments have placed the study of human genetics and personalized medicine firmly on the social policy agenda, raising a vast amount of public interest as well as close scrutiny of its promises and actual impact on patient care.

Pharmacogenomics is a term introduced in late 1990s and is broadly defined as the study of variability in drug safety and efficacy using information from the entire genome of a patient. Variations in both gene sequence and expression are of interest to pharmacogenomic inquiries. By contrast, the term pharmacogenetics has been established since 1950s and refers to investigations on specific candidate genes in relation to individual differences in drug effects. Candidate genes in pharmacogenetic studies are selected based on a priori observations of disease susceptibility, drug absorption, metabolism, transport, and excretion as well as drug targets, as opposed to the genome-wide hypothesis-free approach in pharmacogenomics. Despite these differences, there is also interdependency between the two disciplines. Once the genes or genetic markers relevant to mechanism of drug action or safety are identified through the genome-wide pharmacogenomics search, each individual gene requires further clinical validation by focused and hypothesis-driven pharmacogenetic approaches before they can be routinely applied at point of care in the clinic. We herein chose to use the term pharmacogenomics but many of the ensuing discussion and concepts will also be applicable to pharmacogenetics.

The aim of the present chapter is to introduce the reader to (i) broad pharmacological, genetic and societal drivers as well as the promise of personalized medicine, (ii) specific pharmacogenomic strategies to individualize drug therapy early in drug discovery, clinical development and during routine therapy at point of care in the clinic, and (iii) conceptual and practical barriers to pharmacogenomic-guided personalized medicine and the broader ethical issues associated with customized therapies.

Drivers and Promise of Personalized Medicine

Rationale for Customized Drug Therapy: Variability and the Present State of Drug Safety and Efficacy in the Clinic

Most current medications and the recommended dosing regimens come with a significant risk of drug toxicity or treatment-failure in the clinic. Drug-related morbidity and mortality were estimated to cost up to $137 billion annually in the United States. A recent meta-analysis of prospective studies in the United States suggests that serious and fatal ADRs occur in 6.7% and 0.32% of hospitalized patients, respectively. This translates into more than two million serious ADRs and an annual death rate of 106,000 patients in the United States alone. These estimates rank ADRs as the fourth leading cause of death, ahead of accidents, diabetes and pneumonia. Subsequent extended analysis of pharmaco-epidemiology data in 32 non-U.S. studies from industrialized countries support the contention that fatal ADRs are a significant public health problem in many countries around the world. It is noteworthy that the serious ADRs noted above were observed during treatment with usual doses of drugs that had already been introduced for clinical use and despite the exclusion of cases due to intentional or accidental overdose, human errors in drug administration or non-compliance, drug abuse, and therapeutic failures. Similarly, an independent study of 2227 ADRs in hospitalized patients showed that about 50% had no readily discernible or preventable cause. Nearly 16% of the 1232 pharmaceutical products listed in the Physicians' Desk Reference in the U.S. were deemed to carry a significant ADR risk to warrant a "*black box*" warning on the drug label.

Table 7.1. Response rates of patients to major drug classes in selected therapeutic areas

Therapeutic area	*Efficacy rate (%)*
Alzheimer's	30
Analgesics (Cox-2)	80
Asthma	60
Cardiac arrhythmias	60
Depression (SSRI)	62
Diabetes	57
HIV	47
Incontinence	40
Migraine (acute)	52
Migraine (prophylaxis)	50
Oncology	25
Osteoporosis	48
Rheumatoid arthritis	50
Schizophrenia	60

The societal and global burden of ADRs can be compounded further by consideration of drug morbidity and mortality in ambulatory settings and nursing homes as well as non-industrialized countries. Collectively, these epidemiological observations suggest that more fundamental and previously unaccounted reasons, possibly genetic in nature, may underlie a significant portion of such unpreventable and apparently idiosyncratic ADRs in the clinic. Consistent with this hypothesis, a detailed analysis of 27 drugs frequently cited in ADR studies found that 59% are metabolized by one or more enzyme with a variant allele associated with deficient metabolism. By contrast, only 7–22% of drugs selected at random were influenced by a genetically polymorphic metabolic pathway. Although drug safety has traditionally received much research and media attention, drug efficacy is an equally important and yet, often overlooked dimension of pharmacotherapy. In comparison to ADRs, the public health consequences and economic costs of therapeutic-failure associated with drugs have not been well investigated. A recent review of published data on the efficacy of major drugs used in several important diseases is instructive in this regard. Spear et al. concluded that the response rates vary markedly across various therapeutic areas with 80% of patients responding to Cox-2 inhibitors while the response rate was as low as 25% in cancer chemotherapy and 30% in Alzheimer's disease. Overall, it appears that only about 50% of patients respond to drugs in major therapeutic classes (or conversely, 50% of patients, on average, do not respond to pharmacotherapy).

While drugs are often life-saving in some patients, the existing armamentarium of drugs, taken together, are only moderately effective in the general population and carry significant liabilities in the form of serious and fatal ADRs. The traditional notion of blockbuster drugs overlooks this interindividual variability in drug efficacy and safety despite its adverse public health consequences and economic burden on society at large. In fact, one may argue, in light of the pharmacovigilance data noted above, that there are really very few robust examples of blockbuster drugs in the clinic. The term "*blockbuster drug*" has more economic underpinnings and relates to the commercial promise of a medication. Unfortunately, this term is often misused in a scientific context to refer to a broad array of drugs that are assumed to work in most members of the population with optimal safety whereas, in essence, it indicates the pharmaceutical products that are developed and marketed with the general population in mind. The predicaments associated with safety and efficacy of the existing medications clearly call for more focused science-based therapeutics and rational approaches to selection of drugs and their dosing regimens to customize pharmacotherapy based on, for example, individual patient genetic make-up. Understanding the mechanisms and cause–effect relationships for apparently unpreventable and idiosyncratic ADRs and treatment-failures is crucial for early identification and prevention of such drug related problems in the 21st century healthcare.

Rationale for Genetics: Can it Explain and Predict Variability in Drug Efficacy and Safety?

A prerequisite implicit assumption for any pharmacogenomic study is that the targeted pharmacological trait (or phenotype) is subject to appreciable genetic control. To this end, it is important to recognize that drug effects are usually elicited against the background of disease phenomena. Many of the human diseases display genetic components with varying degrees. Further, some of the biological pathways underlying diseases may serve as targets for drug interventions or alternatively, hold the potential to modify, or counteract the direct pharmacological effects of drugs via homeostatic mechanisms. Thus, genetic regulation of diseases or physiological pathways may indirectly influence variability in drug effects.

More direct evidence for the role of heredity in pharmacology can be observed in pharmacokinetic processes. The origins of pharmacogenomics date to the 1950s when monogenic variations in drug metabolism were the primary focus of research interest. Early on, a number of seminal twin studies in healthy volunteers under uniform basal environmental conditions demonstrated a markedly higher reproducibility of pharmacokinetic indices in monozygotic twins (nearly 100% identity in the genome) compared to dizygotic twins who share, on average, only 50% of their genome. These observations provided the first unequivocal evidence that heredity plays a prominent role in drug metabolism, despite the multitude of other environmental and clinical factors that may potentially influence variability in drug exposure. Subsequently, the debrisoquine/sparteine (CYP2D6) polymorphism was first identified by Smith in London, England and Eichelbaum in Bonn, Germany. Since then, numerous genetic polymorphisms have been firmly documented and functionally characterized in various drug metabolizing enzymes and drug transporters. Most experts in the field of pharmacogenomics now agree that hereditary factors play an important role in drug disposition.

Although the focus of studies on the clinical relevance of genetic variations in pharmacokinetic pathways has been mostly on drug safety, there is both theoretical basis and empirical evidence to suggest that drug efficacy can also be influenced. In this regard, an early anecdotal observation made by Smith during the discovery of debrisoquine polymorphism can be instructive. In a pharmacokinetic study of debrisoquine in 1970s, a subtherapeutic dose resulted in unexpected and profound decrease in blood pressure of a subject, who, in fact, was one of the study investigators. Implicit in this historical account is that the side effect (hypotension) experienced by Smith himself is essentially an extension of the primary intended pharmacological effect of the antihypertensive drug debrisoquine. Such ADRs typified by an augmentation of the primary "*therapeutic*" effect of a drug are classified as Type A drug reactions. Type A reactions are common, dose- or concentration-dependent and also include ADRs due to overdose as well as drug–drug interactions. Thus, drug efficacy and toxicity are usually observed on a successive concentration gradient. This means that any genetic or environmental factor that can influence drug concentrations may also explain individual variations in both efficacy and safety. Dramatic differences in cure rates of helicobacter pylori infection and peptic ulcer with omeprazole (a CYP2C19 substrate) and amoxacillin among patients with different CYP2C19 genotypes further attest to the relevance of pharmacogenomic variability in drug metabolism with respect to drug efficacy.

Genetic variations in receptors, ion channels and other types of drug targets constitute a more recent but growing body of evidence in favor of heredity and its role in drug efficacy and safety. Already, there are accumulating data, for example, documenting the clinical significance of variations in genes encoding arachidonate 5-lipoxygenase (ALOX5) and β_2-adrenoreceptor for response to ALOX5 inhibitors and β_2-agonists, respectively, in asthma; serotonin receptors in response to atypical antipsychotic clozapine; and dopamine D3 receptor gene (DRD3) for predisposition to the movement disorder, tardive dyskinesia, induced by typical antipsychotic drugs. We note that the commonly occurring and unpreventable ADRs may be attributable in part to genetic variations in drug targets and/or presently unknown genetic differences in drug disposition, for instance, in phase II drug metabolizing enzymes and drug transporters.

Genes rarely act in isolation and hence, genetic contributions to pharmacological variability are subject to influences by gene–environment interactions as well as epistatic interactions among various genetic loci. Indeed, the most likely scenario is that the underlying basis of genetically determined variability in treatment response and common ADRs is polygenic. It is therefore often difficult to estimate the *composite genetic component* in pharmacological traits. This information is essential before decisions on further molecular pharmacogenomic work can be justified. Typically, heritability estimates are obtained using the twin method. Although twin studies are indeed very useful to establish the baseline heritability figures for common complex diseases, they may have limited applicability in pharmacological responses to drugs and other xenobiotics. Some of these limitations include difficulties in recruitment of twins, obtaining clinical outcome data in both twins (since the twin pairs may not suffer from the same disease at the same time) as well as the financial cost of twin investigations. To circumvent the difficulties associated with dissection of genetic components with the twin approach, a repeated-drug-administration (RDA) method has been earlier proposed wherein between- and within-subject variances in drug efficacy or safety are compared. A relatively larger between-subject variance as measured by the RDA analysis points to significance of hereditary factors in pharmacological variability. Recent applications of the RDA method demonstrate that genetics also plays a paramount role in pharmacological traits hitherto not subjected to pharmacogenomic analysis such as renal drug disposition.

Recognition of Molecular Heterogeneity in Human Diseases: The Need for New Drug Targets

The completion of the HGP 4 years ago provided the reference framework for the sequence of some 30,000–40,000 protein-coding genes in the human genome. At that time, a high-density map of the human genome consisting of 1.42 million single-nucleotide polymorphisms (SNPs) (now >3.7 million) have also been made available. These advances witnessed in parallel the development of high-throughput genomic technologies and the related infrastructure; this was favorably reflected in marked decreases in genotyping costs over the past several years. On the other hand, some of the alternative viewpoints consider the HGP more of an engineering triumph with the development of tools and technologies for genetic research. For translation of the human genome sequence to biology, clinical medicine and science-based therapeutics, a second additional layer of complexity, namely, interindividual and population-to-population variability in the genome will need to be addressed. The latter issue has recently culminated in the launch of the International HapMap project to identify the SNPs and their patterns (haplotypes) on individual chromosomes in various human populations from Africa, Asia and Europe. In the present post-genomic era, the ultimate goal is to utilize the haplotype map of the human genome as a foundation for future genetic association studies of human diseases as well as drug efficacy and safety. A further important consideration is that genetic variants underlying variability in drug effects are unlikely to be limited to the coding elements of genes. Variants in regulatory regions are most likely to be implicated and it is quite feasible that non-coding, intronic elements, which influence gene transcription, have an important role as well. These considerations greatly broaden the scope of genetic influences that will need to be considered.

Why do we need to know the genetic basis of human diseases? And how does this information contribute to rational therapeutics? A recent biochemical classification of drug targets found that the largest group was comprised of receptors (45%) followed primarily by enzymes (28%), hormones and related factors (11%), ion channels (5%), and nuclear receptors (2%). Overall, current drug targets across all therapeutic areas amount to only about 500 molecular targets. Considering the diversity of human diseases, there is no doubt that novel drug targets will be essential to develop drugs with improved efficacy. To this end, identification of the molecular genetic basis of diseases may have three fundamental contributions. First, knowledge of the genes will eventually help discern the identity of the corresponding proteins leading to disease and its clinical manifestations. In some cases, these proteins can serve as direct targets for therapeutic interventions by conventional small molecule drugs (<500 Da molecular weight). On the other hand, it is also reasonable to expect that not all disease-causing genes or their protein products will be druggable.

A second alternative therapeutic strategy in such cases may involve targeting other components of the biological pathway(s) containing the genes associated with disease. Third, in the absence of molecular genetic corollaries of disease, it is noteworthy that entry points for most therapeutic interventions have thus far been at the protein level. The knowledge of a specific disease- causing gene or mutation may allow interventions further upstream in the biological cascade at the level of gene expression before the corresponding proteins of pathophysiological significance are actually synthesized. For example, libraries of small inhibitory RNA (siRNA) molecules are now being investigated in the pharmaceutical and biotechnology industries as potential therapeutic agents to silence the genes whose expression may predispose to disease.

A glance at recent advances in human genetics can be instructive to gain a balanced context on the drivers of pharmacogenomics in the near future. In rare monogenic diseases, a clear pattern of Mendelian inheritance can be discerned wherein human genetic variation in one or both copies of a single gene will predictably lead to clinical manifestations of the attendant disease. Through positional cloning approaches, more than 1400 genes for some 1200 Mendelian traits have been identified by the year 2003. The majority of the mutations associated with monogenic diseases are in-frame amino-acid substitutions and nonsense codons (59%), deletions (22%) and insertions/duplications (7%) while only about 1% of the mutations linked to Mendelian traits were in regulatory regions of human genes. The remarkable success of the positional cloning strategy in monogenic diseases has not been uniformly reproducible upon application to multi- factorial complex human diseases such as diabetes, schizophrenia and non-familial, sporadic forms of common cancers. A hallmark of complex diseases is that a multitude of genetic loci as well as the environment and life-style importantly contribute to disease risk. The

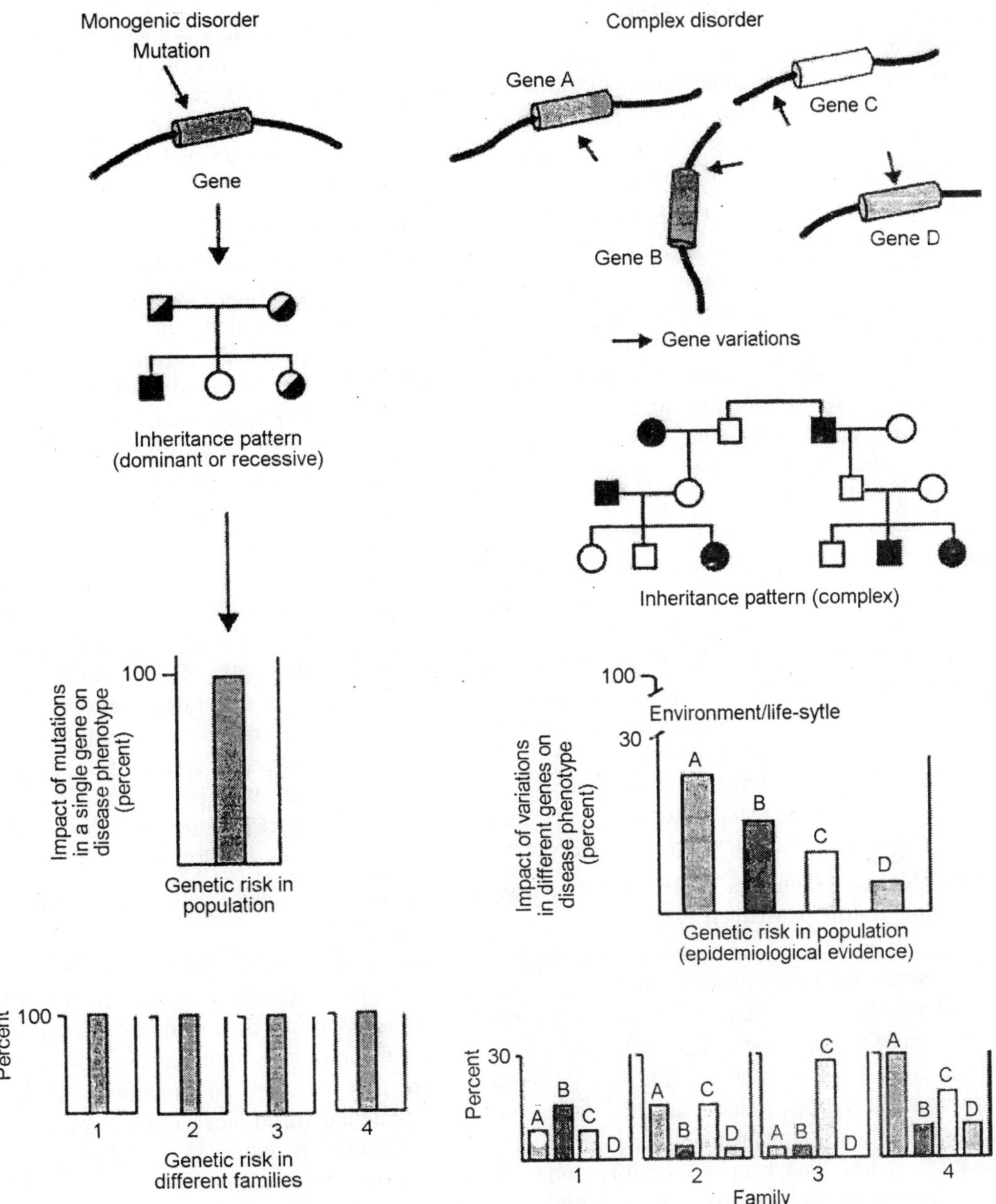

Fig. 7.1. Inheritance of monogenic and complex disorders.

multiplicity of contributory factors and their interactions result in non-Mendelian transmission of disease phenotypes in pedigrees. Further, genetic variations in regulatory regions of the genome that affect gene expression and translationally silent mutations are also likely to play a significant role in predisposition to multifactorial diseases. Hence, current nosologies based on clinical chemistry and symptoms reflect vastly divergent underlying molecular mechanisms leading to the final and ostensibly similar clinical syndromes among patients. This means that effective treatment of patient subpopulations typified by distinct molecular etiologies may require differential therapies with drugs that target a unique complement of biological targets. In the near future, we will therefore likely witness the emergence of genetic tests to assist and complement diagnosis of diseases with clinical nosology. To this end, a synergy between tests for genes associated with disease and drug effects can also be expected. For instance, the APOE4 allele of the APOE gene is associated with predisposition and a lower age of onset for sporadic or late onset familial forms of Alzheimer's disease as well as poor response to acetylcholinesterase enzyme inhibitor tacrine.

Shift in Emphasis on Health Care Policy Toward Disease Prevention

The dictum in the traditional folklore of medicine has been the treatment and alleviation of acute symptoms of disease. Aforementioned advances in our understanding of the risk factors and molecular basis of human diseases are now paving the way to develop medicines that can prevent or slow the progression of disease phenomena. Schizophrenia and some of the neurodegenerative diseases such as Alzheimer's or Parkinson's disease are being investigated in reference to neurodevelopmental theories to develop drugs that can halt the (patho)physiological processes leading to eventual clinical symptoms. The rise of statins and other lipid lowering drugs to prevent long-term cardiovascular morbidity and mortality is another example of preventative pharmacotherapies. It is thus noteworthy that the interest in personalized medicine does not happen in a vacuum and should be viewed within the larger framework of recent changes in health and therapeutic policies over the past decade.

Poised at the threshold of this upcoming and fundamental change in emphasis from treatment to prophylaxis in healthcare policy, pharmacogenomics will likely be shaped in the near future by particular attributes of the pharmacological interventions aimed at disease prevention. For instance, there will be an increasing demand to predict the long-term outcome and benefit-to-risk ratio of preventative therapies. Equally important, adherence to drug treatment by patients will need assurance beyond traditional physician visits and consultations, especially considering that such "future" patients will need to take drugs in the absence of acute symptoms and in the face of a probable disease risk in the far-too-distant future. It is in this very context that predictive pharmacogenomic tests will be essential for patients, physicians and insurers to make informed and rational decisions to subscribe to pharmacogenomically guided and customized therapies that may be offered at premium prices by drug manufacturers.

Asymmetry Between Genetics of Human Diseases and Pharmacological Phenotypes: An Impetus for Pharmacogenomic Research

The fundamental focus of human genetics is to establish the causal links between genes and phenotypes. Since its first introduction in late 1990s, the allure of pharmacogenomics has drawn a considerable number of human geneticists who have previously dealt with complex diseases. This importantly benefited and complemented the classical pharmacological approaches to questions of variability in drug effects. At the same time, a tendency has arisen to view pharmacological responses akin to disease phenotypes. There are however several fundamental differences unique to the field of pharmacology and the attendant phenotypes that may offer a relative advantage in application of genetic methodologies. It has long been known that most chronic human diseases initiate and progress over a considerable period of time before clinical findings become apparent. Thus, human genetics is essentially an observational science wherein molecular genetic markers are correlated with a disease process that is not experimentally controlled or reproducible for obvious ethical and practical reasons. A related corollary is that the scope of gene–environment interactions is often incalculable or difficult to estimate with adequate certainty.

For all the parallels between the disease traits and pharmacological phenotypes, the very difference between the observational nature of study designs in disease genetics and the ability to experimentally produce drug response phenotypes in a setting carefully controlled for environmental factors is perhaps one of the most salient tenets of pharmacology that may offer a marked opportunity to control for gene–environment interactions in pharmacogenomic investigations. For instance, it is feasible to quantify the baseline phenotypes prior to drug administration in humans, which can subsequently be subtracted from drug-induced phenotypes in biological systems. In theory, this can considerably facilitate correlative studies on human genetic variation and pharmacological phenotypes. By contrast, such experimental approaches are not applicable to the study of common multifactorial human diseases. This favorable asymmetry between disease genetics and pharmacogenomics is increasingly being recognized by scientists and clinicians with diverse backgrounds thereby coalescing interest in pharmacogenomics in various medical specialties in academia and the pharmaceutical industry.

Advances in Regulatory Science and Medicolegal Considerations

The transition from a new research idea to actual application in the clinic and drug development is a slow and arduous process. A recent search of the 2000 entries in the Physicians' Desk Reference (year 2003 electronic version) identified only 51 labels containing pharmacogenomic information. Moreover, presentations of the pharmacogenomic data in the labels were generally not in a form that could be readily applied in clinical practice. Although it is difficult to estimate the number of drug labels that should appropriately contain data on host genetic make-up for rational dose titration or choice of medications, the latter example suggests that pharmacogenomic information is likely underrepresented in current drug labels. This is an important issue of relevance for adoption of pharmacogenomics in the clinic because it is not clear whether and to what extent research findings available as off-label scientific publications can be applied in routine medical practice with busy schedules. Still, drug labels do not always reflect the best available evidence. Recent announcement of a guidance document in March 2005 by the U.S. Food and Drug Administration (FDA) to encourage regulatory pharmacogenomics data submission by drug developers is a welcome development in this regard. Advances in regulatory science over the past three decades have been instructive on the critical role of regulatory guidance in widespread implementation of new technologies on practices in the pharmaceutical industry and clinical medicine.

A case in point is the history of development of population pharmacokinetic approaches to explain variability in drug exposure. Despite the theoretical foundations established since the 1970s and the availability of statistical software capable of conducting such advanced pharmacokinetic analyses, the routine use of population pharmacokinetics in clinical drug development has been considerably facilitated in part through recent guidelines developed by regulatory agencies. The present heightened public awareness on societal ramifications of the HGP and the attendant genomic technologies is increasingly prompting governments and policy makers to provide further guidance on pharmacogenomics. Moreover, regulatory consideration may soon be given to drugs already in the clinic. This should further encourage drug manufacturers to adopt pharmacogenomics, with the realization that regulatory review will be applicable at all phases of a medication's life-cycle, both prior and subsequent to introduction for human use. Seen in this light, it is conceivable that developments on the regulatory policy front will importantly shape and drive the application of pharmacogenomics technology in the very near future.

As information on the molecular basis of human diseases and individual variability in drug effects continues to accumulate, a threshold may soon be crossed beyond which the standard of care will include predictive pharmacogenomic testing. Advances in accessibility of pharmacogenomic technologies may thus challenge the traditional questions of ethics and litigation standards. In fact, the clinical significance of genetic variability in certain drug metabolizing enzymes such as thiopurine methyl transferase are already (TPMT) well-established, e.g., in relation to life-threatening toxicity associated with thiopurine anticancer drugs. In such cases where research findings increasingly impact patient care, demands by insurers and government payers as well as legal liability and litigation by patients who suffer from drug toxicity or treatment-failure may set a strong precedent for pharmacogenomic testing by physicians and the pharmaceutical industry. Looking further, it is tempting to suggest that physicians who attend focused continuing medical education courses on pharmacogenomics may presumably be subject to reduced premiums for malpractice insurance in the future. Such complex medicolegal dynamics between patients, insurers, healthcare providers, and drug manufacturers may eventually catalyze the adoption of pharmacogenomics as part of science-based therapeutics.

A recently released survey of American consumers (n = 748) and physicians (n = 400) suggests that nearly 50% of consumers would be agreeable to undergo genetic testing to determine which medication would be most appropriate for them and that they would be willing to pay more for an individually tailored prescription. About 80% of physicians and consumers, on the other hand, expressed views that genetically guided personalized medicine would have a favorable impact on the U.S. healthcare system. It will be of interest to also characterize consumer and physician attitudes in other countries to determine the global patterns of acceptance of pharmacogenomics and the potential barriers to its implementation.

Strategies for Application of Pharmacogenomics to Customize Therapy

Drug Discovery and Preclinical Development

Drug discovery has long relied on serendipitous observations. For drugs introduced in the 1950s and onward, the mode of drug action has been typically discovered after some period of use in the clinic. Over the past two decades, routine application of high-throughput screening (HTS) methods together with combinatorial chemistry and a rich array of chemical libraries significantly accelerated the entry of therapeutic candidates with clearly defined molecular targets to early phase clinical evaluation. Despite these advances, out of 1035 new drug applications approved in the 12-year period from 1989 to 2000 in the United States, a sizable fraction (54%) were differentiated from existing drugs primarily on the basis of dosage form, route of administration, or as a combination product with another active ingredient. Moreover, direct-to-consumer promotions of pharmaceutical products occasionally rely on claims of higher therapeutic "*potency*." An improvement in potency means that the same drug effect can be elicited at a lower drug concentration. This may favorably influence drug selectivity and safety in certain cases.

The excessive emphasis on discovery of more potent compounds overlooks another basic currency of pharmacology: efficacy—the maximal effect that can be produced by a drug. This predicament is best exemplified by the moderate efficacy of current drugs in the clinic. Efficacy is reflected in the asymptotic plateau of concentration–effect curves; it is determined by both the chemical structure of the drug and the biological attributes of the targeted receptor–effector systems. No matter how many structurally diverse hit and lead compounds are synthesized in early discovery, large volumes of compound libraries will not make up for the limited diversity in drug targets (only some 500 at present) thereby markedly constraining the upper limits of therapeutic drug effects in patients. For improvements in drug efficacy, advances made by combinatorial chemistry and HTS need to be complemented by the discovery of novel drug targets, or better characterization of the subtypes of existing targets. Genome-wide association studies of drug response or common human diseases may provide clues for discovery of novel drug targets as well as entry points for the development of first-in-class compounds with unique pharmacological mode(s) of action. In efforts for customized therapies, it is clear that the identification of pharmacogenomic biomarkers should start very early, preferably in drug discovery and phase 2A/2B clinical studies for proof-of-concept.

In the present post-genomic period, another favorable influence of the HGP in drug discovery will likely be seen in preclinical studies of global gene expression before and after drug treatment in animal species. Shared patterns of gene expression among drugs within the same therapeutic class or alternatively, drugs that produce a similar form of toxicity may pave the way to map the attendant biological networks essential for drug efficacy and safety. Further, identification of genes related to common human diseases may contribute towards better preclinical models of drug efficacy, an area that needs much improvement for rational scaling of data obtained in animals to humans.

In the ideal case, the existing HTS processes in drug discovery may soon be tailored to accommodate the specific subtypes of novel or existing drug targets. This can then provide insights on optimal therapeutic candidates prior to clinical trials and create niche subpopulations in whom drugs can be used with greater efficacy and optimal safety. Focused pharmacogenetic testing in the clinic will be essential before such customized drugs can be prescribed. A reverse and complementary approach is to choose the compounds that will bind with high affinity and functionally interact with all subtypes of a given novel drug target. This alternative strategy for drug discovery may alleviate the need for pharmacogenetic testing at point of care: the lead compounds are chosen or customized (instead of the patients), in this case, to accommodate all variants of a biological target. Conversely, these early individualization attempts in drug discovery may be constrained by limits of medicinal and combinatorial chemistry to synthesize compounds that will be versatile enough to bind and activate all drug target subtypes, while demonstrating an adequate safety, bioavailability and drug–drug interaction profile.

All these technical advances and promises of pharmacogenomic-guided drug discovery also come with attendant ethical and social policy challenges. For example, if drugs are discovered and developed only for the most common subtypes of drug targets, this may potentially create therapeutic orphan subpopulations—will there be financial or legislative mechanisms in place to ensure that these individual patients also benefit from novel and mechanism-oriented therapeutic interventions? When developed, genetically tailored medications will likely be available at premium prices. Who will take the responsibility for ethical promotion of such personalized drugs?

It is interesting to note that among 1393 new drugs developed between 1975 and 1999, only 1.1% (16 drugs) was for tropical and other diseases prevalent in developing countries. While one-third of the world population live on less than US$2/day, and occasionally without access to essential drugs, it is foreseeable that some may question how pharmacogenomics may contribute to discovery of drugs that will benefit the patients in the developing world. To this end, it is worthwhile to bear in mind that the genomes from numerous parasitic pathogens, bacteria and viruses have been sequenced and available for the research community. Hence, pharmacogenomics offers much hope for novel drug target discovery and development against infectious agents affecting world's populations. In addition, concepts and technologies developed in parallel to pharmacogenomics may be instrumental for identification of individuals who may be more sensitive or resistant to infectious organisms in developing countries. It is hoped that these promises offered by pharmacogenomics will materialize and will be put into practice with a global public health policy in mind. Finally, although pharmacogenomics will likely revolutionize how new drug candidates are tailored for individual patients, serendipity and keen scientific insights will still continue to play a role in the drug discovery process.

Early Phase Clinical Drug Development

Allometric scaling of preclinical data to humans is often limited by marked interspecies differences in drug disposition, drug targets as well as the inevitable biological contrasts between outbred human populations and the inbred laboratory animals with a homogenous genetic background. First-in-human studies and the subsequent phase 2A/2B proof-of-concept clinical trials of therapeutic candidates in early stages of drug development play a bridging role with drug discovery efforts before large scale and confirmatory phase three clinical studies can be rationalized. The principal aims of these early investigations in humans include estimation of pharmacokinetic variability, the optimal dose ranges and administration schedules, the risk for drug–drug interactions, and provision of evidence on proof-of-concept for drug efficacy (or the lack thereof) and mode of action. Typically, single and multiple ascending doses of a *new molecular entity* (NME) are administered to healthy volunteer subjects and carefully selected groups of patients with a relatively uniform and usually mild to moderate disease state. On the other hand, even though these studies collectively provide preliminary insights into presumed effects of NMEs in humans, the complete range of pharmacokinetic and pharmacodynamic variability within and among human populations is seldom available at the end of phase two drugs development. This predicament, along with the occasional disconnect between the efficacy of NMEs in animal models, and the clinic, have recently stimulated a surge for identification of early indicators or biomarkers of drug activity and mode of action.

Per definitions provided by the U.S. National Institutes of Health expert working group, a biological marker (biomarker) is "a characteristic that is objectively measured and evaluated as an indicator of normal biological processes, pathogenic processes, or pharmacological responses to a therapeutic intervention". A surrogate endpoint represents a special subset of biomarkers that is intended to substitute for a clinical endpoint; this implies a stronger correlation between the surrogate biomarker and clinical outcome (e.g., therapeutic benefit, lack of efficacy, and toxicity). Insofar as the pharmacogenomic biomarkers are concerned, there is growing interest in characterizing changes in the expression of genes that encode known drug targets or other biological elements downstream from the immediate drug target–effector systems. A particular advantage in this regard is that the effects of drug treatment on expression of key pathways related to drug response may precede changes in clinical outcomes; this may alleviate the need for long-term clinical studies and expedite the drug development time frames. Moreover, genomic methodologies typically have a higher throughput than the conventional phenotypic or clinical endpoint-based measures of drug efficacy and safety. This may in effect provide a broader picture of drug effects in various pathophysiological pathways and in some cases, lead to discovery of hitherto unexpected additional mode(s) of drug action and indications for future therapeutic applications. It should be mentioned that all these exploratory and research-oriented applications of pharmacogenomics in early stage development contribute essentially to better characterization of NMEs and their effects in humans. The small study sample sizes in early phase clinical trials, however, are not sufficient to characterize the diagnostic sensitivity and specificity of genetic tests. On the other hand, these early pharmacogenomic investigations, if judiciously analyzed and interpreted, can be invaluable for hypothesis-generation and the initial identification of genetic biomarkers that may later be utilized for customization of drug therapy.

Early stage clinical studies typically describe the pharmacokinetic variability associated with a NME but these estimates, in most cases, remain limited to the study samples. Broader views of pharmacokinetic variations within and among human populations can be obtained only if the mechanisms of variability in drug disposition are discerned. To this end, panel studies in patients representative of the population extremes (e.g., poor metabolizers vs. rapid or ultrarapid metabolizers) for a given drug disposition pathway may help to define the upper limit of contribution of individual CYP450 and Phase II drug metabolizing isozymes or drug transporters to pharmacokinetic variability in the general population. These panel investigations in genetically stratified samples may inform several critical drug development decisions including: (1) extent of variability in dosages required for an optimal response in the targeted population, (2) risk for competitive drug–drug interactions and the list of concomitant medications that may cause a pharmacokinetic interaction upon co-administration with the NME under clinical development, and (3) prioritizing pharmacokinetic studies in different populations.

Pharmacokinetic bridging-studies are usually conducted when regulatory drug approval is sought in various countries. These data provide guidance for registration of new drugs in different populations based on similarities or differences in drug exposure. Consider, e.g., that an NME is found to be metabolized by CYP2C19 in early phase clinical studies. Because CYP2C19 displays marked inter-ethnic differences in the frequency of poor metabolizers (3% in Caucasians and 20–24% in Asians), this would immediately point towards the need to conduct highly focused and comparative pharmacokinetic studies in Asia, North America, Europe, and possibly in other countries. Without knowledge of the precise mechanisms governing interindividual variability in drug exposure, such inter-ethnic differences in drug disposition remain undetected during drug development. If dose adjustments are not made based on genetic or phenotypic differences in CYP450 function early in clinical development, drugs may face the risk of withdrawal from human use after their introduction in the clinic.

A notable application of pharmacogenomics in early phase drug development, which extends beyond personalized medicine, is in proof-of-concept investigations. Phase 2A/2B trials enriched for patients with certain genetic subtypes of drug targets previously shown to confer an increased likelihood of response can facilitate decisions on whether and to what extent a NME is a viable therapeutic candidate. Conversely, an inadequate response to a NME in such enriched samples may serve as an early indication of possible therapeutic failure in the general patient population.

Late Stage Clinical Drug Development—Phase Three Registration Trials

Phase three clinical trials form the centerpiece for overall clinical drug development programs. These pivotal late stage clinical studies are typically conducted in large patient samples and play an important role in registration of therapeutic candidates and confirming their efficacy and safety. This is also the stage of drug development when genetic tests for customization of therapy should be validated with adequate attention to their diagnostic sensitivity and specificity. Any new information learned on subpopulations identified with pharmacogenomic tests at this phase of development can favorably influence the customization of drug labels. Despite investments and enthusiasm for discovery of novel drug targets and pharmacogenomic applications in early phase clinical trials, direct stratification of patients using genetic tests in advanced stages of drug development is still rare. To date, a great majority of the pharmacogenomic biomarker development efforts have taken place in studies that were primarily designed for other purposes: demonstration of drug efficacy and safety.

The highly structured and defined time frames of the latter clinical trials may pose serious limitations for flexibility to accommodate statistical analysis and interpretation of pharmacogenomic data. Also, the high degree of population variability that characterizes the samples recruited for large-scale drug trials adds a further level of complexity to the interpretation of pharmacogenetic data, because of potentially spurious results due. Additionally, the statistical power of the traditional efficacy or safety-oriented clinical investigations may not always be sufficient to identify and validate predictive genetic tests to tailor drug therapy; in cases where epistatic effects are sought (a very likely scenario) there is a high likelihood that most current studies will be vastly underpowered for pharmacogenomic analysis. To achieve personalized medicines in the clinic, commitment to prospective pharmacogenomic testing in phase three trials designed specifically for biomarker validation and development is essential.

Through identification of patient subpopulations that are more likely to display a therapeutic response, pharmacogenomics holds the potential to conduct highly focused clinical trials enriched with "responder" patients. It is anticipated that this may reduce the required sample size and the time to obtain regulatory approval for new drug candidates. If and when successful, pharmacogenomic-guided drug development will also require companion genetic tests to tailor drug dosages or the choice of medicines. It is therefore crucial to coordinate in parallel the timely development of pharmaceutical and diagnostic products.

With the anticipated discovery of genes underlying some of the common complex human diseases over the next decade, we may increasingly witness NMEs with new drug targets and mode of action. These drugs, lacking clinical precedence on the therapeutic value of the targeted novel biological pathways, also bring along a considerable degree of risk for unexpected treatment failure or drug toxicity in the clinic. If predictive pharmacogenomic tests are available, these projected risks and promises associated with such first-in-class drugs can meet with enthusiasm and acceptance by clinicians, patients and drug manufacturers. The recent introduction of Herceptin for the treatment of patients with breast cancer who over-express the HER2 oncogene is a notable example in this regard. These critical drug development decisions can be further influenced by impact of genetic testing on the pharmaceutical patent life-cycle, the commercial promise of therapeutic candidates and the health policies in place for reimbursement of customized medicines and the companion pharmacogenomic diagnostic tests. Adoption of pharmacogenomics in drug development can be anticipated particularly in cases where severe drug toxicity is experienced in a small fraction of patients while the same drug may display adequate or remarkable efficacy in the majority of the patient population. Such therapeutic candidates can be brought to the clinic by genetic testing and identification of patients at risk for severe drug toxicity.

Applications Toward Drugs in the Clinic

A pivotal aim of pharmacogenomics is to provide the clinician with genetic tests that can be applied at relatively low cost in order to predict efficacy and adverse effects. The preceding sections have placed considerable emphasis on the anticipated contribution of pharmacogenomics to the development of new drugs. However, there exists a similarly great need to develop predictive tests that can be applied to existing agents. Antidepressant drugs are a highly illustrative example. Currently several classes of agents are in widespread use—these include specific serotonin uptake blockers, drugs with a putative action on brain norepinephrine as well as serotonergic systems, monoamine oxidase inhibitors and the older tricyclic antidepressants which are widely accepted to be highly effective but impose a significant adverse effects burden. The overall efficacy of all these drug classes is remarkably uniform with approximately 60% of patients meeting response criteria short of full remission and 10–15% less actually remitting. Some of these drugs are true "*blockbusters*" if one considers their annual sales and market share.

It is entirely unclear whether patients who fail to respond to one class of drug will respond to another class and whether there are differences between different drug classes in their efficacy. Patients who do not respond are administered a sequential series of drugs with little information available to the clinician who wishes to make an informed decision based on rational considerations. When response or remission eventually does occur, it is quite possible that this is due to natural termination of the depressive episode, which is ultimately self-limiting in most but not all cases and not to the drug administered at the time. It is highly feasible that response/remission rates to the initial drug could be raised well beyond their current levels by the availability of genetic predictors of response. For this scenario to materialize prospective trials would need to be conducted and it is entirely unclear that the motivation exists for the pharmaceutical industry to support such studies when their targets are drugs that are no longer protected by patents. It is likely that intellectual property issues in this regard have not been sufficiently thought through and there may be possibilities that justify the investment but have not been considered.

Barriers

Cost Factor and Access to Genomic Technologies

Despite the general enthusiasm and belief that pharmacogenomics will benefit drug therapy, the eventual decision to use genetic testing in the clinic may bear in part on cost-effectiveness analyses. This is not an unrealistic assumption because many of the newer therapies customized by genetic tests are anticipated to be offered at premium prices to recover the research and development costs by the pharmaceutical manufacturers. In countries with a publicly funded health care and reimbursement system, cost-effectiveness analyses may particularly be a significant consideration. Similar economical evaluations have contributed in the past to acceptance of molecular genetic tests for the diagnosis of infectious pathogens such as *Chlamydia* and *Mycobacterium tuberculosis* as part of the microbiology services. Insofar as the monogenic variability in drug metabolism is concerned, for example, inpatients in a psychiatry unit who are at extremes for CYP2D6 expression (poor and ultrarapid metabolizers) were found to incur, on average, \$4000–\$6000 higher healthcare costs when treated with drugs eliminated by CYP2D6. By contrast, virtually no pharmacoeconomic data are available concerning the cost of multigenic variability in drug effects.

Veenstra et al. recently proposed five basic requirements that may enhance the cost-effectiveness of a pharmacogenomic test: (i) provision of evidence that severe clinical or economic consequences can be avoided through the use of pharmacogenomics, (ii) current methods of therapeutic drug monitoring are inadequate, (iii) an unequivocal association between genotype and clinical phenotype, (iv) availability of a rapid and relatively inexpensive genetic test, and (v) a relatively common genetic variant. It is foreseeable that the insurers and other third-party payers of pharmacogenomic tests as well as hospital formularies may soon demand pharmacoeconomic data concerning the value and clinical impact of predictive pharmacogenomic testing on hospitalization rates, quality of life and daily functioning of patients, well beyond the direct pharmacological effects of drugs in clinical trials.

It may be argued that the current trends to characterize an increasing number of genetic variants, including the enthusiasm for genome-wide pharmacogenomic association studies, may add to the cost of genetic testing for research purposes, or at point of care as a diagnostic tool. On the other hand, the unit cost of genotyping and other genomic technologies have decreased considerably over the past several years. Additionally, broader inquiries of the human genome recently uncovered regions or blocks characterized by high linkage disequilibrium (LD) interspersed with short segments of very low LD (recombination hotspots). Within the high LD regions, there is limited haplotype diversity and the strong correlation between genetic markers creates redundancy in the informational value of each marker. This led to the recognition that common haplotypes within each block can be discerned with only a fraction of the markers, or a minimal set of SNPs named as haplotype tagging SNPs (htSNPs), present in a haplotype block. These advances may be advantageous to reduce the cost of pharmacogenomic studies further, especially in genome-wide association studies or when highly polymorphic candidate genes are being investigated. By contrast, for diseases that may result from rare haplotypes or in studies of genomic regions with low LD, characterization of all genetic markers may still be necessary. Collectively, it is reasonable to anticipate in the near future that the bottleneck in clinical pharmacogenomic studies will shift towards the rate-limiting step of collection of accurate clinical phenotypic information and relational analyses and interpretations of genetic and clinical datasets.

Pharmacogenomic Testing at Point of Care: Technical Standards and Expectations for Diagnostic Applications

Technical barriers in pharmacogenomic research are increasingly being overcome by declining costs and increased throughput of genotyping (or gene expression) methodologies. To date, much emphasis in pharmacogenomics has been placed on SNPs and their characterization in clinical samples. For genetic testing at point of care to become a reality, a broader scope of human genetic variation will need to be captured, including small insertions/deletions, and nucleotide repeat polymorphisms in the genome. For instance, certain commonly occurring CYF2D6 alleles are typified by insertions/deletion polymorphisms while the slow drug glucuronidation associated with the Gilbert's syndrome is a consequence of dinucleotide (TA) repeat polymorphism in the promoter region of UGT1A1. Attention to rare genetic variants will also be necessary particularly in cases where the test results inform critical decisions on choice of drug prescriptions or dosages. It is noteworthy that the required sensitivity and specificity of molecular genetic assays, in a diagnostic context, are markedly higher than the technical standards acceptable for pharmacogenomic research or biomarker discovery applications.

From a clinical standpoint, if there is a very toxic drug that can be prescribed by means of pharmacogenetic testing and exclusion of at risk patients, the only barrier between a patient and severe toxicity will be the pharmacogenetic test itself. Hence, in cases where the diagnostic sensitivity of the genetic test is not robust, a number of ethical and legal issues will readily emerge. Clinicians who are accustomed to high-throughput of diagnostic tests in clinical chemistry will understandably demand a comparable ease of interpretation of the test results, economic affordability and turn around times within several days or ideally, by the end of each patient's visit. These required standards for diagnostic pharmacogenomic tests at point of care are still not within reach in many countries and genetic testing largely remains restricted to specialized research laboratories or tertiary care medical centers.

Pharmacogenomics and Accelerated Drug Approval: Concerns for Long-Term Drug Safety

A key promise of pharmacogenomics for the pharmaceutical industry is accelerated drug approval in genetically stratified subpopulations or based on genomic surrogate markers of drug activity and efficacy. To be eligible for the accelerated approval program, the FDA however requires that "the medication must treat serious illnesses and show significant benefit over existing therapy for serious or life threatening illness, or provide benefit for serious or life threatening illness for which no therapy exists." The mandate for the latter program was established by the Prescription Drug User Fee Act of 1992 and the FDA Modernization Act of 1997. The published literature over the past 5 years tends to adapt the view that pharmacogenomic biomarkers will markedly reduce the time and number of patients required for drug approval. This is indeed a reasonable expectation but some cautionary restraint is necessary to establish adequate post-approval pharmacovigilance procedures, particularly for drug safety. The standard drug approval process evaluates no more than 3000 patients and healthy volunteers combined; this sample size is able to confirm the primary therapeutic benefits and detect only the common ADRs of new drugs. Rare ADRs (e.g., <1%) are typically detected after introduction of a new medication for routine clinical use. In fact, serious ADRs may be discovered as long as 36 years after regulatory approval.

The concern for drug safety during the post-marketing phase is also supported by the observation that a significant number of drugs carry black box warnings on the label. With this in mind, it is plausible that pharmacogenomic-guided accelerated approval of drugs based on surrogate markers of efficacy in studies with smaller sample sizes may be fraught with safety issues following regulatory approval. In accordance with this, serious ADRs were reported for 79% of accelerated approval cancer or anti-HIV drugs compared with 25% of similar drugs that received standard approval between the years 1996 and 2002. Taken together, this underscores the need to conduct confirmatory studies of efficacy and systematic post-marketing long-term safety evaluations for drugs that are developed by pharmacogenomic guidance. Consistency in definitions and collection of the data on safety endpoints should be planned and envisioned early in the drug development programs. This will ensure that both pre-registration and post-marketing safety data can be pooled to evaluate the broader population-based risks associated with customized therapies.

Clinical Barriers and Attention to Social, Legal, and Ethical Aspects

Studies that yield information relevant to pharmacogenetics might appear easy to perform. Ostensibly, the researcher simply needs to recruit a sample of patients treated with a particular drug, obtain a DNA sample, rate the clinical effect of the drug, document adverse effects and then determine the relationship between genetic variants and the clinical phenotypes of interest. In practice, the situation is considerably more complex. In different populations the frequency of genetic variants can differ greatly, rendering stratification and population admixture major headaches in the interpretation of studies. Stratification and admixture may also exist within samples that are apparently homogeneous from the ethnic standpoint. These considerations require great care in the selection of study populations, the application of tests for admixture and the use of appropriate statistical procedures to account for population differences when samples from different populations are pooled. Studies that take interaction among genes (epistasis) into account, an important requirement when the genetic basis of a phenotype is polygenic, require large samples in order to have sufficient statistical power. Placebo effects are another important consideration. In the absence of a placebo control, apparent association of a gene with a positive therapeutic outcome could represent association with the placebo effect of the drug and not with a true drug effect, as might be the case for the highly studied association of response to antidepressant SSRI drugs with a polymorphism in the serotonin transporter. While the association has been supported by several studies the only study to include a placebo group found an association with response among patients receiving placebo as well as patients receiving the active drug.

Definition of the clinical phenotype that is to be correlated with genetic variation may pose a significant challenge. Potential phenotypes include response to a drug (defined as improvement of symptoms to a predetermined degree), *remission* (defined as complete disappearance of the target disorder for a predetermined minimum time period) and also intermediate phenotypes such as *onset of therapeutic effect* and the *speed of response* or *remission*. It is conceivable that different genes may be implicated in each of these phenotypes particularly when the underlying genetic architecture is polygenic; there may also be varying degrees of overlap. Differentiating and applying these phenotypic definitions can be relatively straightforward, as in the case of cancer therapies but may be complex, as in psychiatric disorders, dementias, and other illness states where the etiology and pathology of the disorders is not known and the mechanisms of action of the drugs used to treat them not well established. Phenotypes may be defined categorically as presence or absence of response/remission or adverse effects or evaluated as continuous variables, the latter approach being more appropriate for analyzing genetic effects as QTLs. Consistent definition of the phenotype is a critical prerequisite for ensuring that studies are comparable and for facilitating meta-analysis which is a critical tool in evaluating the overall significance of ostensibly inconsistent results obtained by smaller, possibly under-powered studies. Thus, definition of the phenotype is a pivotal issue in pharmacogenetics. It needs to be addressed prospectively in the design of studies in order that the required information be collected in the course of the study.

From the social, legal and ethical standpoints the acquisition and storage of DNA samples and genetic information are issues that greatly concern the public. There is no doubt that as with any confidential information regarding an individual, the potential for abuse of genetic information is considerable. The individual has the right to expect that privacy will be strictly maintained and that DNA and genetic information will be used only for the purpose that was intended and for which permission was given. On the other hand there is concern that the steps taken to safeguard the rights of individuals in regard to their DNA and genetic information may be excessive and may impede scientific inquiry and deny important potential benefits. This process has been termed "*genetic exceptionalization*" and it can be discerned in overly stringent rules and regulations that are applied only in the context of genetic research whereas, if justified, they should be applied to other situations as well. In many countries stringent conditions and safeguards that are applied to genetic research by internal review boards are not demanded of non-genetic projects that place the participant at the same or even greater risk.

Many of the ethical concerns raised by pharmacogenomics are shared by genetic research into disease predisposition. Others are specific. The Nuffield Council on Bioethics outlined and discussed some of the major issues. Their report identified four central areas of concern: The first is information.

Since pharmacogenetic tests yield genetic information about individuals this raises issues of consent and confidentiality. The second area identified is resource. Pharmacogenetics may lower the cost of developing and delivering medicines but may also drive it up because of the need to incorporate pharmacogenetic testing at all pivotal stages and to design studies in accordance. The third concern is equity. Pharmacogenetics may significantly improve medical treatment for some people, but it may also result in more people falling into categories for which effective drugs are not developed, because of inadequate financial incentives to develop a drug that may be effective for only a small population, or for a large but economically poor population.

The fourth general category identified by the Nuffield Council is control. Who should decide whether a patient takes a pharmacogenetic test? Should patients be entitled to a drug if they do not wish to take an associated test? In their report the Nuffield Council addresses a comprehensive series of specific questions that are subsumed by these general areas of concern. Among the issues addressed are informed consent, privacy and confidentiality, regulation of pharmacogenetic tests, re-instatement of withdrawn medicines based on pharmacogenetic information, allocation of resources, stratification and the development of new medicines, implications for racial groups, and pivotal aspects of the implementation of pharmacogenetics in clinical practice.

Future Perspectives

Medical therapeutics has long followed an empirical tradition based on average values of pharmacological effects in the population. Unfortunately, this approach does not lend itself to predictable and science-based therapeutics due to marked variations in drug effects among patients and populations. An alternative and preferred strategy to achieve optimal drug safety and efficacy is to elucidate the mechanisms underlying variability in therapeutic outcomes which can inform the rational choice of drugs and their dosages in individual patients or subpopulations.

Pharmacogenomics provides the necessary conceptual framework and technical infrastructure to identify the previously unaccounted host-specific genetic factors underlying common (or rare) medication side effects and therapeutic failure otherwise attributed to idiosyncratic reasons. In this regard, the initial methodological approach was comprised of hypothesis- driven candidate gene studies of drug disposition, safety, or mode of action. Over the past several years, genome-wide hypothesis-free clinical pharmacogenomic association studies and analysis of gene expression before and after drug treatment have been increasingly utilized for discovery of unprecedented biological pathways of relevance to pharmacology and human diseases. It is interesting to note that tangible examples of customized therapies with novel modes of action are still limited in the clinic. However, a lag period should normally be anticipated before any new technology or scientific paradigm bears fruits. New drug development usually takes 10–15 years and for therapeutic candidates with novel molecular targets identified through pharmacogenomic approaches, it would be reasonable to see the first examples in the clinic over the next 10-year period. By contrast, for drugs that are already available for clinical use, it should be feasible to develop genetically customized treatment guidelines within a relatively shorter time frame. It is difficult to verify the practical validity of this theoretical prediction since it is uncertain whether and to what extent the pharmaceutical industry will be willing to adopt pharmacogenomic testing for therapeutic agents in the clinic.

Although patents provide protection for market exclusivity of a given pharmaceutical product, pharmacogenomic diagnostic tests for the same compound can be developed by more than one investigator or institution thereby limiting the economic promise of a genetic test. Because most drug effects are subject to polygenic control, it is foreseeable that a multitude of genetic tests may eventually be developed in various populations by different private or academic not-for-profit interest groups. Although this is certainly an advantageous situation for patients and consumers of pharmacogenomic tests, it may potentially decrease the interest on the part of the pharmaceutical industry to pursue customized therapies once a drug is available for human use. It remains to be seen how, and under which conditions, research funding will be available for pharmacogenomic investigations involving drugs available in the clinic. As aptly stated by several investigators in the field, "the promise of pharmacogenomics is already here—the reality is getting closer."

Customization of drug therapy by pharmacogenomics is an arduous but worthwhile task that requires commitment of substantial research and economic resources before tangible results at point of care can be obtained. During this process, it is crucial to adopt a longer term vision, beyond the immediate goal of obtaining regulatory approval, to enhance the entire life cycle, and quality of a medicinal product: i.e., both prompt and timely introduction of new drugs to patients as well as their sustainable use in the clinic, without post-registration withdrawal or black box warnings, should be taken into account as part of the evaluations on the overall success of pharmacogenomic-guided drug development programs. There will be several additional and foreseeable challenges on the path to targeted therapies. Pharmacogenomic biomarkers will likely be population-specific; divergent sets of genes and epistatic interactions may influence drug effects in different populations. Another crucial consideration is the recognition that the role of genetics in pharmacology depends on the environment (temporal, geographic, or therapeutic) in which drugs are being administered. Thus, the genetic components in pharmacological variability are not physical constants; their magnitude can vary depending on the gene-environment interactions at the time of a pharmaceutical intervention. Drug effects that are apparently under strong genetic control in a certain therapeutic setting may be controlled entirely by environmental factors in another context. This means that environmental components of pharmacological variability, along with the attendant genetic factors, have to be identified in concert to develop unequivocal diagnostic genetic tests and customized therapies in the clinic. The broader philosophical questions surrounding gene patents, commercial genetic testing in the clinic and how best to bring capital, morality and knowledge into a productive, and ethical relationship still need to be resolved. Despite these challenges, the next 10 years will be an exciting and yet decisive period for pharmacogenomics. The gains will be achieved in small but significant increments and will favorably influence therapeutics as a science.

8

Clinical Pharmacokinetics

Clinical response to medication in an individual patient is the net result of the interaction of a number of complex processes. These processes can be categorized into two broad areas: those affecting pharmacokinetics or the relationship between the administered dose and the concentrations of the drug in the systemic circulation, and those affecting pharmacodynamics or the relationship between concentrations of the drug in the systemic circulation and the observed pharmacologic response. Absorption, distribution, metabolism, and excretion of a drug determine its pharmacokinetics. Drug–receptor interactions, concentrations of the drug at the receptor, and homeostatic compensatory mechanisms determine a drug's pharmacodynamics. Pharmacokinetics and pharmacodynamics are affected by a number of patient-specific factors including age, sex, ethnicity, genetics, disease processes, and prior and present drug exposure. This chapter focuses on the effects of advanced age on pharmacokinetics.

In clinical decision-making for the elderly patient it is important to recognize that the elderly may also experience an unexpected clinical response to a medication owing to the impact of factors other than their age, such as concurrent diseases and coadministered medications. Despite the fact that much less is known about pharmacodynamic changes in the elderly than changes in pharmacokinetics, the potential for altered pharmacodynamics must also be considered.

Definition of "Elderly"

"*Elderly*" has generally been defined as age 65 yr or older, although many other chronological definitions have been applied. Some researchers have enrolled patients as young as 50 yr old as "elderly" whereas others have studied only those patients in their 80s or older as "elderly." Although a chronological age is most often used to define elderly, it is important to recognize that the elderly are a heterogeneous group, with individuals aging at varying rates. Interindividual variation is much larger in the elderly than in the young. The aging process has been described as a condition of "*incipient disease*" with a variety of deteriorative changes taking place. When decline occurs more obviously in one organ system than another, a disease is diagnosed.

It is therefore difficult to distinguish between normal age-related changes and pathological states. Biological or physiological definitions of elderly have proved difficult to formulate, so chronological definitions of elderly remain the standard. The Food and Drug Administration's "Guideline for Industry Studies in Support of Special Populations: Geriatrics" arbitrarily defines the geriatric population as comprising patients aged 65 yr or older, although the inclusion of older patients is encouraged to the extent possible.

Elderly Patient

Although many older adults age successfully and lead healthy, productive lives well into their later years, the elderly as a group are more likely to suffer from chronic diseases and take more medications than their younger counterparts. The aging process itself is associated with changes in physiology that may alter drug pharmacokinetics and pharmacodynamics. When applying general knowledge of pharmacokinetic alterations in the elderly to the care of an individual patient in the clinical setting, it is necessary to consider the patient's overall condition, "*physiologic age*," disease states, and concurrent medications.

The elderly are especially vulnerable to adverse reactions to medications. The incidence of adverse drug reactions is two to three times that found in younger adults but may be underestimated because of lack of detection and underreporting. Many adverse reactions are preventable. Examples of preventable adverse effects include consequences of known drug–drug interactions or prescribing an inappropriate dosage for the elderly. The increased incidence of adverse reactions in the elderly results from altered pharmacokinetics, altered pharmacodynamics, increased opportunity for drug interactions, and inappropriate prescribing. While the changes in pharmacokinetics and pharmacodynamics are well recognized, age-related differences in dosing often are not noted in compendia such as the *Physician's Desk Reference* (*PDR*) that are used by prescribers. One recent study found many examples of evidence-based recommendations for dose alterations in the elderly that were reported in the literature but were not noted in the product labeling included in the *PDR*. This could explain, in part, the significant increase in adverse events in the elderly. Knowledge of basic pharmacokinetic differences in the elderly associated with age-related changes in physiology can be used to choose appropriate dosing regimens for the elderly and avoid preventable adverse drug reactions.

Pharmacokinetic Studies in the Elderly

Almost all of the information known about age-related changes in humans, including pharmacokinetics, has been obtained from cross-sectional studies. In these studies, the variable under investigation is measured in groups of subjects of different ages at a single point in time. Age differences are then inferred from a comparison of the mean values for each group or from a regression of the variable on age. The cross-sectional approach assumes that average differences between age groups reflect the change that occurs in an individual with the passage of time, which may or may not be valid.

When studying chronological changes in a particular variable, there are three primary time-related factors that must be considered: the effects of age, the effects of an environmental change or historical event at a specified period in time (period effects), and the effects of being part of the group or cohort of individuals born at a particular time (birth cohort). Cross-sectional studies often confound age effects with birth cohort effects. Findings in a group of individuals aged 65 today may differ from those in a group of 65-yr-olds studied 25 yr from now. These groups would be the same age but from different birth cohorts with different group experiences. Cross-sectional studies can also suffer from selective mortality effects, because the oldest study cohorts include only those individuals who survived to reach old age, and these individuals may be unique regarding the variable of interest.

Another approach to studying age-related changes is longitudinal studies. In these studies repeated measurements of a variable are made on the same individual at various points in time. This approach measures individual rates of aging for the specified variable, rather than differences between age groups as in cross-sectional studies. Although the results of longitudinal studies may be a more reliable approach to studying age-related changes, longitudinal studies tend to confound age effects with the effects of an environmental change or historical event at a specified period in time (period effects). These studies are also very difficult to conduct, taking many years to complete. For this reason, pharmacokinetic studies are virtually always cross-sectional in design.

Two general cross-sectional approaches are used to study pharmacokinetics in the elderly. The first is a formal pharmacokinetic study conducted either in healthy geriatric subjects or in elderly patient volunteers with the disease the drug is intended to treat. A relatively small group of subjects is studied using intensive blood sampling in each individual. In this approach, very healthy elderly people are selected for participation in an attempt to ensure that advanced age, and not disease, is the primary factor under investigation. Often these studies include only relatively young geriatric subjects that can meet the stringent inclusion criteria, limiting the generalizability of the results to the very old or frail patient. Results of these studies must be considered along with pharmacokinetic studies in other populations, such as patients with renal impairment, when making therapy decisions for individual patients.

The second cross-sectional approach is the pharmacokinetic screening or population pharmacokinetic study. These studies are typically conducted in conjunction with the main Phase III (or Phase II) clinical trials program. Under steady-state conditions, a small number of samples for drug level determinations are collected and analyzed. When appropriately designed, the influence of demographic and disease factors on pharmacokinetics can be examined in this type of study. Although the data analysis is more difficult, the advantage to this approach is that age and other factors, as well as their interactions, can be evaluated.

General Pharmacokinetic Changes Associated with Aging

Normal aging is associated with changes in human physiology, and many of these changes contribute to altered pharmacokinetics in the elderly. These changes are even more evident in frail or very old patients. Drug absorption and bioavailability, distribution, metabolism, and renal excretion may be altered in geriatric patients. If these changes are not considered when dosing elderly patients, preventable medication-related problems may result.

Absorption and Bioavailability

The bioavailability of a drug is defined as the fraction of drug reaching the systemic circulation after drug administration. Age-related changes in bioavailability depend on the route of drug administration, age-associated changes in the gastrointestinal tract and other organs of drug absorption, and age-associated changes in metabolism during the first pass through the liver or intestine. Despite changes in physiology with age, oral absorption and bioavailability of most drugs appear to remain unchanged in the elderly owing in part to the large functional reserve capacity of the gastrointestinal tract.

Gastric pH, gastrointestinal blood flow, active transport processes, and gastrointestinal motility have been reported to be altered in the elderly to a variable extent. Atrophic changes in the gastric mucosa may result in decreased acid secretion. The resulting increase in gastric pH could affect the ionization and solubility of some drugs. Decreased perfusion of the gastrointestinal tract and diminished active membrane transport processes could result in decreased rate or extent of drug absorption. These effects may be offset, however, by longer gastrointestinal transit times, with decreased gastrointestinal motility resulting in increased contact time for drug absorption. Most drug absorption in the gastrointestinal tract occurs by passive diffusion, and the majority of studies indicate that there are no clinically significant changes in the rate or extent of drug absorption from the gastrointestinal tract.

Intragastric metabolism and hepatic first-pass metabolism may be reduced in the elderly, resulting in increased drug bioavailability. Studies with levodopa, for example, have shown that the elderly experience a threefold increase in availability of levodopa related to a reduction in gastric wall content of dopa decarboxylase. Intestinal metabolism of verapamil, however, was well preserved in the elderly. Drugs that undergo a high rate of first-pass metabolism, such as propranolol, demonstrate increased bioavailability owing to decreased first-pass extraction.

Absorption and bioavailability for nonoral routes of administration (intramuscular, rectal, buccal, transdermal) and sustained release dosage forms have not been as well studied in the elderly. The rate of intramuscular absorption of antibiotics may be reduced in the elderly, but there are insufficient data to draw conclusions regarding the potential for age- related changes in drug absorption and bioavailability by these routes.

Distribution

Age-related changes in body composition and plasma protein binding may affect drug distribution in the elderly. The elderly tend to have decreased lean body mass, increased body fat, and decreased total body water. Interestingly, elderly individuals with high levels of physical activity are not different from those with low activity levels with respect to fat-free mass and fat mass. Lipid-soluble drugs may show an increased volume of distribution and water-soluble drugs may show a decreased volume of distribution in elderly patients related to these changes in body composition. For example, the elderly have an approx 20% lower volume of distribution for ethanol, which distributes in body water, than young individuals. Changes in body composition resulting in changes in volume of distribution may necessitate changes in loading doses of some drugs for the elderly.

Age-related changes in protein binding do not generally result in clinically significant changes in drug therapy for elderly patients. Generally, plasma protein binding of drugs remains unchanged or is decreased in the elderly. Serum albumin concentrations may be decreased in the elderly by 15–20%, but this is often related to renal dysfunction, hepatic disease, or frailty.

Hepatic Metabolism

Hepatic metabolism is one of the major routes of drug clearance in humans. The rate and extent of hepatic drug biotransformation depend on hepatic blood flow and hepatic enzyme content, affinity, and activity rate. Hepatic inactivation of drugs and environmental toxins occurs through phase I oxidative pathways (oxidation, deamination, or hydroxylation) or phase II conjugative pathways (acetylation, glucuronidation, or sulfation). Not all pathways of hepatic drug metabolism are equally efficient. Hepatic biotransformation results in a metabolite, which may be pharmacologically active or inactive, and may be eliminated from the body or further metabolized before elimination.

Interest in potential age-associated changes in drug metabolism is significant because of the need to reduce the risk of adverse drug reactions and drug interactions in the elderly. A number of age-related changes in physiology that may impact hepatic drug metabolism in elderly patients have been reported, but the effect of age on hepatic metabolism remains controversial. Much of the literature in this area has been conflicting. Early studies attributed observed changes in drug clearance in the elderly to changes in hepatic enzyme activity, and more recently to decreased liver size and hepatic blood flow. In vitro tests of enzyme have been inconsistent with results of in vivo studies. Despite these controversies, several generally accepted principles of the affect of aging on hepatic drug metabolism have emerged.

Hepatic blood flow has been shown to decline by approx 40% with age, in parallel with a decline in cardiac output. For drugs with a high hepatic extraction ratio, where clearance depends primarily on the rate of drug presentation to the liver through hepatic blood flow, aging is associated with decreased drug clearance. Phase I oxidative metabolism of some drugs appears to decline with aging, despite the fact that in vitro hepatic enzyme activity does not appear to be altered by age. Reduction in hepatic oxygen diffusion resulting from age-related changes in hepatocyte volume and surface membrane permeability and conformation is one proposed explanation for reduced oxidative drug metabolism observed with aging. Hepatic enzymes can be inhibited and induced by drugs and other compounds. Changes in hepatic enzyme induction with aging remain controversial. Phase II conjugative metabolic pathways appear to be unchanged with aging.

When prescribing for the elderly patient, age-related changes in drug metabolism should be considered. From a pharmacokinetic point of view, drugs that are metabolized exclusively by phase II conjugative mechanisms are preferred in the elderly. For oxidatively metabolized drugs with a high extraction ratio (high clearance drugs), dosages should generally be reduced owing to decreased hepatic blood flow. Dosages for drugs with a low extraction ratio (low clearance drugs) should be reduced as well. After initial dosing, doses can be adjusted based on patient response and tolerability. The potential for significant drug interactions, particularly resulting from hepatic enzyme inhibition in elderly patients on multiple medications, must be carefully considered.

Renal Excretion

Altered renal elimination of drugs is the most clinically important pharmacokinetic difference between elderly and young patients. Renal clearance depends, in part, on renal blood flow, which delivers drugs and metabolites to the kidneys for elimination. Elimination from the kidneys then occurs through glomerular filtration, tubular secretion, and tubular reabsorption. With aging, renal blood flow declines as cardiac output declines, resulting in decreased glomerular filtration rate as measured by creatinine clearance in the elderly. Although there is considerable interindividual variability, declining creatinine clearance with age (about 10% per decade after age 20) is consistently reported in the literature. Changes in the kidneys that occur with aging include a decrease in kidney weight, a thickening of the intrarenal vascular intima, sclerogenous changes of the glomeruli, and fibrosis and infiltration of chronic inflammatory cells in the stroma. Altered tubular function may also be present in advanced age.

The most important aspect of renal function to monitor clinically is the glomerular filtration rate (GFR). Most decisions about drug dosing for renally excreted drugs can be made based on the estimated GFR. Clinically, creatinine clearance is used to estimate GFR. Serum creatinine alone is not a good indicator of renal function in the elderly population because muscle mass, and therefore creatinine production, declines with age. A normal serum creatinine can result when both creatinine formation and elimination are reduced. Several algorithms have been proposed to estimate creatinine clearance. One frequently used method was developed by Cockcroft and Gault, where creatinine clearance (CL_{cr}) is calculated based on the patient's age, weight, and serum creatinine concentration:

$$CL_{cr} = \frac{(140 - \text{age in yr}) \times \text{weight (kg)}}{72 \times \text{serum creatine (mg / 100 mL)}} \qquad \ldots(1)$$

For women, the result is multiplied by 0.85. This formula is less accurate for estimates in the very high or low range and when renal function is changing rapidly. For frail elderly patients with chronic muscle atrophy, an alternative formula has been proposed that takes into account serum albumin levels as well.

For men:

$$CL_{cr} = \frac{\{[19 \times \text{serum albumin (g / dL)}] + 32\} \times \text{body weight (kg)}}{100 \times \text{serum creatine (mg / dL)}} \qquad \ldots(2)$$

For women:

$$CL_{cr} = \frac{\{[13 \times \text{serum albumin (g / dL)}] + 29\} \times \text{body weight (kg)}}{100 \times \text{serum creatine (mg / dL)}} \qquad \ldots(3)$$

This approach provides more accurate and less biased estimates of CL_{cr} than the Cockcroft and Gault method in elderly patients with renal insufficiency or serum albumin levels < 2.8 g/dL.

EFFECTS OF AGE ON THE PHARMACOKINETICS OF CHEMOTHERAPEUTICS

Old age is playing an increasing role in the treatment of cancer, as the prevalence of cancer in elderly patients is high and increasing: 60% of all cancers occur in patients aged 65 yr and above, and the elderly constitute a growing portion of the overall population, with 20% of the population expected to be > 65 yr by the year 2030.

This will lead to an increased use of anticancer agents by elderly patients. In addition to the physiological effects that aging may have on the pharmacokinetic characteristics of these agents, it has to be noted that the likelihood of polypharmacy due to noncancer, age-related chronic illnesses may lead to an increased incidence of drug–drug interactions. Quite a few of these interactions are pharmacokinetically based, for example, inhibition of hepatic metabolism (cytochrome P450-dependent, CYP) by concurrent medications.

Examples

Previous articles have reviewed the primary literature describing the effects of aging on the pharmacokinetic properties of chemotherapeutic agents. Most of these clinical studies were small, cross-sectional trials and assess plasma concentrations of the drug of interest, and in some cases, their active metabolites. A large portion of these studies reports changes in systemic exposure (e.g., peak plasma concentration, area under the curve, and terminal half-life) rather than more meaningful pharmacokinetic parameters such as volume of distribution, specific organ clearances, and oral bioavailability, if appropriate. Therefore, as pointed out earlier, it is sometimes difficult to assess whether physiological aging, concurrent medications or other confounding covariates are responsible for the observed age differences in systemic exposure. In addition, it is sometimes very difficult to interpret the results mechanistically, that is, what pharmacokinetic process is affected by age-related changes.

Based on these general properties, individual drugs whose pharmacokinetics are known to be affected by age, the likely mechanism of that age effect, and the need for dose modification in the elderly. Note that f_e indicates the fraction of the total dose renally eliminated unchanged. The major reason for dose modification in the elderly is the age-related impairment in renal excretory function. Therefore, the dose modifications based on renal function for selected anticancer agents. Overall, it is apparent that age-related renal impairment is the major cause of dose modifications in the elderly, and the (estimated) creatinine clearance serves as a good predictor for a patient-individualized dosing regimen. Apparent age-related effects on hepatic metabolism/biliary excretion have been observed, but usually do not lead to dose adjustments. Age-related effects on absorption are rare since most agents are given intravenously, while age effects on drug distribution are difficult to observe and are unlikely to result in dose modifications. This overall conclusion may change in the future when cancer treatment will involve chemoprevention and disease modification, with the agents given orally and less likely to be renally eliminated. Furthermore, owing to polypharmacy the likelihood of clinically significant drug–drug interactions at the level of drug absorption, first-pass, and systemic metabolism will increase.

9

Clinical Practices

The Good Clinical Practice (GCP) regulations section in the Code of Federal Regulations (CFR) (21 CFR 312) outlines the respective responsibilities of the clinical investigator, the drug sponsor, and the clinical study monitor involved in investigational new product development. These obligations, along with each participant's moral and ethical responsibilities for the safety of subjects who participate in clinical studies, comprise the essence of GCPs. GCPs have long been the norm for the investigator, as written in the 1572 Form; however, the first proposed regulations pertaining to investigator, sponsor, and monitor were first circulated in 1977 and 1978. In 1987, 10 years later, GCPs were published as final regulations in the CFR. Today, investigators, sponsors, and monitors are obligated by law to follow these GCPs. To conduct clinical research that meets the requirements of the FDA for new product approval, it is essential to understand GCP regulations and their subsequent impact on the clinical development process of drugs, devices, and biologics.

The 1987, Investigational New Drug (IND), regulations specified within the current CFR identify (more clearly than in previously proposed GCP guidelines) the delegation of responsibilities in the conduct of clinical trials. Not only do investigators have a key responsibility in assessing patients' efficacy and safety response to new drugs, devices, or biologics, but the sponsor and monitor also have equal responsibility for the patients' safety and welfare. The key players who are obligated under GCP regulations are described below and will be referenced throughout this article:

Investigator. An investigator is the individual who conducts a clinical investigation (i.e., under whose immediate direction the drug is administered or dispensed to the subject). If an investigation involves many physicians at a particular institution, one physician is designated as the Prinicple Investigator (PI) and they are the responsible leader of the team of investigators. The subinvestigator is any other individual member of that team as identified by the PI. These individuals are usually licensed physicians or individuals working under a licensed physician.

Sponsor/Investigator. A sponsor/investigator is an individual who both initiates and conducts an investigation (i.e., under whose immediate direction the investigational drug is administered or dispensed). This category refers mostly to physician investigators who are conducting clinical research under an investigator IND.

Sponsor. A sponsor is an individual or organization that takes responsibility for and initiates a clinical investigation. This may be an individual, pharmaceutical company, governmental agency, academic institution, or a private or other organization.

Monitor. A monitor is the person selected by the sponsor who is qualified by training experience to facilitate and oversee the progress of the investigation.

Investigator Obligations

In 21 CFR 312.53, the regulations deal with the descriptive information provided on form FDA 1572, the Statement of Investigator form. Also included in 21 CFR 312.53 are the selection requirements for clinical investigators. Previously, to conduct studies designated as Phases 1 and 2, investigators were required to complete a Statement of Investigator form FDA 1572; investigators conducting studies designated as phase 3 or phase 4 completed a different Statement of Investigator form, which was known as form FDA 1573. As a result of the IND rewrite regulations, form FDA 1573 is no longer used for any clinical studies. At present, for Phases 1–4, only the Statement of Investigator form FDA 1572 is required. This document states the obligations of investigators conducting clinical research. In addition to the general information on the 1572, new information includes the following: the name and address of any clinical laboratory facility, the address of the Institutional Review Board (IRB) responsible for the review and approval of the protocol, the patient consent form, and the individual investigators participating in the study. This document also states that the sponsor is charged with the responsibility of selecting qualified investigators, who are defined as those who are capable of conducting the study by virtue of their training and experience. By using the phrase "training and experience," the FDA means that clinical investigators conducting a study of a particular disease should have enough experience in that clinical specialty to observe correctly the signs, symptoms, and progress of the disease being treated with a new investigational drug. For example, if a new drug is designed for an Obstetrics/ Gynecology practice, a pediatrician would not be expected to have the expertise to assess this drug, nor would a cardiologist have expertise in evaluating a gastrointestinal drug.

Investigators are defined as those who have signed and completed form FDA 1572 or sub- or coinvestigators listed on that form, who are considered to have the academic and experiential qualifications for participating in the clinical program.

The "fine print" on the reverse side of form FDA 1572 is a written agreement whereby the investigators assure the sponsor that they will conduct the study in accordance with the appropriate study plan (i.e., the protocol) and will observe the GCP tenets. Implicit in this agreement is the fact that the Investigator will have obtained signed Informed Consent (IC) forms from patients or subjects participating in the clinical research under their jurisdiction. Form 1572 also charges the investigator with the reporting of adverse experiences that occur during the investigation and provides assurance that the investigator has read and understood the investigator's brochure. In addition, he or she assures that all individuals participating in the supervision of any clinical study, under the direction of the investigator, are aware of their responsibilities. Once form 1572 has been signed by the investigator, he or she further assures compliance with the requirements of providing study materials, protocols, and other pertinent information to an authorized IRB for review. This information, along with a curriculum vitae, should be provided along with the assurance that the investigational plan set forth in the study protocol will be complied with.

To summarize, the primary responsibilities of investigators in clinical trials are the ethical and moral obligations to all the participating patients and subjects in the study. Investigators must provide a measure of safety for each participant in the study so that the patient is protected ethically and morally from any endangerment that might occur during a trial using an investigational drug. After the investigator's responsibilities are outlined and he or she has signed form FDA 1572, any additional information from the sponsor that might be necessary should be requested and any concerns regarding procedures should be raised. An investigator is responsible for: (1) ensuring that an investigation is conducted according to the signed investigator statement, the investigational plan, and applicable regulations; and (2) for protecting the rights, safety, and welfare of subjects participating in a clinical investigation on any unapproved product. Also, the investigators must maintain complete control and accountability of the experimental products under investigation. An investigator shall obtain the informed consent of each human subject to whom the drug is administered and shall administer the drug only to subjects under the investigator's supervision or under the supervision of a subinvestigator responsible to the investigator. The investigator shall not supply the investigational drug to any person not participating in the clinical program.

The investigators are required to maintain adequate records of the disposition of the experimental medications, including dates, quantity, and use by subjects. If the investigation is terminated, suspended, discontinued, or completed, the investigator shall account for and return the unused supplies to the sponsor, or otherwise provide written documentation for disposition of the unused supplies of the drug. An investigator is required to maintain accurate case histories designed to record all observations and other pertinent data on each individual treated with the investigational drug. (Usually, this is accomplished by completing case report forms and maintaining medical records).

All investigators shall retain records of all subjects enlisted in investigational trials for 2 years after a new drug application (NDA) is approved for the indication for which the drug is being investigated. If no application is to be filed or if the application is not approved for such indication, records must be maintained 2 years after the investigation is discontinued or the IND is closed and the FDA has notified the sponsor of the status of the application. The investigator shall furnish all reports to the sponsor of the drug. The sponsor is responsible for collecting and evaluating the results obtained. The sponsor also is required to submit annual reports to the FDA on the progress of the clinical investigations. Investigators shall promptly report to the sponsor any adverse effect that may reasonably be regarded as caused by, or probably caused by, the investigational drug. If the adverse effect is serious the investigator shall report the adverse effect immediately. An investigator shall provide the sponsor with an adequate report shortly after completion of the investigator's participation in the study.

Other Investigator Responsibilities

The investigator must assure that an IRB complies with the regulations established in the CFR and that the IRB is responsible for the initial and continuing review and approval of the proposed clinical study. The investigator must also assure that he or she will promptly report all changes in the research activity and all unanticipated problems involving risk to human subjects Adverse Reactions (ADRs) or others to the IRB. In addition, the investigator will not make any changes in the research protocol without IRB approval, except where necessary to eliminate apparent immediate hazards to human subjects.

An investigator will on request from any properly authorized officer or employee of the FDA, at reasonable times, permit such officer or employee to have access to, copy, and verify any records or reports made by the investigator. The investigator is not required to divulge subject names, unless the records of particular individuals require a more detailed study of the cases or unless there is reason to believe that the records do not represent actual case studies or do not represent actual results obtained.

Sponsor Obligations

The sponsor's primary responsibility is clearly delineated in 21 CFR 312.50 and ensures that clinical studies are conducted in compliance with FDA regulations. The sponsor is responsible for selecting qualified investigators and for providing them with the information they need to conduct an investigation in accordance with the published regulations. Usually, the sponsor accomplishes this task by supplying the potential investigator with an investigator's brochure and a protocol of the clinical investigation on the agent to be investigated. An investigator's brochure contains all information from non-clinical studies and reports and any previous human efficacy and safety study reports that reflect previous experiences of patients of the investigational agent. Of primary interest in the obligations is the option of a sponsor to transfer total or partial responsibility for the conduct of a clinical study to a Contract Research

Organization (CRO). During the last decade, CROs have played a significant role in new drug development. However, CROs who contract with sponsor companies are obligated under the same GCP regulations as defined in this chapter. A CRO may be the sponsor or the monitor with equal obligations as defined in 21 CFR 312. The current regulations noted in 21 CFR 312.52 are specific and require that any transfer, whether in total or in part, be described in writing and agreed to by both parties. The FDA states that any obligations not specifically described by the sponsor in the written transfer of responsibilities will be considered as not transferred to the CRO; the liability for these undefined responsibilities, therefore, remains with the sponsor. The FDA further requires the CRO (once any transfer of responsibilities has been made by the sponsor) to comply with all applicable regulations and notes that the CRO is subject to the same regulatory actions as a sponsor if a CRO does not satisfy FDA regulations in the fulfillment of its contracted duties. As a result of these regulations, it is possible for a CRO to act on behalf of a sponsor once this legal transfer of obligations has been completed. Although the CRO must assure complete compliance with the responsibilities assigned, it remains the sponsor's responsibility to ensure the quality and integrity of data generated under the supervision of a CRO. In this situation, the sponsor would be expected to act as a quality assurance auditor of the data, even though assignment for the conduct of a study has been delegated to the CRO. It is important to note the following: that any such transfer shall be described in writing; if not all obligations are transferred, the description of the specific obligations being assumed by the CRO must be clearly stated. Any obligation not covered by the written description shall be deemed not to have been transferred. The regulations also charge the sponsor with responsibility for the inventory and control of the drug. Only investigators participating in a clinical trial may receive and have access to investigational drug and materials.

Sponsor and Monitor Obligations

One of the most important responsibilities of the sponsor is to monitor the progress of every clinical investigation conducted under its direction (21 CFR 312.56). A monitor's obligations, under the auspices of the sponsor, are to ensure that the deficiencies created during the conduct of clinical investigations are corrected or justified by the investigator and that the investigator adheres to the investigational plan. The appointed monitors for any clinical investigation conducted under a sponsor's IND have an obligation to assure that an investigator is complying with the signed Form FDA 1572 and the general investigational plan and that the clinical protocol is being followed. If an investigator does not correct his or her errors and mistakes and no improvement is noted in the progress of the study, the monitor shall promptly secure compliance or discontinue shipment of the investigational new drug to the investigator and end the investigator's participation in the clinical program. In addition the monitors, while monitoring the progress of a clinical investigation, must evaluate the evidence relating to safety and effectiveness. At the same time, sponsors shall make such reports to the FDA regarding information relevant to the safety of the drug, as they are required to do under section 312.32 of the FDA regulations.

When a monitor reports an adverse effect to a sponsor during an investigational study, it is the sponsor's obligation to determine whether there is an unreasonable and significant risk to the subject or patient. At that time, the sponsor must determine if the investigational study is to be discontinued. Important among the procedures of reporting adverse effects is the sponsor's obligation to the FDA, the IRB, and to all investigators who, at any time, participate in clinical studies and who are prescribing the experimental drug. Subsequent to this, the sponsor should furnish the FDA with a full report of the sponsor's actions and shall determine whether or not to discontinue the investigation. If the decision to discontinue is made, based on the seriousness of the ADRs reported, the studies should be terminated as soon as possible and no later than 7 days after making the decision.

It is important to understand that the obligations of monitors include the responsibility for assuring that all records and data recorded on case report forms reflect valid data gathered by the investigator and that they coincide with corresponding medical and hospital records of the candidate participating in the investigational study. Detailed auditing and documentation assure the sponsor that the monitor is overseeing the clinical data collected by the investigator and that GCPs are being followed. One misconception of many monitors who audit clinical investigations is that their only task is to assure correct entry of data. In fact, it is of extreme importance among the monitor's obligations to note any adverse effects or any deviations in laboratory values that could signify a safety problem to investigational study subjects. This is especially true in large multiclinic studies, in which many centers are conducting investigational studies following the same protocol and many monitors are auditing data. If any abnormal reactions or laboratory deviations are noted from center to center, the monitors should compare observations and assess an accumulative percentage of occurrence of these deviations. At times, a sporadic, apparently minor deviation can turn out to be a significant deviation when calculated across all centers. If monitors are astute, they can often prevent recurrence of adverse events that might jeopardize the safety of the subjects participating in investigational drug studies.

Another responsibility of the monitor is to assure maintenance of accurate records showing the receipt, shipment, or other disposition of the investigational drug. These records are required to include, as appropriate, the name of the investigator to whom the drug is shipped, the date, the quantity, and the batch number of each shipment. The monitor/sponsor shall also assure the return of all unused supplies of the investigational drug from each investigator whose participation in the investigation is discontinued or terminated. The sponsor may authorize an alternative disposition of unused supplies of the investigational drug, provided this alternative disposition does not expose humans to risks. Although the overall responsibilities are assigned to sponsors, it is the monitors' underlying responsibility for drug accountability.

In turn, the investigators, during experimental research, are also responsible for record retention similar to that of the sponsor. They are required to maintain adequate records of the disposition of the drug, including dates, quantity, and use by the subjects or patients. The investigator is also obligated, if he or she is terminated, suspended, or discontinued or if he or she has completed a study, to return all unused supplies of the drug to the sponsor or otherwise provide documentation of how the unused supplies of the drug were disposed. (It is recommended always to return the unused study medication to the sponsor). An investigator is required to prepare and maintain adequate and accurate case histories (designed to record all observations and other data pertinent to the investigation) on each individual treated with the investigational drug. The monitor should assure that all the previous procedures are adhered to and reported in a timely fashion.

An often-neglected investigator responsibility is the requirement to submit periodic reports to the sponsor. An investigator should be prepared to provide the sponsor with progress reports. These should include an update of the ongoing investigational trial. Annual reports to the FDA on the progress of the clinical investigations are required to be submitted by the sponsor. These reports contain information based on the investigators' progress reports. Safety reports are another issue. An investigator should promptly report to the sponsor any adverse events that may reasonably be regarded as caused by or likely caused by the investigational drug. Alarming adverse events (i.e., severe adverse reactions that jeopardize a patient's safety in any way) must be reported immediately by the investigator to the sponsor. Lastly, when an investigator has completed or terminated an investigational study, a final report shall be provided to the sponsor. This comprehensive report should be submitted to the sponsor shortly after completion of an investigator's participation in the investigation. The report summarizes the final observations of the study and any adverse events that occurred during the course of the clinical investigation. Monitors should also be responsible for encouraging investigators to complete and submit all the reports listed above. Constant follow-up may be necessary by the monitor if these investigator responsibilities are to be fulfilled. In most cases, the clinical monitor usually will provide the investigator with these reports.

Legal repercussions can occur from any neglect of the obligations by investigators, sponsors, or monitors. The CFR stipulates in 21 CFR 312.58 that the FDA can inspect the sponsor's records or reports on request from any properly authorized officer or employee of the FDA. These inspections normally occur at reasonable times and permit the FDA to have access to copy and verify any records and reports relating to a clinical investigation conducted under an IND. On written request by the FDA, the sponsor may be asked to submit the records, reports, or copies of them to the FDA. Under these regulations, the sponsor is also obligated to discontinue shipments of the drug to any investigator who has failed to maintain or make available records or reports of the investigation. Subsequently, an investigator may, on request from any properly authorized officer or employee of the FDA, at reasonable times, permit such an officer or employee to have access to or copy and verify any records or reports made by the investigator. The investigator is not required to divulge subject or patient names unless the records of particular individuals require a more detailed study of the cases.

GCP Non-compliance

What are the consequences if an investigator has repeatedly or deliberately either failed to comply with these GCP requirements or has submitted false information in any report to the sponsor. Initially, the Center for Drug Evaluation and Research (CDER) or the Center for Biologics Evaluation and Research (CBER) will furnish the investigator with written notice of the matter complained of and offer the investigator an opportunity to explain the matter in writing or at the option of the investigator, grant an informal conference. If the explanation offered by the investigator is not accepted by the CDER or the CBER, the investigator will then be given an opportunity for a regulatory hearing. At this hearing, the issue of whether the investigator is entitled to receive investigational drugs will be addressed. After evaluating all available information, including any explanation presented by the investigator, the FDA commissioner determines whether the investigator has repeatedly or deliberately failed to comply with the GCP requirements or has deliberately or repeatedly submitted false information to the sponsor in any required report.

The commissioner will then notify the investigator and the sponsor of any investigation in which the investigator has been named as a participant that the investigator is not entitled to receive investigational drugs. The investigation can not be terminated without reasonable cause as set forth by the commissioner and committee. Sponsor can also suspend shipment of drugs to the investigator for non-compliance to the protocol. If there is reasonable cause for this action, the investigator becomes subject to further investigation for each IND and each approved application submitted to the FDA containing data reported by this investigator. Therefore, every investigational study conducted by this investigator will be examined to determine whether the investigator has submitted unreliable data. Other investigations that are conducted under the same protocol will be temporarily put on hold. Conversely, the commissioner may determine, after eliminating the unreliable data by the investigator, that the remaining data justify continuing other of the same investigations at other sites.

However, if a danger to the public health exists, the commissioner will terminate the IND immediately; the sponsor will be notified and will have an opportunity for a regulatory hearing before the FDA on the question of whether the IND should be reinstated. If the commissioner determines that the data submitted are unreliable and that the data submitted by the investigator cannot be justified, the commissioner will proceed to withdraw approval of the drug product in accordance with the provisions of the Food and Drug Cosmetic Act (FD&C). As a result, an investigator who has been deemed to be ineligible to receive investigational drugs will be blacklisted and unable to participate in any experimental studies. The investigator may be reinstated when the commissioner determines that the investigator has presented adequate assurances that the investigator will use investigational drugs in compliance with FDA regulations. In conclusion, before an investigator accepts the responsibilities to conduct a clinical investigation with an IND drug, he or she must be aware of the legal obligations he or she has agreed to when form FDA 1572 is signed. Investigators must comply with the protocol and the rules, regulations, and guidelines of GCPs. Investigators must realize that they are subject to a federal offense and can jeopardize their reputation and, ultimately, their ability to conduct further clinical research. Investigators must know that the precise collection of data is mandatory in the conduct of clinical research. Research must be designed to assess the efficacy of the product and, above all, to assure that the safety of the patient remains the primary concern.

Sponsors' and monitors' responsibilities in complying with GCPs are also subject to serious repercussions under 21CFR 312.58. FDA inspectors are allowed to examine sponsors' files and the interventions of monitors' site visits to assure that GCP compliance was executed. Case report forms and clinical results are subjected to the same scrutiny that are applied to the investigators' responsibilities. If during an FDA inspection discrepancies are found in any form among the investigator, sponsor, and, when appropriate, the CRO (i.e., its documents), all three parties will be held responsible, and the IND will be placed on hold until the findings are resolved. Investigators', sponsors', and monitors' obligations must be fulfilled by complying with GCP rules and regulations. Sponsors' and monitors' consistent and persistent managing roles are vital in assuring that each person involved in conducting clinical studies meet his or her legal obligations. The success of any clinical program will depend on the cooperation, understanding, and compliance of this triad working together. With this agreement of responsibilities and a well-organized clinical plan, the results can only conclude valid data in support of a new drug application.

10

Laboratory Practices

The Good Laboratory Practice Guidelines (GLP) have been in existence for non-clinical safety studies since 1976. They have progressed through various transitional phases to become guidelines in some countries and regulatory/statutory instruments in others. The current document is the Organisation for Economic Co-operation and Development (OECD) Principles of GLP and is currently accepted as the industry standard. This was reviewed and published in January 1997 but must be used in conjunction with the appropriate Scientific Guidelines for the scientific side of the study, i.e., the OECD Toxicology Guidelines etc. This sets out to cover all non-clinical safety studies and gives guidance as to how these studies should be conducted in conjunction with the appropriate regulatory toxicology guidelines and, on that basis, when encompassed in the various Directives of the European Union (EU) or in other Memorandum of Understanding, allow data generated under this program to be mutually accepted by other OECD countries. One must not forget, however, the other equally important Guidelines and Regulations of other countries, such as those of the U.S. Food and Drug Administration (FDA) and the U.S. Environmental Protection Agency (EPA), and similar organizations in Japan. All have basically similar rules and, being members of the OECD, data generated to the OECD principles will generally be accepted in the United States and Japan. The EPA regulations used to be quite different and were applied to agrochemical and pesticide products. However, having been revised recently, they have been brought in line with the documents of other agencies.

The guidelines themselves, with the exception of those in countries where they are featured as regulations, are, as stated, guidelines to the conduct of the study and aim to cover compliance with the GLP principles but in no way do they dictate how the science will be performed. It must be remembered that compliance is monitored by adherence to GLP, whereas the regulatory authority and the receiving authority of the dossier when submitted for the application of a marketing permit or similar document review the science.

Objective of the Guidelines

The general objective of the guidelines originates in the very early 1970s, when one pharmaceutical company in particular and a contract research organization (CRO) generated data that, when submitted to the FDA, gave them cause for concern in the accuracy of the data presented and, in certain instances, the honesty of the submission. At that time, a full review of companies and institutions conducting non-clinical safety studies (toxicology) was undertaken by the FDA and although, in general, the industry was found to be credible, one company was found to be generating extremely poor-quality data, in many instances, in a fraudulent manner. This, therefore, caused the FDA to put together and implement the GLPs.

Over the next 10 years, many countries introduced similar good-practices guidelines. The EU in general produced its guidelines and eventually, despite the fact that the world was operating according to similar principles, a standard document was produced by the OECD in the early 1980s and became the industry standard. The reason this was of benefit to the whole industry was because this now precluded the fact that every submitting company would have to be inspected by each relevant monitoring authority and, when implemented into several directives and legal statutes within the OECD, this allowed data generated by one company to be accepted by several receiving authorities without further inspection.

The objective of the GLPs is to ensure that a standard approach is undertaken covering traceability and accountability and, while still allowing freedom for the scientists, to impose certain restrictions on the generation of data and the experimental work.

It must be remembered that GLP is merely common sense in a formal environment. The key phrases that are currently seen in a GLP environment include good documentation, good training, maintenance and calibration of all equipment, the archiving and storing of data in a formal and retrievable manner, and the use of high-quality, validated equipment and accredited test systems (animals).

This in general is merely good science, and the GLPs have further enhanced this by the addition of an independent Quality Assurance Unit (QAU) and a study director/principal investigator who jointly controls and oversees the project and involves the management in putting together adequate resources and assuming overall responsibility for the study. This can be seen as good science, with several slight enhancements. The details of these individual subjects are addressed later in this article.

WHO DOES IT AFFECT?

Any company or institution performing non-clinical safety studies for the submission of data for a new chemical entity; a new biological, immunological, pesticide, veterinary or agrochemical product; or, for that matter, a similar product that will eventually appear in the marketplace and be consumed by the general public must adhere to GLP in the conduct of their non-clinical safety study experimentation. Within a company, every person from senior management to the junior technician is bound by these GLPs and must exhibit clear understanding and training in these practices.

To ensure that the practices are followed, a regulatory inspection takes place on a 2 year basis in most countries, and the objective of this is to review, as an independent group, how these good practices are being followed. Certification or a guarantee that the company is operating according to these standards is the benchmark standard. This is also addressed later in this article. As we move into the twenty-first century, it is quite apparent that the industry will shrink as mergers and acquisitions take place, and, with this, the emergence of the now familiar CRO will become ever more popular in the conduct of non-clinical safety studies. It is, therefore, very important that, in this area, the sponsor has the assurance that these facilities are operating not only to the highest standard of science but also in compliance with GLP and that, as a subcontractor, the data they generate will be equally accepted as if the data were generated by the company itself.

WHY HAVE IT?

In general terms, for companies conducting non- clinical safety studies, it is, a regulatory requirement, and without this certificate or certification of compliance, data will generally not be accepted by the receiving/regulatory authorities. However, one should not embark on the process of obtaining or working to GLP with this sole aim in mind. It should be used as an ongoing improving and quality standard for the laboratory.

In fact, it is the author's experience over the past 5 years, that many companies have gone far beyond the requirements of GLP compliance and that the overall concept of good scientific design and good science has been superseded by the desire merely to obtain compliance. It is quite often seen that an extremely poor quality scientific study has been conducted in complete compliance with GLP. It has been seen on several occasions in a laboratory, for example, where the refrigerator has been located far from its permitted limits; where the temperature has been diligently recorded, signed, and dated as required by GLP, but where no attempt has been made to either document the excursions outside the accepted range or to rectify the problem. The operative was merely under the impression that as long as temperature is recorded, this is GLP despite the damage that excursions outside the temperature range may have caused to any investigational product stored in the refrigerator.

Over the years, those scientists who have worked according to the principles of GLP now readily admit without any prompting that they are unsure how they conducted scientific studies before the advent of these good practices. The ability to reconstruct studies, to work to a standard format across several differing laboratories or countries, and to be able to prove beyond reasonable doubt that these were the values obtained and the results submitted. Certainly, data with a GLP compliance statement are being accepted more readily by the receiving authorities, which has led to fewer repeated studies. This, in turn, is helping to achieve the aim of all scientists in reducing the use of animals. From a company's point of view, working according to the principles of GLP shows that it has an attitude that is both ethical and moral to the production of scientific data with products that will eventually enter the human food chain or be of benefit to mankind.

How is It Enforced?

In the OECD countries, for at least 14 years, an Inspectorate has been set up, varying in inspector numbers from several hundred in the United States to one or two in countries not conducting a great deal of scientific non-clinical research. All countries, however, have a regulatory group that, in some instances, also acts as the receiving authority for the review of data, and reports to the GLP Monitoring Authority. This regulatory group visits on a 2-year basis or, in Germany, a 4 year basis, those companies that have claimed compliance and will then be on a rolling program of review.

Unlike its role in many areas of regulatory compliance, it is still the responsibility of the sponsoring company to claim compliance from the Monitoring Authority. This claim is made for a particular company, laboratory, and/or series of tests. From the date of compliance when a letter is written to the Monitoring Authority, data generated from then are assumed by that company to be in compliance with GLP. This claim in then verified in a visit from the regulatory inspector. The inspection may be performed by one or two persons for 1 to 5 days. At the end of the inspection, an exit meeting is held, and the company is usually given an indication of its performance. Noncompliance points are noted in writing and discussed, and a report is then prepared. In view of the findings, three levels of compliance can be obtained:

1. Sufficient deviations have been seen to question the integrity of the data and, therefore, a complete rejection of the claim of compliance is made, with a revisit necessary.
2. Minor points of compliance have been seen that can be handled in a specified period in which case, the laboratory is placed under the category, of pending compliance.
3. Very minor points of compliance have been seen, which, when addressed in writing by the management in a 1 month period with supportive paperwork, etc., lead to the company being given a Statement of Compliance, a Certificate of Compliance, or an indication that the laboratory is in compliance. It depends on the specific country whether a Certificate of Compliance is given. If a certificate is given, it generally states that on the particular day that the inspection took place, the laboratory was found to be in compliance with the OECD Principles of GLP. Also, the address of the facility is given as well as a listing of areas in which compliance has been confirmed. This could be stated as analytical support facilities, acute toxicology, mutagenicity, or similar designations.

Naturally, the benchmark standard is either the OECD Guidelines or similar standards in Japan or the United States. The Inspectorate carries out inspections against these documents. It could be said that often it is merely a review of the procedure and an opinion of compliance given by the inspector versus the interpretation of the individual conducting the experimental work. To try to overcome this criticism and to ensure that all inspectors work according to a standard format, over the past 4 years, the OECD has instituted a series of mutual joint visits (MJVs).

The process of an MJV is that a company is inspected by its local inspector and that the inspector is accompanied by inspectors from two other countries as observers. At the conclusion of the inspection, the company is given their findings by its local inspector and, outside that meeting, a review of the performance of the inspector with positive and negative points is given by the two observing inspectors. To ensure continuity, one of these three inspectors would then be on the next MJV.

In the past, Memorandums of Understanding (MoUs) have been instituted between certain major countries, such as Japan and the UK, the United States and Japan or Canada, etc. However, these have generally fallen into non-use for a variety of reasons, especially in Europe, where it is now, or has been for some time, not possible for a country to negotiate directly with another country. Brussels, however, being the center of the European Community, has to carry out that discussion with a proposed partner in another country. As such, at the time of producing this overview, very few MoUs are currently in force.

What is GLP?

As noted in the Overview, GLP is a series of guidelines that cover the conduct and data production for non-clinical safety studies. The OECD covers a series of activities and personnel. Responsibilities, training, quality assurance (QA), standard operating procedures (SOPs), study plans and study reports, data production and recording, equipment maintenance and calibration, computers and validation, test systems and test substances, and archiving are the primary areas covered by the GLPs. A very brief overview of each of these areas is given hereafter.

Responsibilities

The prime players in a GLP scenario would be the management, the sponsor, the study director, the principal investigator, and the QA. In a hierarchical structure, management would be totally responsible for the conduct of the work and for the assurance that resources have been made available and that an active role is played by these people in overseeing the conduct of scientific research.

The sponsor is the company that places a contract with a CRO or requests from within a company that work in another department be undertaken. The sponsor is the person who is supplying the money and the request for the work.

The study director is the prime player and is ultimately responsible for the production of the study plan, the conduct of the study, and the overseeing or production of the final report. Naturally, a large amount of delegation may take place; however, this must always be in writing, and the overall responsibility for the conduct of the study; the daily contact with the study staff; the prevention of recording of problems and the assurance that the study has been conducted in line with the study plan, the GLP, and the scientific guidelines solely belongs to this individual.

The Principal Investigator is the next in line of responsibility after the Study Director in a multisite study. For example, they could be the person seen in a field study situation where the crop-spraying, for example, may be undertaken at a place remote from the GLP designated site where the study director works. The principal investigator is therefore the person responsible initially for that portion of the work, although under the direct control of the study director. It may also be that, within a company, work is subcontracted to the Analytical Department, for example, for the analysis of formulated material. The person responsible for this particular aspect of the scientific work is the principal investigator, who is involved in the study plan and responsible to the study director. Another typical scenario is work conducted in a CRO under the control of the study director, where samples of plasma are taken for toxicokinetics, for example, and these samples analyzed by the sponsor. The sponsor's analyst, therefore, may well be designated the principal investigator.

Quality assurance

This is an independent group that does not become involved in the conduct of the study but merely reviews the data, experimental work, and documents produced to ensure compliance with the SOPs, the study plans, and GLP. Other activities such as training and assistance in interpreting GLPs, etc., may be the responsibility of the QAU.

Training and recording

It is the responsibility of the management to ensure that training takes place and the responsibility of the Study Director to assure that the individuals conducting the work are adequately trained and have adequate records. At a minimum, there must be a CV, a training record, and a very clear job description. Specifically, with regard to a study director, there must be explicit details of how the study director position can be met and the responsibilities of that individual in carrying out the relevant duties. There should be procedures detailing how the training will take place; recording of the training must be made on a regular basis, the records must be stored in archives and regularly updated, and a complete and historical review of the trainee's activities, previous training, and ability to conduct the work according to GLP must be documented.

Quality Assurance

This function, as has already been stated, is an independent review. The responsibilities here start with a review of the study plan and continue through the review of the study in the in-life phase, data audits, and the final study report audit. In addition to these, systems audits and process audits can be undertaken. The aim of QA is to assure the management that compliance with GLP is maintained throughout the entire study, that the data integrity is maintained, and that compliance with the SOPs and the study plan is adhered to by all experimental study staff. The study audit is a specific audit of the study in direct relation to the study plan. A systems audit, however, rather than proceeding in a vertical line, takes a horizontal line across all studies and would include such tasks as archiving, training, SOPs, general computer validation, animal house operation, and management activities. These are but a few areas that would constitute a systems audit but, hopefully, gives an idea of the type of activities across studies that would be audited.

Process audits, on the other hand, have specifically been addressed in the revised 1997 GLPs, and these are basically aimed at auditing short-term studies of a repetitive nature, generally undertaken by similar teams of people. Here, that the system is working and that parts of the process are reviewed over a quoted period in the QA SOP are assured. The aim is to ensure that all critical aspects of this process are reviewed through different studies over a period of time. This, then, does not necessitate QA review of all short-term studies on every occasion, nor does it require the review of such areas as analytical analysis on a batch-by-batch basis or the analysis of hematology or biochemistry samples each time these come up for analysis.

QA itself is required to produce SOPs that clearly detail operation, method of selection of critical phases, and studies and to report its results to the management.

After every audit, a report is produced that is then discussed with the study director and circulated to the management with the overall agreement from the study director relating to the audit findings and their explanation of the resolution.

Standard Operating Procedures (SOPs)

These generally have been likened to a complete documented history of the entire aspect of conducting non- safety studies. Any activity needs to be described in one of these documents. There may be a compilation of activities, or they may address single items such as the calibration and use of an electronic balançe. They must be produced by the individual most familiar with the task, agreed on by the management, and counter-signed by a person senior to the author.

Once produced, SOPs must be reviewed on a regular basis, (approximately every 2 years) and any changes to these procedures must be made in writing, with the agreement of all parties and circulated to each owner or user of the SOP. The SOP itself must be filed in the archive and additional copies produced. An SOP management system must be set up, whereby a responsible person knows the whereabouts of all SOPs and can retrieve and replace them with amended or superseded revesions and can make sure that they are reviewed regularly and disposed of when no longer required.

The SOP must appear immediately in the area adjacent to the workplace to be readily available to all persons. Frequently, SOPs are the basis of training, and most companies now have SOP-based training schemes. The content and receipt of the SOP should be acknowledged immediately on receipt and a training program set up whereby confirmation of the understanding and the ability to perform the duties stated in the SOP is documented in the appropriate training record.

SOPs should be adequately controlled to prevent unauthorized photocopying, which may lead to the possibilities of a superseded copy not being administered to the known recipients. Someone making an illegal photocopy would not be on the distribution list and, therefore, would not always receive updated versions, with the possibility that an outdated method could be used.

The requirement for archiving historical copies is one of the key attributes of GLP in that traceability can be seen as originating at the archive. The dates and historical record of the SOPs can prove irrevocably that a particular action was the method in use at the time.

SOPs can be paper-based or electronic. The trend toward electronic record-keeping is becoming more common in laboratories. The only requirement made by the inspectorate is that accurate, controlled copies are available on the electronic media and that prevention of copying or unauthorized changing are built into the SOP system.

Study Plans and Reports

Before any study can be undertaken satisfactorily, a study plan must be produced. The study plan is merely an indication of all of the activities that will take place, resources required, time frames, and objectives. The study plan can be likened to a road map that, when given to all the participants, will allow them to start at the beginning and to proceed through the various mazes to the final completion point indicated by the study report. The one golden rule in GLP is one study plan, one study director, and one report. The study report itself is a mirror image of all the headings in the study plan and serves to confirm that the objectives of the study have been met and that the results and discussions of the data presented give an indication of the outcome of the particular experimental work. Both the study plan and the report are audited by QA, and each study plan and report are generally determined by the company's format.

Data

Raw data, or source data, are generally considered the first records made, either electronically in computer-readable form, or records created the first time that the "pen hits the paper."

These should be original signed and dated recordings that may be on any type of media. Cases in which media such as heat-sensitive paper contain the result, should be photocopied in the event of deterioration over a time.

Electronic data can be regarded as the disk, CD-ROM, or similar media provided that this material, when reintroduced to the computer and the software, can generate the images stored on the disk or electronic media in a 100% readable form. There are many types of electronic media, machines, and source data or raw data within the toxicological environment. However, ironically, the most common storage media and the most common raw data are paper. Paper and its storage partner, microfilm, have been around for many years, and their stability and reproducibility are well known. Other electronic media, however, do not have the same capability of reproduction known over a long period, and, thus, most industries and companies prefer paper. In regard to the data they should be recorded promptly, legibly, and signed and dated, and any corrections should be made in a format to allow the original record to be seen, the change described and justified where applicable, and the change signed and dated by the individual making the revision. This procedure, whether on paper or via computer, should have the same standards. With use of the computer, an audit trail is necessary to identify the change and the person making it, along with the reason.

Equipment

As can be imagined, equipment in a toxicological study may be varied, simple, or complex. As such, it is difficult to describe each individual type of equipment in this limited space.

GLP requires that equipment be maintained, calibrated, and generally demonstrated as fit for use.

Equipment such as high-pressure liquid chromatography (HPLC) should have system-suitability checks, installation qualifications, and operational qualifications performed at a minimum.

Other equipment such as centrifuges and balances should be maintained and calibrated and, with regard to the latter, regular checks should be made with known, standardized, regularly calibrated weights. These should be placed on the balance with a frequency to guarantee that data from the machine are accurate. Even if the balance is an electronic calibrating balance, regular manual check weights should be applied.

Each piece of equipment should have a log book that gives a historical record of its use, breakdown, repair, and service. Generally, it is acceptable that these log books be placed by the equipment generating critical data to be presented in the final report.

All equipment should be clearly identified as to the time that it started producing raw data for experimental use and, when no longer required, the equipment should be removed from the laboratory or suitably labeled "not for GLP use."

The calibration and validation of equipment have been addressed extensively but, equipment that can be shown as "fit for use," within the GLP environment is generally acceptable to most regulatory inspectors.

Computers

Over the past few years, computers have played a very important role in many aspects of toxicology. The general trend in the industry and particularly from the Inspectorate is to ensure that they are fully validated.

Validation, however, means different things to different people. Some companies and their Information Technology Group (ITG) will dismantle the computer and its software components, reconfigure them, test them, and then reinstall them. Others will take a more realistic approach and work on the basis that the computer was brought in for a specific task and, is considered validated provided that task is completed with the aid of the computer in a reproducible and acceptable manner.

However, in the most simplistic form, validation could be covered by "evidence that the computer will perform the task for which it was purchased and, more importantly, continue to perform that task for the foreseeable future." In other words, as with other equipment, is the computer fit for purpose?

Several documents have been written from a regulatory standpoint, the most useful being Monograph 10 of the OECD Principles, Application of GLP to Computer Systems. Many books are available and vary in detail and content to cover everything that one would wish to know about computers, but were afraid to ask, down to the simple documentation giving the essentials for validation and providing a disk with the SOPs to comply with GLP!

The prime concern of the Inspectorate is that the user responsible for performing the validation and producing the report is in control of the equipment and can ensure and prove the integrity of the data when entered into the computer and regenerated in some other form.

It is generally accepted in the industry that acceptance testing is perfectly satisfactory for most computers and assures that the computer, when installed on company premises, will perform the function for which it was purchased. However, each computer must be viewed in the role it will play in the company and suitable testing must be conducted to ensure that the data and integrity are of the highest quality and that total control over output is maintained.

As with all equipment, computer maintenance and calibration records are of paramount importance. If in-house software programs are produced, they are tested and validated, and the source code is made available. One of the key elements required in the computer record-keeping is that of change control and password protection and training. One very important rule is that the electronic signatures rule, and it must be observed when data are signed off electronically. This FDA requirement became effective August 20th, 1997, and covers all data for which signatures are made electronically and requires that the FDA is officially notified.

Test Systems

This really is a slightly complex name for what is generally considered the animal subject. Test system, however, has been utilized because in many instances in toxicology, GLP now applies to such subjects as ground water, soil, insects such as earthworms and honey bees, and microorganisms such as daphnia and, therefore, the use of the word animal is not always applicable.

The main criteria are that the origin of the test system is known with its breeding history, where applicable, that these are purchased from well-known and, if possible, accredited suppliers, and that the quarantine period is observed to ensure that test systems are of high quality and fit for use.

Care, husbandry, intermediate sacrifice if the test system is found to be "in extremis," and humane sacrifice before necropsy are essentials for the test system. Separate housing among species and experimentation is critical, and all aspects of manipulation of the animal from clinical observations, dosing, and special tests such as electrocardiogram (ECG) need to be well documented and outlined in SOPs.

Animal husbandry itself, the animal room, and the animal room diary giving an indication of exactly what occurred in the room and to the animal are essential items of documentation. Unique identification is also of paramount importance with the animals, cages, and the location of the cages.

Full and documented history of heating and ventilation are required and, in barrier-maintained rooms, signed and dated records of positive to negative pressures are to be kept. These records should also reference any malfunction and its rectification. Furthermore, excursions outside the permitted range must be documented, and the effect on the study and data integrity must be identified and addressed by the study director in the final report.

Test Substance

In most instances, the test substance can be the new chemical entity (NCE) or an existing product; a comparator, pharmaceutical, veterinary, or agrochemical product; or even a device. Knowledge of the composition, characterization, stability, and other physiochemical properties is essential. Stability, however, may be determined as the short-term studies progress, with the proviso that the overall stability is known, along with full characterization, by the time long-term toxicity studies are carried out. Stability testing may well be carried out in parallel as long as the stability of the active ingredient and formulated product is known sufficiently to allow for control of the dosing to be done within the period of stability known at that time.

One of the key elements of test substance control is accountability. A record of the amount received for toxicity testing should be accurately recorded, and 100% accountability of that product throughout the life of the testing is an essential element of GLP.

Again, formulation of the product is required to be covered in detail, and, in many companies, the elements of GLP are the benchmark standards when dealing with test substance. Use of the test substance in the animal facility, the maintenance of homogenity of suspensions, the mixing of the product in feed, and the testing of the product are all essential. This is one particular area in which within the toxicology testing area, support functions such as analytical studies then come under GLP. These functions will be required to test formulations and feedstuffs, etc. to ensure that the correct amount of the active ingredient is present as determined by the study plan for the various dosing groups. This requires that a validated method be available before any work is carried out, with the ability to analyze samples of the formulated product or plasma samples for toxicokinetics as the study progresses.

It is required that a reserve or retention sample of the active ingredient is retained. This should be retained for as long as it affords reasonable testing and within the expiry period determined by the analytical facility. It is also required that a retention sample be retained for studies that are not considered to be short term. This is one particular area in which revision of the GLPs is sometime not well-thought through. Originally, it had been stated that reserve samples should be taken for studies exceeding 4 weeks. This was subsequently revised to specify "studies that are not considered to be short-term." The glossary in the GLPs defines a short-term study as "a study of short duration with repetitive processes." This, one must admit, does not give a lot of guidance!

Archives

Having addressed all the various aspects of the study, one can see that much documentation, tissues, slides, and wax blocks could well be accumulating. The requirement is to store this material for "a period of time." Again, very little guidance is given in the GLP, and one is referred to the national guidelines for the storage of data. However, it is of great importance that this material is maintained in good condition in a retrievable format for at least 15 years for or 2 years past the availability of "the product," whichever is longer.

Generally, companies themselves are maintaining that material for far longer, or for 2 years past the availability of the product.

All the material must be retained in a secure location for easy access, under the responsibility of a management-designated archivist and deputy. The security aspect of the archive should preclude damage from outside sources, fire, water, rodents, etc. The entire aspect of archiving is basically one of common sense, and guidance on how to archive these materials can be obtained from government agencies that store personnel records or from libraries.

How can compliance be Maintained within a Facility?

Compliance, having been granted after an inspection, should be monitored on a daily basis. However, it is the author's opinion that many companies standards of compliance relax after the initial certificate has been granted only to find that, 2 years later, for example, an enormous rush 1 month before an announced inspection is required to generate the appropriate documentation and to update the system.

It is suggested that QC reviews be carried out on a regular basis to ensure that points likely to detract from the overall compliance are reviewed regularly and that project meetings be held where QA is invited to give a precis of the regular points seen during audits so that these can be addressed and rationalized.

Training and retraining, along with an awareness of the requirement to comply with GLP, are of immense importance. New equipment, major SOP revisions, and transfer of technicians or scientists among departments are always good signs that additional training be carried out. It must be remembered that GLP is team work. It is no good considering that there are the scientists and technicians on the one hand and, QA on the other. There is also no point in considering that whatever happens and however little QC is carried out, QA will discover all the mistakes in the final report and review. Remember, it is not QA's problem; that department's role is to ensure that compliance has been maintained; QC and data-checking are the responsibilities of every member of the staff team.

Improvement targets should be set in line with quality-control manuals used in other accreditation systems. It is always a good point to review internally and on a regular basis: (1) problems that have been encountered in experimentation; (2) audit findings; (3) ways to improve work by looking at new systems and reviewing SOPs to ensure that these are current; and (4) and areas where improvements can be made.

An example can be taken from the accreditation systems, in which, in addition to QA audits, departments become involved in self-inspection. Each department can identify a QA representative whose daily responsibility is to review compliance issues, to look at the overall quality policy of the company, and to ensure that between QA audits, self-inspection is performed and that a departmental review is made of these findings with action points and a time plan identified.

The primary impetus for the maintenance of compliance, however, is the regular external inspection by the Inspectorate. In addition, it is now becoming frequent for independent consultants to be brought in to do pre-regulatory inspections. Whichever way one views the system, whether through consultation or by assigning a department to perform inspections in one area and to conduct audits in another, the regular review of compliance should be maintained.

When using CROs, the whole aspect of auditing takes on a different light. Here, subcontracting is usually performed because of internal pressures, shortage of space, or lack of in-house expertise. Dealing with CROs is no different than setting up an in-house GLP system. The CRO should be regarded as an extension of the facility in which the sponsor is conducting its own research.

Pitfalls and Benefits

In conclusion, it is worthwhile to address the pitfalls and benefits of operating according to the principles of GLP. A pitfall could be seen as a restriction on the scientist against performing free research. It could also be seen as an intrusion by an independent body looking at why problems occur and at the sorts of problems that occur and carrying out regular reviews with senior management about these problems. Costs will increase because of time pressures and the necessity of involving third-party reviews. The recording of data will now be subject to more QC, more required approvals, extra costs, and, generally, more data presented. Time must be taken to write and review SOPs. This in itself can be a very costly exercise; the author knows of one company that, having spent more than 6 months writing its SOPs, classed them as capital pieces of equipment and put a value of $5500 on that volume.

Other companies and personnel may encounter similar pitfalls. The list is not intended to be exhaustive but merely to indicate areas in which additional time, money, and resources will be allocated. However, on the positive side, benefits can be seen immediately.

In talking to many people who have operated under the GLP system for the past 20 years, it is generally heard that the system allows for a better standard of research, less repeated work, the ability to have full accountability and traceability of everything within the experimental phase, and the knowledge that all documentation produced at the end of the study is now safe and secure in the archive and can be readily accessed for regulatory review or inspection.

Fewer studies are being repeated, and, therefore, the immediate benefit is the lowering of subject usage. The fact that data, when generated with a certificate or a compliance statement, will now be accepted by all OECD member countries means that once the study is completed and the regulatory submission made, the time for acceptance several countries (if submissions are made in a multistate procedure) will be reduced dramatically. Finally, it is considered that the initial bureaucratic straitjacket of GLP when thrust on the international research community in 1976 has rapidly turned full circle and now is seen as the quality standard to which all companies in all countries want to aspire. From that point of view, all non-clinical safety studies, when conducted according to the principles of GLP and adequately addressing science as well as compliance, can achieve a very high success rate both in the outcome of the science and in the acceptance of data for a regulatory submission

11

MANUFACTURING PRACTICES

The Current Good Manufacturing Practice (cGMP) regulations for finished pharmaceuticals that have been promulgated by the U.S. Food and Drug Administration (FDA) have been a subject of active discussion since they were first published with the passage of the Kefauver–Harris Drug Amendments in 1962. GMPs were intended to establish minimum manufacturing and control practices for the pharmaceutical industry and focus on what needed to be done rather than how it should be done. Failure to comply with the current Good Manufacturing Practice regulations as set forth in the "Code of Federal Regulations," 21 CFR Parts 210 and 211, constitutes adulteration of a drug that is entered into interstate commerce and is therefore subject to regulatory action. These requirements apply to human and animal drugs. The regulations in Part 210 are introductory in nature; Part 211 contains the more detailed and descriptive regulations.

In the late 1970s, the FDA organized a task force to study the GMPs. Revised GMPs were published in September 1978, and became official in March 1979. At that time, the FDA also considered establishing more specific GMP regulations for products such as small-volume parenterals, medicinal gases and drug substances, to supplement the existing umbrella regulations.

Today, separate GMPs are in effect for biologics and foods but have not yet been promulgated for small-volume parenterals, medicinal gases or drug substances. In attempting to create regulations for specific products, the FDA concluded that it would be better to first issue guidances and guidelines rather than to revise regulations. Thus, what is put forth in 21 CFR Part 211 is supplemented with a number of guidances, guidelines and Compliance Policy Guides. There remain some differences, however, between guidances and guidelines from the Center for Biologics Evaluation and Research (CBER), the Center for Drug Evaluation and Research (CDER), and the Compliance Policy Guides, sometimes leaving a firm's cGMP status subject to the interpretation of a field investigator.

Based on the amount of time needed to promulgate a revision of the regulations, it is understandable that it is preferable to work with guidances, guidelines, and compliance policy guides. Current GMPs are supposed to be, as their title indicates, a description of the current manufacturing and control practices that are acceptable for a pharmaceutical company selling products in the United States. Although these cGMPs are not enforced in some foreign countries, an FDA inspection in a foreign country, based on current GMPs, can be the key to importing and marketing a product in the United States.

The FDA is required to inspect a firm every 2 years for compliance to cGMPs. With the advent of programs such as the new drug preapproval inspection program implemented in 1990, inspections may be more frequent and have expanded into areas not previously investigated regularly by the FDA, such as clinical manufacturing. An unsatisfactory inspection can delay approval of new products and lead to further regulatory action by the FDA, such as seizure and injunction, for existing products. The penalties can apply to the individual or both the firm and individuals.

The GMPs as set forth in 21 CFR Part 211 also have been applied to drug substances and clinical products. Guidelines and guidances have been issued to describe the FDA interpretation of 21 CFR Part 211 pertaining to drug substances and the production of investigational drugs and reinforce the agency's understanding that cGMPs are applicable. The FDA has reinforced the connection between registration of drugs and the manufacture of active pharmaceutical ingredients by the issuance of guides to industry. Recently, the FDA has issued for comment a draft guidance for "Good Manufacturing Practice for the Manufacturing, Processing, and Holding of an Active Pharmaceutical Ingredient." Finalization of these draft cGMP principles is being written into a guideline that is being coordinated through the International Conference on Harmonization of Technical Requirements for the Registration of Pharmaceuticals for Human Use (ICH) toward publication of a guidance for active pharmaceutical ingredients that will be standardized and followed by manufacturers in the United States, Europe, and Japan. As a sidenote, active pharmaceutical ingredients have also been called drug substances and bulk pharmaceutical chemicals. The "Status of Current Good Manufacturing Practice Regulations for Finished Pharmaceuticals" is as follows:

(a) The regulations set forth in this part and in parts 211 through 226 of this chapter contain the minimum current good manufacturing practice for methods to be used in, and the facilities or controls to be used for, the manufacture, processing, packing, or holding of a drug to assure that such drug meets the requirements of the act as to safety, and has the identity and strength and meets the quality and purity characteristics that it purports or is represented to possess.

(b) The failure to comply with any regulation set forth in this part and in parts 211 through 226 of this chapter in the manufacture, processing, packing, or holding of a drug shall render such drug to be adulterated under section 501(a)(2)(B) of the act and such drug, as well as the person who is responsible for the failure to comply, shall be subject to regulatory action.

The "Applicability of Current Good Manufacturing Practice Regulations for Finished Pharmaceuticals" is as follows:

(a) The regulations in this part and in parts 211 through 226 of this chapter as they may pertain to a drug and in parts 600 through 680 of this chapter as they may pertain to a biological product for human use, shall be considered to supplement, not supersede, each other, unless the regulations explicitly provide otherwise. In the event that it is impossible to comply with all applicable regulations in these parts, the regulations specifically applicable to the drug in question shall supersede the more general.

(b) If a person engages in only some operations subject to the regulations in this part and in parts 211 through 226 and parts 600 through 680 of this chapter, and not in others, that person need only comply with those regulations applicable to the operations in which he or she is engaged.

This article reviews Part 211, Current Good Manufacturing Practice for Finished Pharmaceuticals. Title 21, Parts 600 through 680 for biological products, supplement but do not supersede the regulations in this part, unless the regulations explicitly provide otherwise. The focus of Good Manufacturing Practice for all products is on a quality control unit that has the responsibility and authority to approve or reject all components, drug product containers, closures, in- process materials, finished product, and production and control documentation. "Quality Control Unit" refers to any person or organizational element designated by the firm to be responsible for the duties relating to quality control. Specific subparts of Part 211 are summarized and described later. This article is not intended to reproduce the complete GMPs, but certain parts are excerpted for emphasis.

Organization and Personnel

Responsibilities of Quality Control Unit

(a) There shall be a quality control unit that shall have the responsibility and authority to approve or reject all components, drug product containers, closures, in-process materials, packaging material, labeling, and drug products, and the authority to review production records to assure that no errors have occurred or, if errors have occurred, that they have been fully investigated. The quality control unit shall be responsible for approving or rejecting drug products manufactured, processed, packed, or held under contract by another company.

(b) Adequate laboratory facilities for the testing and approval (or rejection) of components, drug product containers, closures, packaging materials, in-process materials, and drug products shall be available to the quality control unit.

(c) The quality control unit shall have the responsibility for approving or rejecting all procedures or specifications impacting on the identity, strength, quality, and purity of the drug product.

(d) The responsibilities and procedures applicable to the quality control unit shall be in writing; such written procedures shall be followed.

The intent of this subpart is to ensure that there is a group within the organization that can review and judge the acceptability of procedures used to produce pharmaceutical products on an independent basis, as well as judging the products themselves, before they are entered into interstate commerce. The FDA has emphasized separation of the quality control unit from production (organizationally). In addition, the FDA considers the organizational level to which the quality control unit reports very important. From a legal perspective, the chief executive officer (CEO) or president of a firm is considered the most responsible official and thereby becomes the most liable. Therefore, he is subject to criminal prosecution should the organization be found to violate the Food, Drug and Cosmetic (FDC) Act. One of the most serious infractions is fraud, that is, the intent to mislead the FDA. Hence, it is incumbent on the CEO to have well-qualified personnel in the organization and an organizational structure that reinforces quality.

Personnel Qualifications

This section emphasizes the training of personnel both in cGMP and in their specific responsibilities with regard to manufacturing, processing, packing or holding of a drug product and functions to provide assurance that the drug product has the safety, identity, strength, quality, and purity that it purports or is represented to possess. This section also requires that there be a sufficient number of qualified personnel.

(a) Each person engaged in the manufacture, processing, packing, or holding of a drug product shall have education, training, and experience, or any combination thereof, to enable that person to perform the assigned functions. Training shall be in the particular operations that the employee performs and in current good manufacturing practice (including the current good manufacturing practice regulations in this chapter and written procedures required by these regulations) as they relate to the employee's functions. Training in current good manufacturing practice shall be conducted by qualified individuals on a continuing basis and with sufficient frequency to assure that employees remain familiar with cGMP requirements applicable to them.

(b) Each person responsible for supervising the manufacture, processing, packing, or holding of a drug product shall have the education, training, and experience, or any combination thereof, to perform assigned functions in such a manner as to provide assurance that the drug product has the safety, identity, strength, quality, and purity that it purports or is represented to possess.

(c) There shall be an adequate number of qualified personnel to perform and supervise the manufacture, processing, packing, or holding of each drug product.

This section makes it clear that the quality control unit is not the only group responsible for the quality of products and conformance with GMP. Because the quality of a product must be "built in," control (at the manufacturing level) of raw materials and process control are important.

Buildings and Facilities

This section requires that the buildings and facilities are adequate, provide specifically defined areas for certain operations and are designed to prevent mix-ups. Included are design and construction features; lighting; ventilation, air filtration, air heating and cooling; plumbing; sewage and refuse disposal; washing and toilet facilities; sanitation; and maintenance. Lighting, ventilation, air filtration, and air heating and cooling must be adequate. Again, the word adequate is used frequently. This is where an individual investigator's and firm's interpretations can differ. This section also requires written procedures associated with sanitation and that the facilities should be maintained in a good state of repair. Although it may seem obvious that maintenance should be performed regularly, it can happen that preventative maintenance programs compete with production requirements for attention; however, an in-depth preventative maintenance program should be in place.

Equipment

This section addresses equipment design, size, and location, as well as construction, cleaning and maintenance. Similar to the requirements for buildings and facilities, it is necessary to provide appropriate equipment for the manufacture of a product and ensure that the equipment material of construction is not reactive, additive, or absorptive. In the 1978 version of the GMPs, requirements for equipment cleaning and use logs, as well as written procedures for equipment cleaning and maintenance were added. These requirements aid in the investigation and solution of problems by identifying batches that may also be implicated in a particular problem.

Control of Components and Drug Product Containers and Closures

This section relates to the receipt, identification, storage, handling, sampling, testing, and approval or rejection of components and drug product containers and closures, and the requirements for written procedures for each. It also covers the use of approved materials, retesting of approved material, and prevention of use of rejected materials. Although the requirements of this section indicate that each lot be appropriately identified as to its status and that materials in different statuses be stored separately, the implementation of computerized warehouses has made it possible to eliminate status labels and physical separation of quarantined and approved materials. Rejected materials are usually handled separately. These practices are not to imply that a computerized system can be used without appropriate assurance of controls. The current GMP requirement that materials must be tested or examined for all specifications and released prior to use is in conflict with the philosophy of vendor certification, which is based on a consistent, reliable record of good quality. Only vendors with well-controlled processes and a good record of acceptable batches qualify for such a program. Thus, a material could be put into use based on the quality record of the supplier (vendor), even if testing is only for identification. This section also requires the use of oldest approved stock first, retesting of approved stock "as appropriate," and controls for drug product containers and closures. It prohibits use of rejected components and drug product containers and closures.

Production and Process Controls

This section focuses again on the need for written procedures and formal authorization by the quality control unit for any deviation from written procedures. Areas covered are addition of components;

calculation of yield; equipment identification; sampling and testing of in-process materials and drug products; time limitations on production; control of microbiological contamination; and reprocessing.

Many drug companies are using electronic means of verifying component names or item codes, receiving and control numbers, weights, or measures, and even the verification of component addition to a batch. There is a range of acceptability on the part of the FDA of electronic means of verification and batch documentation; however, the validation of such systems must be performed to accept electronic means of identification and verification.

The process controls required in this section should be based on process capabilities rather than conforming with a checklist based on the regulations. This would mean that tests not typically used for a particular dosage form may be appropriate, whereas other more commonly used tests may be without any value. This not only depends on the validation of the process but also equipment and process qualification. In addition, the need for microbiological controls can be greatly reduced by knowing whether a product supports microbial growth and whether the environment in the production area is maintained at a sufficiently low bioburden. Clearly, certain products require close attention to the production environment because of the ingredients and the end use.

Many firms use the so-called clean-zone concept, in which the restrictions on personnel entering a production area and the required protective clothing are based on the nature of a product—whether the product is prone to the growth of microbes or whether it is required to be sterile. Even for products not required to be sterile or that are not supportive of microbial growth, this concept controls the production environment through reduction of bioburden.

Reprocessing frequently receives considerable attention from the FDA. Over the years, reprocessing appears to have decreased, not only because of FDA pressures, but also because more products and processes are being validated and better controls are being exercised during production. At times, however, there is the need to reprocess, but it requires authorization of the quality control unit.

For a product covered by a New Drug Application (NDA) or Abbreviated New Drug Application (ANDA), provision for reprocessing must be included in the approved registration document. Although it is not always possible in the filing of an NDA or ANDA to foresee all reasons why a product may need to be reprocessed, a procedure for reprocessing can be evaluated and included in the registration document. If not included in the approved registration document, the regulations require submission of a supplemental application and prior approval in order to market a reprocessed batch.

To some people, batch or lot yield may seem to be more of a business concern rather than a regulatory or technical matter. However, GMPs require that yield tolerances be established and that yields outside of the tolerances be investigated. The need for an investigation is to determine that yields outside of normal limits can be an indication of problems during production that would not be evident with routine testing. A minor deviation may be relatively insignificant and could simply mean that the yield tolerances need to be reevaluated, a procedure that should be followed periodically.

It may seem that the identification of equipment in the processing record is also a superfluous burden. If several pieces of equipment have been shown to be used interchangeably, one might question the reason for this additional documentation; however, when a problem arises, it is necessary to know exactly which equipment was used. It may be possible to trace this back by reviewing equipment cleaning and use logs, but the investigation is simplified by having this information in the batch record. Recording variable batch information concerning the equipment, such as tablet compressing speeds, is also necessary.

Packaging and Labeling Controls

This subpart covers one of the aspects of pharmaceutical production that has received much attention because of recalls, including an increase in recalls related to labeling errors or product mix-ups associated with the packaging and labeling operation. Specific requirements identified in this section recently include the following.

Materials Examination and Usage Criteria

1. Use of gang-printed labeling for different drug products, or different strengths or net contents of the same drug product, is prohibited unless the labeling from gang-printed sheets is adequately differentiated by size, shape, or color.
2. If cut labeling is used, packaging, and labeling operations shall include one of the following special control procedures:
   (a) Dedication of labeling and packaging lines to each different strength of each different drug product;
   (b) Use of appropriate electronic or electromechanical equipment to conduct a 100% examination for correct labeling during or after completion of finishing operations; or
   (c) Use of visual inspection to conduct a 100% examination for correct labeling during or after completion of finishing operations for hand- applied labeling. Such examination shall be performed by one person and independently verified by a second person.
4. Printing devices on, or associated with, manufacturing lines used to imprint labeling upon the drug product unit label or case shall be monitored to assure that all imprinting conforms to the print specified in the batch production record.

Labeling Issuance

Procedures shall be utilized to reconcile the quantities of labeling issued, used and returned, and shall require evaluation of discrepancies found between the quantity of drug product finished and the quantity of labeling issued when such discrepancies are outside narrow preset limits based on historical operating data.

Packaging and Labeling Operations

Identification and handling of filled drug product containers that are set aside and held in unlabeled condition for future labeling operations to preclude mislabeling of individual containers, lots, or portions of lots. Identification need not be applied to each individual container but shall be sufficient to determine name, strength, quantity of contents, and lot or control number of each container.

These requirements reflect an increased use of electronic means to ensure correct labeling and tight controls on the practice of filling containers that will be labeled at a later date. A time-consuming operation required in the current GMPs is associated with the reconciliation of labels. The recalls and associated investigations demonstrate that unless 100% accountability can be achieved in the reconciliation process, there will not be an effective means of ensuring correct labeling. Section 211.132 was revised on February 2, 1989, to describe tamper-resistant packaging and labeling requirements for over-the-counter (OTC) human drug products. Compliance Policy Guide 7132a. 17 was issued in 1992 to describe the standardized tamper-resistant packaging requirements. This section also covers information concerning requests for packaging and labeling exemptions. It allows changes in packaging and labeling to comply with the requirements for OTC products subject to approved NDAs to be implemented prior to FDA approval as provided for in Section 314.70(c). Manufacturing changes to provide for sealed capsules require prior FDA approval under Section 314.70(b). Section 211.132 states that none of the requirements for "*special packaging*" (child-resistant packaging), as defined in Section 310.3[1] and required under the Poison Prevention Packaging Act of 1970, are affected. Subpart G also covers drug product inspection and expiration dating. The expiration date that is required in Section 211.137 relates to stability studies performed on the drug product described in 21 CFR 211.166. It requires that expiration dates be related to storage conditions stated on the product labeling.

Furthermore, the programs established are to use stability-indicating methods, under controlled conditions, in the marketed container–closure system and on an adequate number of batches to determine the appropriate expiration date. The FDA has issued guidelines on stability testing which outline in more detail the requirement to establish a stability program to determine and support the expiration date of a product. A new draft guidance for stability testing was published by the FDA in 1998, and discussions with comments to finalize this guidance are still continuing.

Holding and Distribution

This section covers warehousing and distribution and the procedures required for the quarantine of drug products before release by the quality control unit, storage of drug products under appropriate conditions, procedures to ensure use of the oldest approved stock first, and a system for documenting the distribution of each lot of drug product. This is another area where computerized systems are being used extensively. During inspections, the FDA review includes evaluation of the validation of any computerized systems and controls.

Laboratory Controls

This entire section refers to the requirements covering the testing of drug products and their components prior to release for distribution. It also covers stability testing and special testing, including testing for penicillin, if a reasonable possibility exists that a non- penicillin drug product has been exposed to cross- contamination with penicillin and laboratory animals. Additional information can be found in the Good Laboratory Practices, 21 CFR 58. Reserve samples arc required to be maintained for active ingredients and drug products. These specific requirements are elucidated in 211.170. The section on reserve samples also requires that a visual inspection of reserve samples of drug products be conducted at least once a year for evidence of deterioration. Fundamental to the testing requirements is the need for validated methods with established and documented accuracy, sensitivity, specificity, and reproducibility. It is also necessary to have meaningful sampling and testing plans that meet statistical quality control criteria. Judgments made with regard to sampling procedures should be based on the quality of the process control or the reliability of the vendor who supplies a raw material, drug substance, or packaging component.

Records and Reports

This section details the records and reports required to be maintained for pharmaceutical drug products, their components, and the equipment used in the processing of a drug product. Through these records, the entire history of a batch can be traced. The records cover equipment cleaning and use logs; component, container, closure, and labeling records; master production and control records and production record review; laboratory records; distribution records; and complaint files. Because this amount of recordkeeping can be voluminous, Section 211.180(d) allows for microfilm, microfiche, or other accurate reproductions of the original records for storage. Many firms are using the electronic generation of batch and analytical records. It is important to be able to retrieve all of the above records easily during an FDA inspection. Electronic methods must be supplemented with proper procedures to ensure that the records do not deteriorate over a period of time and can be retrieved when the computer systems used to generate the records have been revised or replaced.

This section also requires a master production and control record for each product, from which the batch production and control records are generated. These records must include complete instructions concerning the manufacture of a batch and precautions to be followed. Prior to the commercial distribution of a drug product into interstate commerce, all executed production and control records must be reviewed. If there is a discrepancy or a failure of any batch or any of its components to meet specifications, there must be an investigation and a written report of the findings. The investigation are to extend to other batches of the same or other drug products that may have been associated with the out of specification batch or discrepancy. Another part of this section covers complaint files, which are reviewed regularly during FDA inspections. In fact, a complaint file review may be the sole reason for an inspection if the FDA receives a complaint directly from a pharmacist, which may be a cause for concern. Sometimes the FDA will visit a firm to follow up on a complaint, even though the firm may not have been informed by the complainant. In the event that a complaint is received by a firm, it should be evaluated and a response sent to the complainant. It may be necessary also to conduct an investigation and prompt further action regarding the product or batch in the marketplace.

Returned and Salvaged Drug Products

This section requires that extensive records be maintained on returned drug products including ultimate disposition. Again, if the reason that a drug product is returned implicates other batches, an investigation is to be conducted in accordance with 211.192. Drug product salvaging is not allowed for drug products that have been subjected to improper storage conditions. If there is a question as to whether drug products have been subjected to such conditions, they may be salvaged only if there is evidence from laboratory tests that all applicable standards of identity, strength, quality, and purity have been met. In addition, evidence is required from the inspection of the premises that the drug products and associated packaging were not subjected to improper storage conditions as a result of a disaster or accident. Understandably, the value of the material to be salvaged is taken into consideration when such rigorous requirements exist for salvaging. Compliance with GMP requires that responsible employees in a firm be knowledgeable about the practices that other firms follow in order to comply. FDA investigators visit many firms and find a broad picture of current manufacturing and control practices. Thus, Current Good Manufacturing Practices are "state of the art," constantly changing. To be in regulatory compliance, a firm must review their procedures and systems regularly and revise them as necessary.

12

Drug Interactions

The setting of chemotherapy for cancer is rife with potential for significant drug interactions and this topic has been the subject of several excellent reviews. Most patients receive multidrug combinations for their malignancy. Also, many of these patients are treated with intercurrent medication for co-morbidity or for cancer-related disorders (coagulopathy, infection, pain, seizures, etc.). The clinical significance of these potential drug interactions is also all the more relevant in cancer chemotherapy because the cytotoxic agents traditionally used do not have clear therapeutic windows. That is, the doses selected produce toxicity in a significant proportion of patients without necessarily providing benefit. Drug interactions causing an increased exposure of the patient to the cytotoxic agent may produce more severe side effects, whereas those causing a decreased exposure may jeopardize tumor control. Unfortunately, both the good and bad effects of chemotherapy are unpredictable, and the influence of drug interactions in either eventuality is almost impossible to detect in individual patients. These, however, may be borne out in large-scale studies, or when combined with pharmacokinetic data. Therefore, most drug interactions in cancer chemotherapy may go undetected unless some *a priori* knowledge alerts the clinician or oncology pharmacist to their likelihood.

When we think of drug–drug interactions, we usually think about classical interactions with the cytochrome P450 enzymes, as these have been well recognized and characterized over the last few decades. Certainly, this mechanism remains at the forefront of clinically significant drug–drug interactions. However, the pathways involved in the classical ADME of drug disposition (absorption, distribution, metabolism, and elimination) are all candidates for drug interactions. In particular, our understanding of transporters and their role in the systemic disposition of anticancer drugs has evolved exponentially over the last few years. They are now recognized as a major locus of drug–drug interaction. Also, the routes of metabolism of importance for the elimination of anticancer drugs are almost as diverse as their mechanisms of action, and some unexpected drug interactions have arisen as a result.

The aim of this chapter is to review some of the potential mechanisms of drug–drug interactions and to illustrate these with published data. The focus here is to examine the possible loci of drug interactions that should be considered in the setting of drug development rather than an exhaustive listing of all the known interactions. In addition, the possibility of exploiting drug–drug interactions to improve cancer chemotherapy is raised.

Loci for Drug Interactions: Process by Process

As mentioned briefly in the previous section, any of the traditional processes implicated in drug pharmacokinetics (i.e., ADME) is a potential locus for drug–drug interactions.

Drug Absorption

Drug interactions can occur at the site of absorption by a multitude of mechanisms. Although oral chemotherapy has traditionally been limited in the past, many of the newer agents are being developed with the possibility of oral administration. Part of this challenge has arisen following demonstration that some of the newer "targeted" therapies are likely to require protracted exposure to ensure maximal benefit. Repeated intravenous administration in this context is impractical and there has been a push toward orally bioavailable drugs.

Gastric transit time and environment

For oral drugs, interactions leading to significant pharmacokinetic changes may arise as a result of changes in the gastric emptying time. Food is the most widely accepted factor for increasing gastric transit time, but a number of drug-related factors may have similarly important roles. Drugs may affect directly the rate of gastric emptying with most slowing this process, although some, such as metoclopramide, actually speed it up. Many cancer drugs produce transient nausea and vomiting. Nausea produces a slowing down of gastric emptying and may influence the rate and extent of absorption of oral chemotherapy. Many of the anticancer drugs given orally to date display wide variability in their absorption (e.g., mercaptopurine), which would possibly mask these subtle effects. Small-intestinal transit time is also likely to be an important factor). Certainly, the advent of rationally developed oral chemotherapy may, in the future, require specific consideration of these factors.

Drug interactions during absorption may also follow from alterations in the gastrointestinal environment. For example, the camptothecins are unstable at physiological pH and drugs affecting intragastric pH could be of concern for the administration of these agents by the oral route. This was the basis for a study of oral topotecan with and without ranitidine. Conversely, temozolomide is unstable at low pH and ranitidine was examined for an effect on drug absorption. In neither case was there any significant effect. In some cases, the instability of drugs at acidic pH has led to the direct incorporation of inhibitors of gastric acid production into oral bioavailability studies. Antacids may also be worthy of investigation from this point of view. Other nonspecific interactions that may modulate drug absorption can arise from the coadministration of binding drugs such as cholestyramine. Some parenteral formulations have surfactants to solubilize hydrophobic drugs in aqueous solutions. Although it is attractive to use intravenous formulations to investigate the oral route of administration of these drugs by simply administering these, the nonspecific effects of these agents may significantly modify the absorption of the compound of interest. In the case of paclitaxel, coadministration with its intravenous formulation surfactant, Cremophor EL, was shown to decrease greatly paclitaxel bioavailability whereas polysorbate 80 (Tween 80) had the opposite effect.

Drug metabolism

During their absorption from the gastrointestinal tract, drugs run the gauntlet of gut mucosal and hepatic drug metabolism, the so-called "first-pass effect." As reviewed else where in this book, a multitude of pathways are implicated in the metabolism of anticancer drugs. One of the first drug interactions observed in oncology was that which occurs between 6-mercaptopurine and allopurinol. An important metabolic pathway for the catabolism of 6-mercaptopurine is mediated by xanthine oxidase, which is inhibited by allopurinol. In the study by Zimm et al., administration of allopurinol increased peak concentrations and the area under the concentration–time curve (AUC) of 6-mercaptopurine by fivefold, but only when 6-mercapoturine was administered orally. Methotrexate is another, albeit weaker, known inhibitor of xanthine oxidase.

Inhibition of gut wall and hepatic metabolism may well be a requisite for appreciable absorption of some drugs from oral formulations. For example, the bioavailability of oral 5-fluorouracil (5-FU), which is of the order of 20–30 %, is limited by intestinal and hepatic dihydropyrimidine dehydrogenase (DPD), the major catabolic pathway for 5-FU. Novel oral formulations of fluoropyrimides often contain a DPD inhibitor to minimize this loss of drug to improve bioavailability. In the case of UFT, uracil is added in a 4:1 molar ratio as a competitive inhibitor of DPD with the 5-FU prodrug tegafur. With the DPD inhibitor ethyniluracil, the bioavailability of orally administered 5-FU approaches 100%. These are examples of how drug interactions can be exploited to improve the pharmacokinetic properties of important drugs. Another major class of drug metabolizing enzymes present in the mucosa and liver is the cytochrome P450 (CYP450) superfamily. In general, drug–drug interactions occurring at the CYP450 locus have been documented mostly in the context of parenterally administered cytotoxic drugs and these are discussed later.

Drug transport

There has been a revolution in the pharmacology of drug interactions following the demonstration that several of the ABC transporters, including P-glycoprotein, line the gastrointestinal lumen. Aside from the context of multidrug resistance, there has been the realization that these transporters, in facilitating basal to apical fluxes of drugs, are able to reduce greatly drug absorption following oral administration. This mechanism is now being extensively manipulated in the experimental setting to try and achieve oral chemotherapy of drugs previously considered too poorly absorbed. The taxanes are avid substrates of P-glycoprotein and particularly suitable for testing the concept of modulation of this transporter on drug bioavailability. Cyclosporin A and its nonimmunosuppressive analog PSC833 were some of the first blockers of P-glycoprotein to be tested for this modulation, demonstrating impressive improvements in paclitaxel bioavailability in mice. Results in clinical trials of 60 mg/m^2 of oral paclitaxel combined with 15 mg/kg of oral cyclosporin also showed large increases in oral bioavailability of paclitaxel. The bioavailability of the combination was approx 30%, which may, however, have been under-estimated because of the nonlinearity of paclitaxel kinetics. Nevertheless, targeting relevant concentrations (i.e., those achieved by intravenous administration) may prove difficult although possible. Other P-glycoprotein modulators (e.g., GF120918) are being investigated in this setting.

In the same vein, topotecan is a substrate of both P-glycoprotein and the half-transporter breast-cancer-related protein (BCRP) and both these transporters are expressed in the gut mucosa. The P-glycoprotein modulator GF120918 is also a potent modulator of BCRP and caused a further increase in topotecan bioavailability in the mouse as a result of blocking this second transporter.

Drug Distribution

Transporters

Aside from controlling the transfer of drugs across the gastrointestinal mucosa, the same transporters also control the distribution of drugs into other compartments (e.g., central nervous system, placenta). Inhibition or induction of transporters may therefore have an impact on the distribution of anticancer drugs. An effect of drug distribution would be detectable either from an effect on the volume of distribution of the drug or its pharmacokinetics in a specific compartment (e.g., central nervous system [CNS], cerebrospinal fluid [CSF], etc.). In a study of PSC833, Advani et al. examined the effects of this P-glycoprotein blocker (5 mg/kg po four times per day for 3 d) on a regimen of doxorubicin and paclitaxel. Importantly, this was a crossover study and, although the sequences were not randomized, this design enabled the effect of PSC833 to be observed in each individual. The presence of PSC833 led to a doubling of the terminal half-lives of both doxorubicin and paclitaxel. In the case of paclitaxel, the effect was due primarily to a trebling of the volume of distribution, indicating a substantial interaction with the distribution of this drug. In contrast, in the case of doxorubicin, the effect was attributable mostly to changes in total clearance. Specific compartments may well be targeted by such drug interactions. Indeed, there is the exciting possibility of improving drug distribution into the CNS by coadministration of blockers of P-glycoprotein and other transporters located at the blood–brain barrier. Importantly, however, an increase in CNS toxicity may be a down side to such strategies. Also, issues in relation to the concentrations required need clarification. There are conflicting data in animal models on the potential of cyclosporin A to modulate brain uptake of drugs and this may reflect subtle differences in the probe drugs and their schedules of administration. However, this is a clear area of concern for potential drug–drug interactions.

Protein binding

In theory, the competition by two drugs for a plasma binding protein can lead to an increase in the free concentration of the displaced drug. This, however, depends largely on the physicochemical and pharmacokinetic properties of the drug in question. In most cases, the displaced drug distributes rapidly into tissue compartments and/or is eliminated more rapidly with no net effect on free plasma concentrations. If the tissue compartment contains the tumor or organs of toxicity, then there may be a clinical effect of this displacement. These are, however, relatively rare but may need to be considered for drugs with very high plasma binding and small volumes of distribution. Cyclosporin A has been reported as being able to cause an increase in the unbound fraction of teniposide and increase the myelosuppressant effect of the latter. In such cases, however, it is difficult to discern whether the effect is exclusively pharmacokinetic. Methotrexate is a drug suspected of being the subject of many drug–drug interactions, some of which may possibly be mediated in part through protein-binding alterations. However, the data on this mechanism are relatively sparse, although a significant effect was shown with trimethoprim–sulfamethoxazole in pediatric leukemia patients with the free fraction of methotrexate rising from 37% to 52 % in the presence of the antibiotic. The significance of this modest change is not evident. Other compounds can produce similar effects and these include the salicylates, other nonsteroidal anitiinflammatory drugs (NSAIDs), sulfonamides, phenytoin, tetracycline, chloramphenicol, and *p*-aminobenzoic acid (PABA).

Direct interactions

Thiol protective agents (e.g., amifostine) provide nucleophiles able to react directly with platinum drugs. This could potentially alter the distribution and activity of these drugs. However, studies looking at possible pharmacokinetic interactions have so far not revealed clinically significant interactions with either cisplatin or carboplatin or other drugs for that matter.

Nonspecific effects

Several of the formulation vehicles are membrane-active compounds that may modify drug solubility and disposition. This was discussed briefly earlier in relation to the oral absorption of drugs. Similar effects may be relevant with regard to peripheral distribution of drugs. In fact some of these can be significant and the cause of apparent drug–drug interactions.

Drug Metabolism

Arguably, the most clinically significant drug–drug interactions in medical oncology are caused by interference at this locus. Several specific and nonspecific mechanisms are possible. Although it is beyond the scope of this chapter to explore all the possible enzymatic interactions, it is worth differentiating between some of the major mechanisms.

Competitive inhibition

Competitive inhibition is the dominant mechanism when two drugs compete for the same metabolic enzyme and a reduction of the metabolism of one occurs due to competitive displacement by the other.

Erythromycin and cyclosporin A, for example, are competitive inhibitors of cytochrome P450 3A. A feature of many substrate inhibitors of CYP3A, however, is their ability to form a reversible nitrosoalkane intermediate, which forms a tight complex with the CYP3A heme. Although reversible in theory, this complex is almost impossible to dissociate under physiological conditions. This is true for many of the compounds that undergo *N*-dealkylation reactions such as the macrolide antibiotics (erythromycin, troleandomycin, clarithromycin), some local anesthetics (e.g., lidocaine), diltiazem, fluoxetine, and tamoxifen. The complex typically requires significant preincubation with NADPH and enzyme to form and so may not be detected on a casual screen, in which preincubations with drug are the exception rather than the norm. As a result, the screen may detect only the immediate competitive component and greatly underestimate the possible interaction in vivo. Indeed, this form of complex may explain why some drug interactions with drugs such as erythromycin are much more extensive than predicted from inhibition constants estimated from competitive inhibition experiments. Long-term treatment with such drugs depletes the affected CYP until an equilibrium of CYP synthesis and deactivation occurs. The most potent inhibitors of CYP3A activity are the azole antifungals and some of the HIV protease inhibitors (ritonavir, indinavir, etc.). Although the latter may be problematic in the setting of HIV-related malignancy, interactions with azole antifungals are much more likely in the routine setting where they are sometimes used in antifungal prophylaxis. This may lead to severe, occasionally fatal interactions. The clearance of cyclophosphamide in children receiving fluconazole is reduced by almost 50% relative to controls, and in vitro experiments were in support of a role of decreased CYP metabolism in this interaction.

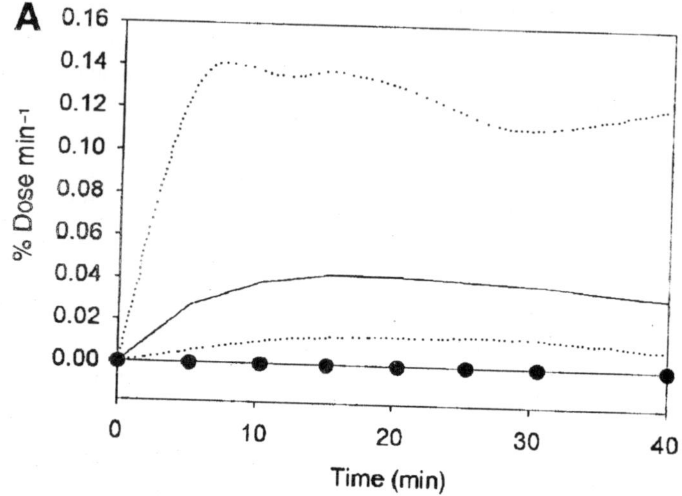

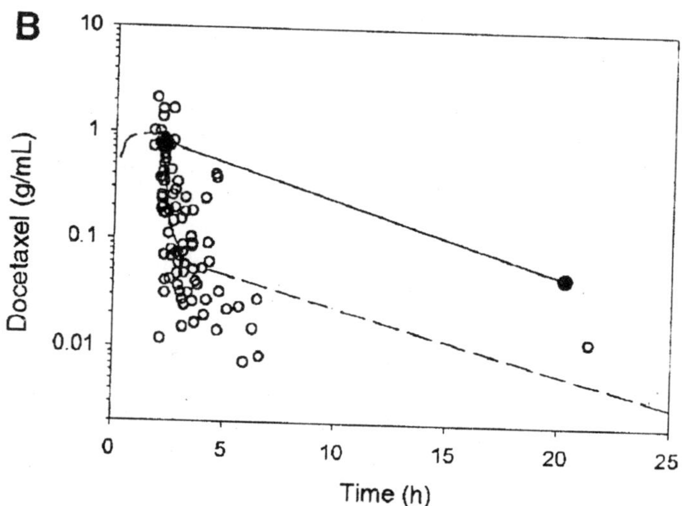

Fig. 12.1. A–The results of the [^{14}C]erythomycin breath test performed on 54 cancer patients prior to treatment with single-agent docetaxel. B–Sparse docetaxel plasma concentration data for the same individuals as in (A)

The azole antifungals are also inhibitors of CYP2C8, albeit at higher concentrations. Paclitaxel is metabolized more avidly by this isoform and an interaction with high-dose ketoconazole was thought possible on the basis of in vitro studies. However, acute administration of ketoconazole after paclitaxel or 200 mg orally 3 h prior to paclitaxel had no pharmacokinetic consequences. Whether this implies safety of paclitaxel with steady-state ketoconazole administration cannot necessarily be implied.

Other drugs metabolized by CYP3A include topotecan, irinotecan, paclitaxel, and docetaxel. With irinotecan, the importance of this pathway was recently made clear in a study of ketoconazole pretreatment. Administration of 200 mg of ketoconazole 1 h prior to and 23 h after the infusion of irinotecan did not impact on the clearance of irinotecan. However, it significantly shifted the metabolic profile away from CYP3A deactivation toward carboxylesterase-mediated activation. The apparent metabolic ratio for CYP3A was decreased approx 10-fold. Therefore, this interaction could provide a significant safety risk to patients receiving this combination.

Ketoconazole and the other azole antifungals are also inhibitors of P-glycoprotein (but possibly not substrates) and Kehrer et al. considered this as a potential factor in the drug interaction with irinotecan. Drug–drug interactions with azole antifungals may therefore be mediated at least partially through modulation of P-glycoprotein transport. For example, as mentioned previously, vinblastine does not readily penetrate into the CNS largely because of P-glycoprotein function, and mdr1a/1b knockout mice are at greater risk of neurotoxicity following administration of this agent. The clinical interaction between itraconazole and vincristine therefore may be due to modulation of CNS distribution of vincristine by P-glycoprotein. Fluconazole, in contrast, is a poor inhibitor of P-glycoprotein and given that doxorubicin is not appreciably metabolized by CYP450, a clinical interaction would not be predicted. This appears to be the case, at least in nonhuman primates.

Conversely, many of the investigated inhibitors of P-glycoprotein are inhibitors of CYP3A4, and this may contribute to drug–drug interactions. This includes some of the later generation inhibitors such as PSC833. The metabolism of thiotepa, which is at least partially mediated by CYP enzymes, has been shown to interfere with that of cyclophosphamide. Significant reductions in the *C*max and AUC of the active 4-hydroxycyclophosphamide metabolite were observed when thiotepa was administered 1 h prior to cyclophosphamide. Recently, it has been demonstrated that thiotepa is a potent, selective inhibitor of CYP 2B6, one of the key pathways in oxazaphosphorine metabolism. One of the issues with investigating drug–drug interactions involving the oxazaphosphorines is the fact that their metabolism is extremely complex, with some pathways responsible for both activation and deactivation reactions. Carmustine, which inhibits human aldehyde dehydrogenase 1, causes a reduction in the deactivation of the aldocyclophosphamide intermediate.

Suicide inhibition

Occasionally, the inhibiting drug is transformed into a highly reactive species by the action of the enzyme, and the two react to form a covalent complex. This type of inhibition is potentially more significant than competitive inhibition because the extent and duration of enzyme inactivation can both be extensive. In Japan, an interaction between an antiviral nucleoside, sorivudine, and 5-FU was suspected as being responsible for a series of 18 deaths. An investigation into the metabolism of sorivudine found that the drug was hydrolyzed into 5-(2-bromovinyl)uracil by intestinal bacteria. The latter is a potent suicide inhibitor of DPD, the major catabolic pathway of 5-FU. Blockage of DPD effectively transforms these patients to a DPD-deficient phenotype with possible lethal consequences. Ironically, 5-(2-bromovinyl)uracil was a well-recognized inhibitor of DPD and had previously been shown to be of benefit when combined with reduced doses of 5-FU in animal models. Indeed, tumoral overexpression of DPD is a recognized mechanism of resistance to fluoropyrimidines, and other suicide inhibitors of DPD have been developed clinically to reduce both the systemic and intratumoural metabolism of 5-FU.

Although suicide inhibition is an attractive mechanism to exploit in cancer chemotherapy (e.g., exemestane and aromatase), the situation with sorivudine exemplifies that drugs that produce suicide inhibition of key catabolic enzymes can have serious consequences unless they are administered for the specific purpose. Preclinical screening of compounds for their potential to inhibit DPD has become commonplace. Several 17α-ethinyl-substituted steroids such as gestodene and ethinylestradiol are suicide inhibitors of CYP3A and this would suggest potentially multiple drug–drug interactions. However, clinical studies looking for such effects with, for example, ethinylestradiol, have not been in support of a major effect under therapeutically relevant conditions.

Enzyme alkylation

Alkylating agents have the potential to interact with most cellular and extracellular macromolecules including enzymes and transporters. For example, the active product of cyclophosphamide, 4-hydroxyphosphoramide, and an eventual byproduct of its metabolism, acrolein, are able to react with cytochrome P450 enzymes. This can be blocked by the addition of thiol protective agents, suggesting a reaction with CYP sulfydryl groups. However, it is unclear what the clinical consequences of this are, if there are indeed any. Likewise, aquated platinum species can react with CYP enzymes leading to inactivation, but although these interactions can be demonstrated in vitro, pharmacokinetic interactions of this nature appear to be minor in vivo, as demonstrated with etoposide. Nevertheless, the demonstration that JM216, another recently developed platinum analog, also inhibits multiple CYP enzymes, indicates that some care should be taken with this class of drugs. Interaction of platinum compounds may extend to other enzyme systems, and, indeed, the clearance of 5-FU is reduced approx 25% by coadministration of oxaliplatin. The effect, however, does not appear to be mediated via an inhibition of DPD.

Reduced expression

Enzyme activity also relates to the expression of the protein and drugs able to modify the expression of the enzyme in question will also potentially lead to drug–drug interactions.

Cytotoxic drugs

Exposure of cells to cytotoxic agents may lead to differential expression of metabolic enzymes. In a rat model, Yoshisue et al. demonstrated that oral administration of 5-FU reduced the activity of several drug-metabolizing enzymes (phases I and II). The loss of activity was apparently mediated by a reduction of these proteins within the cells and displayed little specificity. The effect was more marked in enterocytes than hepatocytes, suggesting that interactions might be more pronounced for orally administered drugs. Certainly, some drug interactions involving fluoropyrimidines have been reported, but these have so far been limited to a handful of substrates, implying greater selectivity of this effect in human subjects. In particular, clinically significant interactions between fluoropyrimidines and substrates of CYP2C9 such as phenytoin and (*S*)warfarin have been reported.

In male rats, the mRNA expression of the sexually dimorphic CYP isoform 2C11 can be repressed by treatment with cisplatin whereas the expression of "female" cytochrome p450s is increased. Similar observations have been made by the same laboratory using cyclophosphamide. The mechanism and clinical relevance of these observations are both unclear and only serve to highlight the species differences that may cloud the investigation of drug–drug interactions in animal models.

Biological agents

Cytokines are able to down-regulate the expression of many cytochrome P450 enzymes, and this may explain the apparent link between inflammatory diseases and decreased metabolic drug clearance observed in several disease states including cancer. Exogenous cytokines can have the same effect and the administration of interferon-α to patients was associated with a significant 37% decrease in cyclophosphamide clearance. This was consistent with a reduction in metabolic activation, because the AUC of the activated metabolite 4-hydroxycyclophosphamide was correspondingly reduced by 45%. Similar data demonstrating a reduction in 5-FU clearance when administered with interferon-α have been reported, but this effect has varied between studies, possibly reflecting differences in schedules and doses.

Enzyme induction

Cytochrome P450s in general are inducible enzymes. In the case of CYP3A4, it is well recognized that glucocorticoids (dexamethasone), barbiturates, rifampicin, and several anticonvulsant agents (phenytoin, carbamazepine) are able to up-regulate enzyme activity transcriptionally. Indeed, drug interactions resulting from increased CYP3A-mediated metabolism following the administration of anticonvulsants and steroids are among the most commonly encountered and problematic drug–drug interactions in medical oncology. Among the CYP3A substrates that have been demonstrated as being affected are the *Vinca* alkaloids, cyclophosphamide, irinotecan, etoposide, and teniposide. In the study of Baker et al., the range of teniposide clearance in six children on anticonvulsants was 21–54 mL/min per m^2 (22 courses) as compared to 7–17 mL/min per m^2 in a control group matched for age and sex. The clearance of topotecan has also been shown to increase by approx 50% when phenytoin is coadministered with concomitant increases in the AUC of the CYP3A metabolite *N*-desmethyltopotecan. Steroids have been reported to induce the metabolism and/or clearance of other drugs, including paclitaxel. Many of these inducers also induce other CYP450 isoforms, including members of the CYP2C superfamily. The oxazaphosphorines ifosfamide and cyclophosphamide display autoinduction of metabolism with unregulated expression of several enzymes in vitro. However, this is a complex effect and its role in drug interactions is not well established. It is complicated by the fact that cyclophosphamide metabolites can also inactivate CYPs, as discussed previously.

A confounding factor for the interpretation of drug–drug interactions with drugs such as the anticonvulsants, steroids, and other CYP-inducing drugs (e.g., rifampin and phenobarbital) is that these compounds can coordinately up-regulate P-glycoprotein and other transporters. Hence, even drugs that are not extensively metabolized by the cytochrome P450 system may have altered pharmacokinetics, presumably through an effect on transporter- mediated excretion.

Excretion

Drug interactions leading to modified drug excretion generally relate to interference with transporter function. Specifically, drug transporters in the proximal tubule of the kidney and the bile canaliculi are most likely involved. A major problem is identifying the tissue and transporter most at play in any observed drug–drug interaction. For example, cyclosporin A is an inhibitor of not only CYP3A but also of the transporters MRP-2 and P-glycoprotein. In addition to the effects on drug distribution discussed previously, cyclosporin also modulates both the renal and nonrenal clearance of several drugs including etoposide.

Renal excretion

Many drugs undergo active tubular secretion in the kidney, and there is the potential for drug interactions at that locus. The interaction between methotrexate and probenecid is one of the best known examples. Several transporters of the *organic anion transporter* (OAT) family are present in the tubular epithelium of the kidney and their inhibition by probenecid, various antibiotics, and NSAIDs is the likely mechanism. These interactions are indeed now being determined at the molecular level, which was not possible until relatively recently. This type of interaction may be important for other antifolate analogues with significant tubular secretion, although there is a paucity of data on this subject. Alterations in tubular secretion may also be modified through less direct effects. For example, Beorlegui et al. reported an apparent interaction between omeprazole and methotrexate. They argued that inhibition of the tubular proton pump by omeprazole caused a reduction in methotrexate secretion because of the requirement for protons by the latter.

Biliary excretion

Biliary excretion is a major route of excretion of many anticancer drugs. As mentioned previously, several transporters are present at the canalicular membrane including P-glycoprotein, MRP1, MRP-2 (cMOAT), and MRP-3. The development and discovery of drugs that act on these transporters has recently enabled the elucidation and exploitation of drug interactions at this locus.

Inhibition of biliary excretion

There are no documented cases of drug interactions specifically involving biliary excretion of anticancer drugs. Mostly, the problem is that measurement of biliary excretion is not routinely possible. Therefore, some of the pharmacokinetic interactions that have been reported might be attributable to this locus, but confirmatory evidence is not available. Preclinical experiments using perfused rat liver preparations have shown that inhibitors of P-glycoprotein may reduce biliary excretion of compounds known to be excreted such as doxorubicin. Using a similar model, Smit et al. demonstrated the potential for interactions between *Vinca* alkaloids and doxorubicin.

Induction of biliary excretion

Transporters, as with metabolic enzymes, can be involved in drug-drug interactions as a result of induction of activity. It is increasingly recognized that the induction of transporters such as P-glycoprotein can be caused by agents that overlap substantially with those capable of inducing CYP3A. As a result, some interactions with anticonvulsants may actually be the results of up-regulation of important transporters. This is a possible mechanism for the interaction between methotrexate and anticonvulsants.

Predicting Interactions

The prediction and evaluation of significant drug-drug interactions has in many instances been a rather piecemeal process. However, significant inroads in our understanding of the loci of these interactions have been made in vitro through to in vivo and there are now instances of systematic screening for these interactions during drug development.

Historical Data

In assessing likely interactions for a new drug, it is enormously useful if the compound has metabolism and excretion similar to those of previously characterized analogs. In the absence of such information, the usual sequential processes of in vitro and preclinical studies need to be carried out. One of the major problems is the manner in which these experiments have been performed often varies significantly from study to study and the data often reported are in different formats. There is therefore a real need for consistent experimental design and reporting in such studies. In the absence of such a platform, however, other groups have assembled electronic databases, which at least should enable some qualitative predictions of potential drug-drug interactions. A drug-drug interaction locus identified in vitro will be relevant only if this pathway represents a major route of elimination for the candidate drug. This is one of the major issues that databases such as the one proposed by Bonnabry et al. are trying to address.

Predicted from In Vitro Experiments

The advantage of being able readily to obtain drug metabolism enzymes from recombinant sources (insect cells, human lymphoblastoid cells, yeast, bacteria) has greatly facilitated the task of establishing the important routes of metabolism likely to be encountered when administered to patients. Similarly, these systems can also be used to search for potential drug interactions. Rapid throughput systems have been developed that use specific fluorogenic substrates to facilitate the large-scale and thorough screening required. The much larger potential problem is that relating to drug transporters. Here, the best systems are likely to be panels of stably transfected cells expressing each known transporter, starting probably with P-glycoprotein, BCRP, and MRP-1 and MRP-2. Alternatively, cells mimicking the relevant in vivo system may be used to test simultaneously the effects of expression of transporters and metabolic enzymes. A specific problem with the in vitro testing of drug interactions with alkylating anticancer drugs relates to the fact that these have complex pharmacology featuring multiple, often unstable species. Comprehensive studies of metabolic interactions with such drugs are difficult to perform and to interpret.

In Silico

Ultimately, the structure–activity relationships for each enzyme/transporter may become sufficiently documented by the use of large databases to enable direct *in silico* predictions of the metabolic and transporter properties of new drugs. These in turn would enable extrapolation of likely in vivo disposition, pharmacogenetics, and possible drug interactions. As mentioned previously, predictions are complicated by the overlap between transporters and metabolism. The interaction of etoposide with cyclosporin reported by Bisogno et al. could, on the basis of other observations discussed above, be the result of interaction with metabolism, biliary and intestinal secretion, and protein binding. Likewise cimetidine, which is often used as a relatively nonselective CYP450 inhibitor, is also an inhibitor of OAT in the kidney. Hence the mechanism for the drug interaction reported between cimetidine and epirubicin is also difficult to identify. Ultimately, therefore, classical in vitro and in vivo approaches for the investigation of drug interactions are required.

Preclinical Studies

Animal models may enable certain drug–drug interactions to be examined in a more physiologically meaningful fashion. However, some major interspecies differences exist with respect to the metabolism and excretion of drugs. For example, rats are relatively deficient in the aldo–keto reductases that metabolize anthracyclines to their corresponding C-13 alcohols. The cytochrome P450 enzymes also often differ markedly between species, not only in terms of their substrate affinities and reaction products but also in their susceptibility to inducers and inhibitors. The regulation of CYP450 is also highly species dependent. For example, induction of CYP3A by rifampicin is pronounced in humans and rabbits but not in rats. Hence, investigations of drug interactions require the use of the most representative animal or in vitro system to ensure relevance.

Clinical Studies

Many of the clinical drug interactions reported have been detected on the basis on comparisons of relatively small patient groups. In most cases, data are compared to historical or case-matched groups. Even less reliable are isolated case reports that report suspected drug interactions on the basis of abnormal drug disposition. Because of the large interindividual differences in metabolism and disposition, many of these studies are underpowered and biased. Ideally, clinical studies should be performed using a randomized crossover design as is normally used in trials to support of registration of compounds. FDA guidelines are available for the design of such trials. However, in medical oncology, many of the drugs are inherently unsafe. Usually drug–drug interactions are investigated because they pose a threat either to the safety or the efficacy of a compound and it becomes ethically difficult to propose such trials in patients who cannot really afford either. One alternative is to incorporate extensive population pharmacokinetics as part of Phase II and III trials of anticancer drugs. This then enables the identification of patients with unusual pharmacokinetic data and the identification of possible interactions. One of the down sides of this approach is that studies may require a very large number of subjects (several hundred) unless the interacting drug is very commonly used in the intended setting (e.g., anticonvulsants in CNS malignancy).

The drug candidates most worthy of further study for possible interactions are obviously those that are likely to be coadministered and for which there is some support from *in silico*, in vitro, preclinical, or clinical data. Other factors to be considered include the doses of the agents, their dosing regimen (single or multiple doses), and the timing of the administration (A before B, A after B, or

A + B). The latter is particularly important when the drug interaction is modulated through alteration of gene expression. For example, a study on the effects of rifampicin on drug clearance would require several days of rifampicin treatment prior to administration of the test drug to ensure maximal induction of the relevant enzyme system.

When the Problem is Not the Drug

In some instances, apparently classical drug–drug interactions have subsequently been shown to have little to do with the drugs involved. Consideration of these alternate mechanisms should be part of the investigation of drug–drug interactions.

Vehicle Effects

Many drugs are not sufficiently soluble to be administered in purely aqueous solvents. Instead a formulation component is frequently a surfactant. These compounds should not be dismissed as inactive and inconsequential. For example, Cremophor EL has some membrane effects and has been investigated for its ability to reverse P-glycoprotein-mediated multidrug resistance. It also modulates differentially the toxicity of cisplatin to marrow and tumor cells. Cremophor EL has been shown to modulate the distribution and elimination of doxorubicin in both preclinical and clinical studies. In the study of Millward et al., 11 patients were randomized to receive either 50 mg/m^2 of doxorubicin alone or in combination with 30 mL/m^2 of Cremophor EL. They were then crossed over to the alternative regimen. Cremophor significantly reduced the clearance of doxorubicin by approx 20%. The metabolite doxorubicinol was present in higher concentrations after Cremophor EL administration, resulting in an almost doubling of its AUC. Cremophor EL is also the likely major component of the interaction between Taxol and anthracyclines. When Taxol is administered immediately prior to a doxorubicin infusion or as an infusion prior to bolus doxorubicin, the clearance of doxorubicin is reduced by 20–30% and concentrations of doxorubicinol are again greatly increased. The latter suggests a possible reduction in the biliary clearance of the metabolite or a redistribution phenomenon secondary to the membrane effects of the Cremophor EL. Indeed, even when paclitaxel is administered 24 h after doxorubicin, sudden rebound profiles of doxorubicinol are observed. The effects of Cremophor EL on the hepatic disposition of paclitaxel itself also appear to be due to nonspecific effects on distribution rather than direct effects on biliary excretion.

Polysorbate 80 (also known as Tween 80) is used in the current formulation of docetaxel and etoposide. The coadministration of polysorbate 80 by itself or in the etoposide formulation had up to a twofold effect on doxorubicin AUC, mainly through increased early tissue distribution. The effect of etoposide on methotrexate pharmacokinetics reported by Paal et al. may also be due to the nonspecific effects of the Tween 80 present in etoposide. Indeed, the rebound profile of plasma methotrexate that occurred a few hours following etopo side is qualitatively similar to the rebound of doxorubicinol concentrations when paclitaxel is administered in Cremophor EL.

Effects of Dose Form

Several drugs are now marketed in liposomal formulations (doxorubicin, daunorubicin, amphotericin B). Theoretically, drugs can self-load into preformed liposomes in the circulation, and this was first demonstrated in a mouse model. When combination therapy includes a liposomal agent, the fact that many anticancer drugs are amphiphilic compounds that can interact with membranes suggests that drug–liposome interactions could take place. By binding to liposomes, it is possible that the release of the encapsulated drug would be modified and this has indeed been demonstrated in vitro. In vivo, however, this appears less likely and the predominant effect appears to be the uptake of the free drug into the circulating liposomes. In the study of Waterhouse et al., mice administered idarubicin and liposomal vincristine had a 3.6-fold increase in circulating concentrations of idarubicin 15 min later.

Effects of Treatmeht Regimens

Apart from aspects of formulation composition, specific treatment regimens require additional procedures to ensure adequate safety. For example, fluid loading is usually undertaken prior to cisplatin or methotrexate to ensure adequate renal function. Therefore, administration of another drug also cleared by the kidneys with either cisplatin or methotrexate might possibly result in altered disposition relative to drug alone. Some data are in support of such an effect. For example, Hudes et al. reported an increase in the renal clearance of trimetrexate when administered with cisplatin. Paradoxically, the urinary recovery of pemitrexed was reduced and its total clearance increased when administered with cisplatin. It is expected that effects of volume loading on renal clearance would be most pronounced in patients with some degree of renal dysfunction. For example, Kaye et al. found greatly increased methotrexate clearance when coadministered with cisplatin and forced diuresis only in a patient with renal clearance < 60 mL/min.

Administration of premedication agents for nausea/vomiting and hypersensitivity reactions may also be implicated. For example, interaction studies of a drug regimen with or without cisplatin might reasonably introduce not only the cisplatin but also antiemetics in the regimen. Ondansetron, for example, has been suggested to cause a slight decrease in the clearance of cyclophosphamide in high-dose regimens as compared to historical controls. Other studies have also noticed similar modest effects on both cyclophosphamide and cisplatin elimination by ondansetron, again when compared to historical controls. Similarly, the requirement for steroid prophylaxis for hypersensitivity reactions with docetaxel has been suggested to be the mechanism behind the interaction between ifosfamide and docetaxel.

When the Cytotoxic Agent is Not the Victim

Because cytotoxic agents are potentially dangerous drugs we are actually more concerned about the effects of concomitant therapy on the cytotoxic drug rather than the reverse. However, many drugs that are used for the intercurrent treatment of the patient may also suffer from small therapeutic windows. As discussed above, there have been reports of perturbed coagulation parameters in patients on warfarin receiving capecitabine. Similarly, blood concentrations of phenytoin are increased under similar circumstances. The effect is unlikely to be mediated by an acute interaction, given that capecitabine does not inhibit the cytochrome involved in the metabolism of warfarin. However, as mentioned previously, it appears that oral fluoropyrimidines can affect the expression and activity of cytochrome P450s.

Can We Exploit Drug Interactions?

Oral Delivery of Drugs

Drug interactions, as shown in the relevant sections above can have both detrimental and beneficial effects in chemotherapy. In particular, the inhibition of gastrointestinal transporters and enzymes greatly improves the bioavailability of oral drugs and enables oral delivery of some drugs that could previously not be administered orally. Poor bioavailability is usually associated with highly variable systemic concentrations and an additional possible benefit could be a reduction in intra- and interpatient variability in pharmacokinetics, although this is unlikely to be reduced to less than that encountered with parenteral administration. An example of successful exploitation of this strategy is the development of orally administered fluoropyrimidines that incorporate an inhibitor of DPD.

Many transport and enzyme modulators are currently being investigated in the setting of oral chemotherapy, although analogues that are specifically not substrates for these pathways provide an alternative route of development. For example, several taxanes that are not P-glycoprotein substrates are currently being evaluated for oral chemotherapy.

Systemic Administration

As previously discussed for the DPD inhibitors, administration of an inhibitor may greatly reduce intratumoral metabolism that in some cases may act as a significant mechanism of resistance in vivo. The second possible advantage of the suicide inhibitors of DPD (e.g., ethinyluracil) is that when coadministered, the elimination of 5-FU is no longer mostly via DPD catabolism but by renal excretion. The latter pathway is inherently less variable and more predictable than DPD, thereby potentially facilitating the dose individualization of treatment, although this has not been exploited in Phase III trials of the combination. Other DPD inhibitors have been developed in combination with oral prodrugs of 5-FU. These combination products include S-1 and UFT. S-1 also contains potassium oxonate as an inhibitor of thymidine kinase, and this assists in reducing activation of the 5-FU in the gastrointestinal mucosa.

The reduction in fluoropyrimidine dose that is made possible with DPD inhibitors underscores another way in which drug interactions can be exploited. In the early years of cyclosporin A use, the interaction between diltiazem was characterized and exploited to enable substantial cost savings. However, interactions based on reversible mechanisms are very difficult to predict because of constantly varying profiles on the target and inhibitor drug. In oncology, because of the limited safety of many of these agents, introduction of an additional variable into the chemotherapy regimen may become counterproductive, and such strategies are used only in the experimental setting. Such interactions also need to be proven from the aspect of activity, and the substantial costs of the additional Phase III trials probably outweigh the savings. Ironically, cyclosporin has now been proposed as a modulator of several agents to improve their pharmacokinetic and pharmacodynamic properties.

Future Directions

From a drug development aspect, the most exciting proposition is that accumulated knowledge about current drugs and their metabolism will enable some *in silico* prediction of likely mechanism of clearance and the potential drug interactions that might arise. This could greatly assist the rational refinement of drug leads and reduce the expense of development. The possibility of using well-characterized drug–drug interactions to enable oral therapy may prove obvious potential advantages, but this has not yet been developed into the routine clinical setting. Finally, genomic advances are likely to advance greatly our understanding of drug–drug interactions, particularly as they relate to instances in which drug metabolism is induced. For example, cytochrome P450 3A expression is extremely sensitive to control from interactions of nuclear receptors with the RXR. Some of the nuclear factors involved (CAR, PXR, and PPAR) have recently been shown to be subject to functional polymorphic variation. The elucidation of genotype/phenotype associations may help ultimately enable prediction of drug–drug interactions in individual subjects.

13

Incretin Modulators

The stimulation of insulin secretion has been a therapeutic principle since the introduction of sulfonylureas in the 1950s, when tolbutamide and carbutamide were introduced. Second- and third-generation sulfonylureas like glibenclamide and glimeperide remain to be among the most commonly used antidiabetic agents, attesting to the fact that promoting β-cell secretory function is a feasible way of controlling plasma glucose in patients with type 2 diabetes. Nevertheless, sulfonylureas are far from ideal as antidiabetic agents, since their use is associated with weight gain and with the provocation of hypoglycemia. The latter is caused by the absence of a strict glucose dependency of the ability to promote insulin secretion, since sulfonylureas per se are able to close the ATP-dependent K^+ channel, even at rather low glucose concentrations.

The incretin concept was developed when it had become obvious that the oral ingestion of nutrients, especially carbohydrates (glucose, starch, etc.) releases insulinotropic hormones from the gut mucosa, which in turn augment the insulin secretory response induced by meal-related glycemic excursions. When the first incretin hormone to be described in detail, Glucose-dependent Insulinotropic Polypeptide (Gastric Inhibitory Polypeptide, GIP) was characterized, one of the remarkable properties was the strict glucose dependency of its insulinotropic actions, both in perfused rat pancreas and in human subjects in vivo. Werner Creutzfeldt, in his 1978 Claude–Bernard lecture to the European Association for the Study of Diabetes, made this characteristic of GIP a core component of the definition of incretin hormones in general. Obviously, with a peptide like GIP, it was impossible to provoke hypoglycemic episodes, even when it was administered at high doses. A natural compound that potently stimulates insulin secretion, however, without a risk of provoking hypoglycemia, attracted attention as a potential candidate parent compound for the development of antidiabetic drugs. Because GIP has lost most of its insulinotropic activity in patients with type 2 diabetes, it was not until the identification of glucagon-like peptide-1 (GLP-1) and the demonstration that GLP-1 had preserved insulinotropic (and additional) activities in patients with type 2 diabetes that the idea of using incretin hormones as the basis for novel antidiabetic drugs could be actively persued.

Definition of the Problem and Basic Pathophysiology

Secretion and Action of Incretin Hormones in Physiology

Physiological roles of gastrointestinal peptide hormones

The ingestion of nutrients elicits the secretion of gastrointestinal hormones intimately involved in the regulation of gut and gallbladder motility, digestive juice secretion, and postprandial carbohydrate metabolism. In particular, incretin hormones stimulate insulin secretion from the endocrine pancreas.

Through the action of incretin hormones, enteral nutrition provides a more potent insulinotropic stimulus relative to an isoglycemic intravenous challenge. This phenomenon is named the "*incretin effect*".

GIP

The first incretin to be identified, GIP, was purified from porcine intestine extracts by virtue of its ability to inhibit gastric acid secretion (therefore, the original name was *gastric inhibitory polypeptide*). Soon, it was discovered that GIP displayed potent insulinotropic actions in animals and in human subjects. GIP was shown to be a 42 amino acid peptide hormone synthesized in duodenal and jejunal enteroendocrine K cells in the proximal small bowel (duodenum and jejunum).

GLP-1

Much later, the second incretin hormone, glucagon-like peptide-1 (GLP-1), was identified as a partial sequence of the cDNAs and genes encoding proglucagon. After posttranslational processing of proglucagon in gut endocrine L-cells, GLP-1 exists in two circulating equipotent molecular forms, GLP- 1 ("glycine-extended GLP-1") and GLP-1 amide ("amidated GLP-1"). The amidated form is more abundant in the circulation following meal ingestion in humans. Although the majority of GLP-1 is synthesized in the distal ileum and colon, plasma levels of GLP-1, like GIP, increase shortly after starting meals. This leaves two possibilities: Either there is an upper gut signal mediating GLP-1 release from more distal stores (i.e. the locations where GLP-1 is most abundant). Alternatively, GLP-1 is predominantly released from the sparse L-cells that are present in the upper gut. Quantitative considerations make it appear feasible that GLP-1 from gut segments coming into direct contact with chyme is the source of postprandial increments in GLP-1 concentrations.

Proteolytic degradation of incretin hormones by dipeptidyl peptidase-4

Plasma levels of total GLP-1 (including proteolytic degradation products) are low ("basal") in the fasted state (approximately 5 pmol/L) and increase rapidly following meal ingestion, reaching levels in plasma of 15–50 pmol/L. Only a minor proportion of circulating GLP-1 (approximately 10–20%) is intact, biologically active GLP-1. This is true after endogenous secretion as well as during exogenous administration, for example, during continuous intravenous infusion or after subcutaneous injection. The major reason is the rapid proteolytic degradation and inactivation by dipeptidyl peptidase-4 (DPP-4), an aminopeptidase recognizing peptides with a proline or alanine in the second aminoterminal position. It removes the first two aminoterminal amino acids, rendering the breakdown products (GLP-1 amide or GLP-1) biologically inactive or even weakly antagonistic. The circulating levels of intact GLP-1 and GIP are further kept low by rapid renal clearance. Whether additional proteases such as human neutral endopeptidase 24.11 are also essential determinants of GLP-1 inactivation remains under active investigation. Mice with targeted inactivation of the DPP-4 gene exhibit increased levels of plasma GIP and GLP-1, increased insulin secretion, and reduced glucose excursion following a glucose challenge.

GIP and GLP-1 receptors

GIP and GLP-1 exert their actions via engagement of structurally distinct G protein-coupled receptors. GIP receptors are predominantly expressed on islet β-cells, and to a lesser extent, in adipose tissue and in the central nervous system. In contrast, GLP-1 receptors are expressed in pancreatic endocrine β-cells and in several peripheral tissues including the central and peripheral nervous system, heart, kidney, lung, and the gastrointestinal tract. Activation of both incretin receptors on β-cells leads to rapid increases in levels of cyclic AMP and intracellular calcium, followed by insulin exocytosis, in a glucose-dependent manner. Incretin receptor signaling is associated with protein kinase A activation, induction of gene transcription, enhanced levels of (pro-)insulin biosynthesis, and the stimulation of β-cell proliferation. GLP-1 and GIP receptor activation protect β-cells against toxin-induced apoptosis (elicited by glucotoxicity – hyperglycemia, lipotoxicity – high concentrations of free fatty acids, streptozotocin, or hydrogen peroxide) and enhanced β-cell survival, findings observed in studies of both rodent and human islets.

Biological activity of GIP and GLP-1

The main functions of GIP are the glucose-dependent augmentation of insulin secretion during periods characterized by physiological hyperglycemia, the incretin function *sensu strictu*. Animal experiments suggest that GIP receptors on adipose tissue are essential for adipocyte triglyceride storage after meal ingestion: GIP receptor knock-out mice do not become obese when fed a high-fat diet.

GLP-1 does not only display glucose-dependent insulinotropic ("incretin") activity, but also inhibits glucagon secretion, decelerates gastric emptying and reduces food ingestion, and promotes enhanced glucose disposal via neural mechanisms involving receptors in the "*hepatoportal*" region. It is of interest that GLP-1 effects on glucagon secretion, like those on insulin secretory responses, are glucose-dependent, whereas counter-regulatory release of glucagon in response to hypoglycemia remains undisturbed even in the presence of pharmacological concentrations of GLP-1.

Effect of incretin receptor knock-out in mice

The physiological importance of endogenous GIP and GLP- 1 for glucose homeostasis can be examined using specific receptor antagonists or knock-out mice. Acute antagonism of either GIP or GLP-1 action lowers insulin secretion and increases plasma glucose following oral glucose ingestion in rodents. Similarly, mice with inactivating mutations in the GIP or GLP-1 receptors exhibit reduced glucose-stimulated insulin secretion and impaired glucose tolerance. GLP-1, but probably not GIP, is essential also for the control of fasting glucose concentrations, as acute antagonism or genetic disruption of GLP-1 action leads to increased levels of fasting glucose in rodents.

Effects of GLP-1 receptor antagonists in human subjects

The GLP-1 receptor antagonist exendin has been used to elucidate the role of endogenously secreted GLP-1 in human volunteers. Administration of exendin leads to a reduction in glucose-stimulated insulin secretion, diminished glucose clearance, and increased glucagon secretion. Indirect evidence suggests more rapid gastric emptying following disruption of GLP-1 action in humans as expected from the activity profile of GLP-1.

Activity of the Entero-Insular Axis and Incretin Hormones in Type 2-Diabetic Patients

Reduced incretin effect in patients with type 2 diabetes

In healthy human subjects oral glucose elicits a considerably higher insulin secretory response than does intravenous glucose (even if leading to the same glycemic increments). This incretin effect is substantially reduced or even completely lost in patients with type 2 diabetes. The reduction in the incretin effect probably is an acquired defect, since it is also found in patients with diabetes secondary to chronic pancreatitis, whereas chronic pancreatitis without diabetes is characterized by a normal incretin effect.

Secretion of incretin hormones in patients with type 2 diabetes

Cross-sectional analyses of larger cohorts suggest that there is a slight reduction in postprandial GLP-1 secretion following the ingestion of a mixed meal in patients with type 2 diabetes. Subjects with impaired glucose tolerance display intermediate results between healthy controls (normal response) and type 2-diabetic patients (reduced response). This is true for both total and intact GLP-1. However, the overall difference is small, and concerns the second and third hour after starting meal ingestion, whereas the characteristic differences in insulin secretory pattern are found in the early period after glucose or meal ingestion. Therefore, it cannot be considered likely that the slight reduction in postprandial GLP-1 secretion in patients with type 2 diabetes has any immediate impact on glycemic control. Along the same lines, any administration of GLP-1 receptor agonists should not be simply considered a replacement of an essential hormone (e.g. GLP-1) that is lacking in patients with type 2 diabetes.

GIP secretion in patients with type 2 diabetes has been reported as exaggerated, normal (on average), or reduced. In all cases, the differences were small in comparison with appropriate control subjects and are not likely to indicate any importance for the pathophysiology of the entero-insular axis in type 2 diabetes. Certainly, there is no complete lack in GIP in patients with type 2 diabetes.

Insulinotropic activity of GIP and GLP-1 in patients with type 2 diabetes

While the interaction of both GIP and GLP-1 with their respective receptors on healthy pancreatic endocrine β-cells leads to cAMP production and the augmentation of glucose-stimulated insulin release in a very similar manner, the insulinotropic activity of GIP is almost completely lost in patients with type 2 diabetes. This does not appear to indicate a lack of expression of GIP receptors on type 2-diabetic β-cells, since a bolus injection of GIP still elicits some insulin secretory response. However, prolonged infusion, even of highly pharmacological doses of GIP, is unable to meaningfully stimulate insulin secretion. This certainly is the fundamental defect underlying the reduced incretin effect in patients with type 2 diabetes.

On the other hand, a considerable proportion of the insulinotropic activity of GLP-1 as found in healthy subjects is preserved in patients with type 2 diabetes. Physiological concentrations of GLP-1 (as found after meal ingestion), however, have little if any effect on insulin secretion in patients with type 2 diabetes.

Upon a closer look, the insulinotropic activity of GLP-1 is also somewhat reduced in patients with type 2 diabetes compared with healthy control subjects. However, even a relatively low dose of GLP-1 can acutely restore the ability of β-cells to respond to increasing glucose concentrations with an insulin secretory response similar to healthy subjects. Nevertheless, the insulin response remains at approximately 20–25% relative to the effect in healthy subjects exposed to the same GLP-1 doses and concentrations. This partial preservation of insulin secretory effects is sufficient to make GLP-1 a potent insulinotropic agent in patients with type 2 diabetes.

Pharmacological doses of GLP-1 display the full spectrum of activities also in patients with type 2 diabetes. This includes effects on insulin and glucagon secretion, gastric emptying, appetite, and meal size. As a consequence, antidiabetic properties of pharmacological doses of GLP-1 have been examined in patients with type 2 diabetes.

Therapeutic Potential of Incretin Hormones

Owing to their pivotal role in the postprandial regulation of insulin secretion, both GIP and GLP-1 have been suggested as potential antidiabetic drug candidates. However, no significant reduction in glycemia could be achieved in studies with intravenous infusions of the GIP in hyperglycemic patients with type 2 diabetes. Indeed, while GIP exhibits potent insulinotropic properties in healthy subjects and probably mediates the major proportion of the incretin effect under physiological circumstances, its insulinotropic effect is markedly diminished in patients with type 2 diabetes. It is a current matter of debate whether this loss of incretin activity in type 2 diabetes is due to a specific defect, for example, in GIP signaling on pancreatic β-cells, or whether it goes along with a general decline in β-cell mass and function in such patients. In support of the latter hypothesis, the insuliotropic effect of GIP is not only reduced in patients with type 2 diabetes, but also in individuals with other forms of diabetes, such as MODY or type 1 diabetes. A number of GIP analogues exhibiting prolonged biological half-lives due to the chemical modifications, mostly at the N-terminal end of the peptide chain, have been proposed as potential drug candidates for the pharmacotherapy of type 2 diabetes, but as yet none of these compounds has been tested in patients with diabetes. Given the obvious inefficacy of native GIP in such patients, it is questionable whether GIP analogues will indeed exhibit a significant antihyperglycemic potential. Furthermore, unlike GLP-1, GIP even stimulates glucagon secretion, thereby potentially counteracting its insulinotropic effect.

Antidiabetic Actions of GLP-1

Short-term intravenous infusions of GLP-1 (approximately 1.2 pmol/kg/min, leading to pharmacological plasma concentrations of total GLP-1 of approximately 100 pmol/L, and intact biologically active GLP-1 of approximately 15 pmol/L) lower blood glucose in human subjects with type 2 diabetes through a transient glucose-dependent stimulation of insulin and suppression of glucagon secretion and gastric emptying. A 6-week subcutaneous infusion of GLP-1 in patients with type 2 diabetes achieving plasma levels of total GLP-1 of around 65 pmol/L was followed by a substantial improvement in insulin secretory capacity, insulin sensitivity, a reduction in HbA_{1c} by 1.2%, and weight loss. Although intravenous or subcutaneous GLP-1 infusions may be useful for the short-term control of hyperglycemia under a variety of clinical conditions, the long-term treatment of type 2 diabetes requires a more feasible approach for achieving sustained GLP-1 receptor activation. The proof-of-principle that GLP-1 can help lower, even normalize plasma glucose in a substantial number of patients with type 2 diabetes, has paved the way to explore the clinical efficacy of (i) peptides that act as GLP-1 receptor agonists, but have more suitable pharmacokinetic properties than are characteristic for the parent compound, GLP-1, and (ii) DPP-4 inhibitors (small molecules with substantial oral bioavailability).

Therapeutical Approach of Relevant Drugs, Understanding and Pinpointing Clinical Pharmacology, Critical Evaluation of Drugs

GLP-1 Receptor Agonists

Exenatide (synthetic exendin-4)

Exenatide (synthetic exendin-4) was isolated from the salivary gland of the gila monster, a lizard found in the deserts of Arizona. Due to an ~50% amino acid homology with native human GLP-1, this peptide acts as a potent agonist at the mammalian GLP-1 receptor, but is not substrate to proteolytic cleavage by DPP-4. This leads to a circulating plasma half-life of 2–4 h, with exenatide levels being raised for ~6 h after a single subcutaneous injection.

The clinical effects of exenatide in the treatment of type 2 diabetes have been examined in phase 3 trials. In these studies, exenatide (5 or 10 μg s.c. twice daily) was added to an existing therapy with metformin, sulfonylureas, a combination of both, or thiazolidinediones. HbA_{1c}-reductions achieved after exenatide treatment over 30 weeks ranged from 0.8% to 1.0%, with HbA_{1c}-levels at baseline ranging between 8.2% and 8.6%. In addition, body weight was reduced by ~1-3 kg after 30 weeks (baseline weight: ~100 kg), and patients continuing in an open-label extension study for 80 weeks exhibited a total weight loss averaging ~4.5 kg. The latter effect is remarkable in that all other insulinotropic drugs (sulfonylureas and glinides) as well as insulin itself typically cause weight gain during long-term administration.

In an open-label comparison of exenatide with insulin glargine in diabetic patients suboptimally controlled with metformin and sulfonylurea, both treatment regimens led to a reduction in HbA_{1c} levels by ~1.1% after 26 weeks (baseline: 8.2%). However, while fasting glucose concentrations were reduced to a greater extent with insulin glargine, exenatide treatment elicited greater reductions in postprandial glycemia. The most striking differences between both treatment regimens were observed in body weight. Thus, patients treated with insulin glargine experienced a weight gain of 1.8 kg, whereas patients on exenatide lost on average 2.3 kg over the treatment period. Similar findings have been reported for the comparison of exenatide and premixed insulin aspart, both injected subcutaneously twice daily.

In April 2005, exenatide (trade name, Byetta) was approved by the FDA for the treatment of type 2 diabetic patients who have not achieved adequate glycemic control on maximally tolerated doses of metformin and/or a sulfonylurea. In Europe, exenatide was approved in November 2006.

Liraglutide

Liraglutide (NN221 1; Arg34, Lys26-[*N*-∈ (γ-Glu[*N*-α-hexadecanoyl])]-GLP-1) is a GLP-1 derivative developed by Novo Nordisk, which is currently undergoing phase 3 clinical trials. The plasma half-life of this compound has been extended to ~10–14 h through an amino acid substitution (Arg_{34}→Lys) and the attachment of a glutamic acid and a 16-C-free fatty acid addition to Lys_{26}. The acyl moiety induces non-covalent binding to albumin with ~1–2% of Liraglutide circulating as the non-albumin bound, "free" peptide. These modified pharmacokinetic properties make the compound suitable for once-daily s.c. administration. In clinical studies in patients with type 2 diabetes, liraglutide reduced HbA_{1c} levels by up to 1.75%. Liraglutide induced a moderate weight loss during chronic administration, similar to the effects of native GLP-1 and exenatide.

Long-acting GLP-1 receptor agonists

As a single subcutaneous injection of exenatide does not produce effective glucose control for more than 6–8 h, there is considerable interest in the development of longer-acting GLP- 1 receptor agonists, which require less frequent parenteral administration. Exenatide LAR ("*long-acting release*") is a poly-lactide-glycolide microsphere suspension containing 3% exendin-4 peptide, which exhibits sustained dose-dependent glycemic control in diabetic fatty Zucker rats for up to 28 days following a single subcutaneous injection. Preliminary experience with exenatide LAR in 45 subjects with type 2 diabetes mellitus indicates a much greater reduction in fasting glucose concentrations and HbA_{1c} following once-weekly administrations of exenatide LAR for 15 weeks. However, long-term experience with exenatide LAR in larger numbers of patients has not yet been reported. Exenatide LAR is currently being examined in a Phase 3 trial head to head against twice-daily exenatide.

Additional strategies for development of long-acting GLP-1 receptor agonists include the use of chemical linkers to form covalent bonds between GLP-1 (CJC-1131) or exendin-4 (CJC-1134). Similarly, recombinant albumin-GLP-1 proteins (e.g., "albugon") have been developed, which mimic the full spectrum of GLP-1 actions in preclinical studies. Although these drugs are expected to exhibit a prolonged pharmacokinetic profile suitable for once-weekly dosing in diabetic patients, only limited clinical information is available about the efficacy and safety of these albumin-based drugs in human subjects.

DPP-4 Inhibitors

The therapeutic use of GLP-1 is primarily limited by its rapid in vivo degradation by the enzyme DPP-4. DPP-4 is a ubiquitous membrane-spanning cell-surface amino-peptidase widely expressed in many tissues including liver, lung, kidney, intestinal brush-border membranes, lymphocytes, and endothelial cells, which can also be found circulating in plasma. DPP-4 nonspecifically cleaves peptides displaying a proline or alanine residue in the second amino-terminal position, thereby making a number of gastrointestinal hormones, including GIP, GLP-1, GLP-2, PACAP, Neuropeptide Y, and Peptide YY substrates to DPP-4 degradation.

Endogenous GLP- 1 plasma levels typically increase by ~2–3-fold after meal ingestion and return to baseline values within ~3–6 h. Inhibiting DPP-4 activity extents the circulating half-life of the incretin hormone, thereby raising intact GLP-1 levels for up to 5 h after meal ingestion. While DPP-4 inhibitors primarily lower postprandial glycemic excursions, there is now evidence that basal concentrations of intact GLP-1 are also raised to some extent by DPP-4 inhibition, which may explain their (modest) effects on fasting glycemia. As a rule, DPP-4 inhibitors mimic many of the actions of native GLP- 1, such as the stimulation of insulin and inhibition of glucagon secretion. However, unlike

GLP-1 and its analogues, DPP-4 inhibitors do not typically influence body weight or gastric emptying. These discrepancies might be due to the nonspecific mode of action of the DPP-4 inhibitors, which also prevent the degradation of other peptides, especially GIP and NPY, which might exert opposite effects on gastric motility and the central nervous control of appetite. As an alternative explanation, it seems possible that the modest elevations in intact GLP-1 levels (approximately doubled) seen after DPP-4 inhibition are of insufficient magnitude to elicit significant effects on gastric emptying and food intake. A number of small molecule DPP-4 inhibitors suitable for oral administration are currently undergoing clinical trials. This article focuses on the two major compounds with available reports regarding phase 3 clinical trials.

Sitagliptin

The DPP-4 inhibitor sitagliptin has been developed by Merck Pharmaceuticals and was recently approved for the therapy of type 2 diabetes by the FDA under the name Januvia. The elimination half-life of sitagliptin is 12–14 h, thereby allowing for once-daily administration. In phase 3 trials enrolling drug-naïve patients with type 2 diabetes, sitagliptin led to HbA_{1c} reductions of 0.79% and 0.94% a dose of 100 and 200 mg, respectively (baseline: 8.0%). In diabetic patients inadequately controlled with metformin (baseline HbA_{1c}: 8.0%), HbA_{1c}-levels were reduced by 0.65% after 24 weeks of sitagliptin treatment. Likewise, patients pretreated with pioglitazone (baseline HbA_{1c}: 8.1%) exhibited a 0.7% HbA_{1c}-reduction after 24 weeks of sitaglitin treatment. Regarding the control of glycemia (HbA_{1c}), sitagliptin was equipotent to the sulfonylurea glipizide, when added to metformin pretreatment. Glipizide, however, caused significant weight gain. Similar to vildaglitin, sitagliptin does not have any systematic effect on body weight.

Vildagliptin

The DPP-4 inhibitor vildagliptin has been developed by Novartis Pharma and is currently awaiting approval. Vildagliptin has been studied at doses between 50 and 100 mg administered once or twice daily per os. In a study over 4 weeks, once-daily administration of 100 mg vildagliptin reduced fasting glucose by 0.70 mmol/L, and post-prandial glucose excursions by 1.45 mmol/L. This effect was accompanied by a significant reduction glucagon levels, whereas plasma insulin remained rather unchanged. However, similar insulin profiles at lower glucose concentrations indicate an improvement in glucose-stimulated insulin secretion. Consistent with this, indirect evidence from mathematical modeling studies suggested a significant improvement in β-cell function during vildagliptin treatment.

In metformin-treated patients with type 2 diabetes, the addition of vildagliptin led to a reduction of HbA_{1c} by ~0.8% (baseline: 7.7%), and this effect was maintained during an open-label extension for 52 weeks. Recent studies in patients with type 2 diabetes treated with the twice-daily administration of 50 mg vildagliptin also demonstrated a significant improvement in postprandial plasma triglyceride and apolipoprotein B-48-containing triglyceride-rich lipoprotein particle metabolism, suggesting that this compound might exert antiatherogenic effects beyond its glucose-lowering actions.

In a direct comparison, vildagliptin did not quite achieve noninferiority in comparison with metformin in terms of lowering HbA_{1c}-levels, but was associated with a lower frequency of GI-side effects. When compared with rosiglitazone, vildagliptin treatment elicited a similar reduction in HbA_{1c}-levels, but did not cause a similar increase in body weight.

Contrasting Properties of GLP-1 Receptor Agonists and DPP-4 Inhibitors

Twice-daily exenatide administered via subcutaneous injection is currently indicated for the treatment of patients with type 2 diabetes mellitus failing one or more oral agents, often as an alternative to institution of insulin therapy. In contrast, once-daily DPP-4 inhibitors may find use as first-line therapy or as add-on therapy to patients failing one or more oral agents. Although there does not appear to be a great difference in the HbA_{1c}-lowering capacity of GLP-1 receptor agonists versus DPP-4 inhibitors, the obvious difference between these classes of drugs is their effect on body weight. Weight loss is a common outcome of therapy with native GLP-1, exenatide, and liraglutide, whereas therapy with DPP-4 inhibitors is associated with prevention of weight gain. In contrast, gastrointestinal side effects, predominantly nausea, are frequently reported following treatment with injectable incretin mimetics, but have not been described with DPP-4 inhibition. These differences may be explained in part by the relatively modest stabilization of postprandial GLP-1 seen after DPP-4 inhibition versus the pharmacological increases in circulating levels of incretin mimetics exemplified by exenatide. Although nausea is a common side effect of exenatide therapy, many patients experience weight loss independent of nausea. Consistent with the above differences in circulating levels of GLP-1, incretin mimetics, but not DPP-4 inhibitors, profoundly decelerate gastric emptying.

Practical Outline in the Management

In this chapter, a suggestion will be developed on how incretin mimetics and DPP-4 inhibitors will fit into established treatment algorithms for glycemic control in patients with type 2 diabetes.

Choice of Patients

Incretin mimetics

Since incretin mimetics are injectable antidiabetic drugs, their use will most likely be considered, when oral antidiabetic agents in combinations do no longer assure glycemic control of the required quality. This is the moment, when – according to current guidelines – the start of insulin treatment would be considered according to most recommendations. However, such guidelines have, until now, not considered the availability of incretin mimetics or DPP-4 inhibitors. An attempt has been made to incorporate these novel antidiabetic treatment choices into a more complex algorithm.

Incretin mimetics (e.g. exenatide) would have some advantages over using insulin. In particular, they promote weight loss, whereas the initiation of insulin treatment must be expected to be associated with weight gain. This difference has been demonstrated in two head-to-head studies comparing twice-daily exenatide injections either with once-daily insulin *glargine* or twice-daily premixed insulin. It is, however, not known whether the resulting weight difference (approximately 5 kg) represents a significant health benefit in terms of cardiovascular risk or even outcome. Longer-term studies examining cardiovascular endpoints will be necessary to clarify this point. It can, however, be foreseen that for the obese type 2-diabetic patients, who has struggled to lose weight, an agent that will provide a good chance to lose rather than to gain body weight is an attractive choice. Along these lines, for patients in whom insulin therapy had been initiated recently, and in whom this has led to considerable weight gain, switching to incretin mimetics might be a reasonable alternative. However, studies examining the consequences of changing therapy from insulin to incretin mimetics in this particular situation are not yet available.

DPP-4 inhibitors

Given the fact that metformin is the established first-line drug for the anti-hyperglycemic treatment of obese type 2 diabetes, especially considering the reduction in the incidence of acute myocardial infarction and related mortality demonstrated in the UKPDS, the use of DPP-4 inhibitors may be considered, when metformin alone has failed to maintain adequate glycemic control, or is not likely to achieve treatment goals unless combined with additional agents. An early initiation of anti-hyperglycemic combination treatment is supported by the recent finding that metformin and sitagliptin achieved a higher likelihood of treatment success when given in combination to patients with type 2 diabetes not previously treated with oral agents. As a second oral antidiabetic agent, the use of DPP-4 inhibitors has to be weighed against the alternatives, sulfonylureas, glitazones, α-glucosidase inhibitors, and (basal, "bedtime") insulin. All other treatment choices (except acarbose or miglitol) will cause weight gain, whereas DPP-4 inhibitors generally can be considered weight-neutral. Sulfonylureas can provoke hypoglycemic episodes, and glitazones may precipitate fluid retention and congestive heart failure. Given the comparable antidiabetic potency of sitagliptin relative to the sulfonylurea glipizide and of vildagliptine in comparison with the thiazolidindione rosiglitazone, their weight-neutrality and unremarkable side-effect profile make DPP-4 inhibitors a serious contender for the second oral antidiabetic agent to be added to metformin treatment.

Given the fact that incretins (both GIP and GLP-1) are eliminated via the kidneys and that patients with impaired renal function have elevated circulating concentrations of GIP and GLP-1, treatment with usual doses of DPP-4 inhibitors might lead to further elevations in incretin plasma levels, potentially causing adverse events. Therefore, lower doses of DPP-4 inhibitors may be appropriate in such patients. Like in the case of renal functional impairment, not much is known on the use of DPP-4 inhibitors in patients with type 2 diabetes and associated diseases leading to severe organ failure (liver cirrhosis, heart failure, pulmonary disorders, etc.).

Initiation of Treatment

Incretin mimetics

Since starting exenatide injections may be associated with the provocation of nausea, it is better to start treatment at a lower dose (5 μg per injection, twice daily subcutaneously) and to increase the dose to 10 μg twice daily after 4 weeks. This has been shown to make the 10-μg dose more tolerable. Following this regimen has been associated with low withdrawal rates in studies using 10 μg twice daily. Initial studies using liraglutide had identified 0.75 mg once daily as a subcutaneous dose close to the maximum tolerated dose upon a single injection into treatment-naive subjects or patients. Later, a regimen starting at 0.5 mg once daily, and increasing the dose by 0.5 mg on a weekly basis, was used to extend the final dosage to 2 mg once daily for the majority of patients. Therefore, it appears advisable to start liraglutide at a low dose and titrate the daily dose up to the 2-mg range. The most recent trial has reported the use of 0.65, 1.25, and 1.9 mg once daily.

DPP-4 inhibitors

DPP-4 inhibitors can immediately be started at the target dose, since the initiation of treatment has not been associated with any untoward responses. Since studies examining effects of sitagliptin and vildagliptin at single (100 mg once daily orally) or divided doses (e.g., 50 mg twice daily orally) have not consistently resulted in different efficacy, once-daily dosing will probably be the standard.

Choice of Dose and Timing

Incretin mimetics

In studies examining the dose–response relationships for exenatide, 10 μg twice daily has uniformly been more effective than 5 μg twice daily. Therefore, for the majority of patients, exploiting the efficacy of 10 μg twice daily will be necessary to reach treatment targets. For those patients achieving their goals already at 5 μg twice daily, continuing at this dosage is an option.

Given the pharmacokinetics of exenatide injected subcutaneously into human subjects, a single injection is likely to be clinically effective over a period of 6–8 h. This can be inferred from the fact that the glycemic rise after breakfast and dinner is almost completely abolished when injecting exenatide before breakfast and dinner, whereas there remains a glucose excursion after lunch.

One consequence of the rather short duration of action of a single injection of exenatide is that timing the injection relative to meals is of some importance. Linnebjerg et al. demonstrated that exenatide should be injected within 60 min before starting meals. This appears plausible, since one important mode of action of exenatide is the deceleration of gastric emptying. Further, the question arises whether more frequent injections of exenatide (three or four per day) would provide even better glycemic control, including a more profound effect on fasting glucose concentrations and lunch-time glycemic control. One study had not found advantages of three over two injections. Rather than increasing the number of injections per day, the development has been in the direction of more extended-acting preparations of exenatide.

Preliminary results of using exenatide LAR indicate that doses of 0.8 and 2.0 mg per week (injected subcutaneously) are effective in reducing HbA_{1c} considerably. Interestingly, only the higher dose significantly reduced body weight, while the effect on HbA_{1c} after 15 weeks was relatively similar. This raises the question whether the dose–response relationship is different for glycemic control and for the reduction in body weight. If this were true, higher doses should be used, if weight reduction is among the treatment goals. Similarly, liraglutide reduced HbA_{1c} at doses of 0.65, 1.25, and 1.9 mg injected once daily subcutaneously, to a rather similar extent, while only the higher dose(s) significantly reduced body weight. Perhaps, the upper end of the dose–response relationship for weight reduction has not been characterized, and doses even higher than 2 mg daily would have more profound effects on body weight. Like with exenatide, the choice of the dose should consider whether or not weight loss is among the individual treatment goals.

DPP-4 inhibitors

Sitagliptin and vildagliptin exert their antidiabetic activity by inhibiting DPP-4 enzymatic activity. Since a single dose of 100 mg inhibits DPP-4 activity by >90% for most of a 24-h period, there is no obvious reason why higher doses should be more effective. As a consequence, a dose of 100 mg once daily will most likely be used rather uniformly, both for sitagliptin and vildagliptin, unless they are combined with other antidiabetic agents (like metformin), which are usually administered twice daily. Reduced doses may be necessary for patients with renal functional impairment.

Choice of Antidiabetic Agents to be Used in Combination

Incretin mimetics

Based on available clinical studies, a combining exenatide with metformin has the most obvious advantages: A substantial reduction in HbA1c is associated with the numerically largest weight loss (compared with combinations including sulfonylureas) and no increased risk of hypoglycemia (despite better glycemic control). Addition to thiazolidinediones is similarly possible. If exenatide is to be combined with sulfonylureas, the benefit of better glycemic control has to be weighed against the risk of hypoglycemia and less weight reduction. A combination of a short-acting incretin mimetic (to control postprandial rises in glycemia) and a long-acting insulin (to titrate fasting glucose into the target range) may theoretically appear to make sense, but no studies are available to report experience with this particular combination.

DPP-4 inhibitors

DPP-4 inhibitors can safely be combined with metformin and thiazolidinediones. A combination with sulfonylureas does not suggest particular advantages, since both agents, through different mechanisms, enhance insulin secretion. This combination would, most likely, not be as safe regarding hypoglycemic episodes. No studies are available regarding a potential combination with α-glucosidase inhibitors or insulin treatment.

Measures to Assure Metabolic Control (Self-Blood-Glucose Monitoring)

Although exenatide was approved by the FDA and introduced for use in the USA in 2005 (and other countries since) and sitagliptin has been approved in the USA and elsewhere in late 2006, no recommendations regarding metabolic control have been issued. The following suggestions, therefore, are based on the known properties of incretin mimetics and DPP-4 inhibitors.

Incretin mimetics

Since incretin mimetics will be used at fairly standardized doses (vide supra), and not based on individual titration (like in the case of insulin), and since incretin mimetics alone do not provoke hypoglycemic episodes, there will be a rather limited need for blood-glucose self-control in addition to regular determinations of HbA_{1c}. The frequency of glucose control will primarily depend on other antidiabetic agents used in combination and their potential to elicit hypoglycemia. Certainly, in comparison with any insulin regimen, the requirement for blood glucose-self control will be much smaller. This could affect the acceptability of such treatment regimens to patients and on the overall cost–benefit relationship.

DPP-4 inhibitors

DPP-4 inhibitors, in their most likely use, in combination with metformin, do not require additional measures of blood-glucose self-control, since they are administered at a standard dosage and do not provoke hypoglycemia. Thus, only occasional profiles to assess glycemic control are adequate.

Discontinuation of Treatment

With randomized clinical trials concerning incretin mimetics and DPP-4 inhibitors lasting up to 1 year, and open-label follow-up reported up to 2 years, it is obvious that these studies cannot provide an estimate of how long treatment with incretin mimetics and DPP-4 inhibitors can meaningfully control glycemia. It is, however, obvious that not all patients treated with such agents achieve their glycemic target, even within the time frame of the studies that have been reported. Therefore, preliminary thoughts on when incretin mimetics or DPP-4 inhibitors should be discontinued, and what the treatment alternatives would be, seem adequate, even in the absence of studies that would provide any firm guidance.

Incretin mimetics

Treatment with exenatide results in fairly stable fasting glucose and HbA_{1c} concentrations after approximately 3 months. If by then HbA_{1c} targets (e.g., <7.0%) have not been met, intensification of treatment has to be considered. Since weight loss associated with the use of exenatide progresses at least up to a duration of 2 years, a secondary improvement of glycemic control appears possible with further weight reduction, although this is not clearly confirmed by serial HbA_{1c} measurements. Certainly, once weight becomes stable and HbA1c remains outside the target range, antidiabetic therapy needs to be intensified.

Adding more or other oral antidiabetic agents at this stage of type 2 diabetes does not seem to be helpful in achieving adequate glycemic control. Rather, insulin-based treatment regimens will most likely be needed. Since there is no reported experience with a combination of exenatide and insulin, this cannot be recommended. Established treatment regimens ranging from a combination of once-daily basal insulin and oral agents, twice-daily premixed insulin, or intensified regimens with multiple daily insulin injections should be initiated instead.

DPP-4 inhibitors

When a DPP-4 inhibitor added to metformin no longer adequately controls glycemia, the options for intensifying therapy include the start of basal insulin or an incretin mimetic. It is not known what continued treatment with DPP-4 inhibitors would add to a combination of metformin (continued) and basal insulin (newly initiated). In addition, there has been no published experience with a combination of a DPP-4 inhibitor and an incretin mimetic. Such studies are needed to justify a continuation of DPP-4 inhibitor treatment under these circumstances. Since there have been no head-to-head comparisons of the anti-hyperglycemic efficacy between DPP-4 inhibitors and incretin mimetics, one can only speculate whether switching from a DPP-4 to an incretin mimetic would improve glycemic control. Based on comparisons of the effects on fasting glucose and HbA_{1c} concentrations, one might assume that longer-acting incretin mimetics (exenatide LAR, liraglutide) would probably provide a better glycemic control than a DPP-4 inhibitor.

Side Effects of Treatment

Side Effects of Incretin Mimetics

Side effects of exenatide

As is typical for the administration of native GLP-1, a considerable proportion of patients receiving exenatide experience gastrointestinal side effects, such as nausea and more rarely vomiting or diarrhea. In the phase 3 trials with exenatide, the frequence of these adverse effects was reported to be as high as 48% during treatment with 10 μg of exenatide. However, it should be noted that, though frequent, these side effects were mostly mild to moderate in intensity and usually transient. Overall, the percentage of patients who discontinued exenatide treatment as a result of side effects was low. When considering all patients enrolled in the exenatide phase 3 trials, there also seemed to be an increase in the frequency of hypoglycemic events, but this was limited to the patients receiving additional treatment with sulfonylurea drugs. In contrast, the incidence of hypoglycemia was unchanged in patients treated with metformin.

Antibody formation has been reported in ~40–50% of patients receiving Exenatide treatment. However, these antibodies seemed to exhibit a weak binding affinity and have not been associated with severely impaired antidiabetic effectiveness of exenatide in the majority of treated subjects.

Side effects of liraglutide

In the published phase 2 trials with liraglutide, nausea, vomiting, and diarrhea were the most frequent adverse events reported, with the incidence of events being dose-related. Only a small proportion of patients (<5%) discontinued treatment due to these side effects. The frequency of hypoglycemia was not increased during liraglutide treatment. Side reactions of urticarial injection were reported in 1 out of 135 patients exposed to liraglutide in one trial and did not occur in the other published studies. No antibody formation has been reported after exposure to liraglutide.

Side Effects of DPP-4 Inhibitors (Sitagliptin and Vildagliptin)

A number of theoretical concerns have been expressed regarding potential adverse effects of DPP-4 inhibitors. In particular, the large number of physiological substrates of DPP-4 gave rise to speculations that inhibiting the action of this protease might interfere with numerous other hormonal axes, thereby potentially causing adverse reactions. Furthermore, since DPP-4 is also expressed on T-lymphocytes as CD26, it was speculated that chronic DPP-4 inhibition might alter immune functions. Against these theoretical considerations, the DPP-4 inhibitors have so far proven to be safe and well tolerated in clinical studies, and no characteristic pattern of adverse events has been observed. Thus, in patients with diabetes pretreated with metformin, the incidence of adverse effects during 12 weeks of treatment with sitagliptin was similar to the placebo group. Likewise, the frequency of side effects was not different from the placebo group in diabetic patients previously treated with a dietary regimen. With sitagliptin, the frequency of gastrointestinal side effects was slightly higher compared with placebo in one, but not all studies. Overall, the gastrointestinal side effects typically reported during the treatment with GLP-1 analogues do not represent a problem during DPP-4 inhibitor administration. Nevertheless, further long-term studies will be required to confirm the absence of a potential to cause clinically important adverse reactions before these drugs can unequivocally be accepted as safe, especially with regard to their potential effects on other hormonal axes and immune functions.

Key Issues in the Treatment Strategy

Based on presently available study results, the clinical benefit of using incretin mimetics is determined by their ability to control glycemia (i.e., lower HbA_{1c}), their inability to cause hypoglycemia unless combined with other antidiabetic agents that have the potential to initiate hypoglycemia, their weight effects (promotion of weight loss in the case of incretin mimetics, weight neutrality in the case of DPP-4 inhibitors), and their safety and tolerability, especially the absence of a potential to cause specific severe adverse events.

The novel classes of antidiabetic agents, incretin mimetics and DPP-4 inhibitors, may hold two additional promises: A reduction in cardiovascular complications typically associated with type 2 diabetes and the metabolic syndrome, and a positive influence on the natural history of type 2 diabetes, which with current treatment options is characterized by a steady loss of β-cell function, which in turn determines a rather short "*durability*" of successful glycemic control with any choice of antidiabetic agents.

Possible Effects of Incretin Mimetics and DPP-4 Inhibitors on β-Cell Mass

Both type 1 and type 2 diabetes are caused by a significant deficit in β-cell mass, caused by increased β-cell apoptosis. Strategies to inhibit β-cell apoptosis and/or increase the rate of β-cell replication may therefore allow for the prevention or even reversal of diabetes. A number of studies have suggested that GLP-1 might exhibit such properties. Thus, in β-cell lines (INS-1 cells), GLP-1 increased the rate of proliferation through induction of phosphatidylinositol 3-kinase, protein kinase C zeta, and activation of PDX1 gene expression. In rodent models of diabetes, GLP-1 led to an increase in β-cell replication, a stimulation of islet neogenesis, and an inhibition of β-cell apoptosis. An inhibition of β-cell apoptosis by GLP-1 was also noted in isolated human islets. These actions therefore raised hopes that GLP-1 analogues and DPP-4 inhibitors might halt or even reverse the progression of diabetes.

With exenatide, an increase in β-cell replication and neogenesis resulting in increased β-cell mass has been reported after partial pancreatectomy in rats, and a diminished recovery of β-cell mass after partial pancreatectomy was shown in GLP-1 receptor knock-out mice. Likewise, exendin-4 stimulated β-cell neogenesis in streptozotocin-induced diabetic rats as well as in Goto–Kakizaki diabetic rats. The effects of liraglutide on β-cell mass and turnover were studied as well. In db/db mice, liraglutide treatment significantly increased β-cell mass and proliferation resulting in improved diabetes control. In addition, liraglutide inhibited both cytokine- and free fatty acid-induced apoptosis in isolated rat islets.

Not only GLP-1 and its analogues, but also the DPP-4 inhibitors have been shown to exert beneficial effects on β-cell mass and turnover. Along these lines, Pospisilik and colleagues reported a significant increase in β-cell mass in strepozotocin-induced diabetic rats following 7 weeks of treatment with the DPP-4 inhibitor P32/98, and recently a significant increase in β-cell mass was reported after treatment with des-fluoro-sitagliptin in high-fat diet (HFD)/streptozotocin (STZ)-induced diabetic mice.

Taken together, these studies suggest that both incretin mimetics and DPP-4 inhibitors might indeed have a potential to induce β-cell regeneration in patients with diabetes during long-term treatment. It is, however, difficult to draw firm conclusions from these studies in rodents or in vitro for the situation in humans. In fact, the rates of β-cell turnover seem to be much lower in humans than in rodents, and the overall capacity for islet regeneration in humans appears to be limited. Furthermore, it is yet impossible to directly measure changes in β-cell mass or turnover, since the human pancreas are inaccessible for repeated biopsy sampling, and since the functional assessment of insulin secretion might only partly relate to the actual β-cell mass. Therefore, while current evidence strongly suggest that the GLP-1 analogues and DPP-4 inhibitors will indeed induce β-cell regeneration in patients with diabetes, this question will ultimately have to be answered in further long-term trials.

The recommendation of an extended and perhaps earlier use of incretin mimetics, for example, starting an injection therapy instead of using oral antidiabetic agents although oral agents would provide adequate glycemic control, would require the demonstration of unique benefits. In principle, the demonstration that exenatide and liraglutide, like GLP-1, can inhibit β-cell apoptosis and increase β-cell mass in isolated pancreatic islets and rodents, would provide a rationale to counteract the progressive loss of β-cell function (and presumably, β-cell mass) typical of type 2 diabetes. However, although some experiments with human islets or islet cell precursors have reported similar findings, only preliminary hints have been gained from clinical studies examining the long-term effect of incretin mimetics on parameters of "β-cell health."

Whether the reported decreases in the proportion of proinsulin (relative to insulin) can be used as makers of improvements in "functional β-cell mass," and whether these changes reflect specific actions of the treatment with incretin mimetics or mainly the removal of glucolipotoxicity as a consequence of improved metabolic control, remain to be demonstrated in long-term studies. Islet and β-cell turnover appear to be much slower in human subjects than in rodents. Certainly, the demonstration of profound improvements in β-cell mass and function, possibly associated with a longer durability of anti-hyperglycemic effects of incretin mimetics relative to other antidiabetic agents, would suggest their use at earlier stages of type 2 diabetes, perhaps even including prediabetes.

A similar reasoning seem to apply to DPP-4 inhibitors: In selected animal models, effects of using sitagliptin or vildagliptin on the rate of β-cell apoptosis and β-cell mass have been demonstrated. In one clinical study an improvement in meal-related β-cell function after a year of treatment has been reported. If substantial benefits in terms of "β-cell health" could be demonstrated, this could broaden the indications for the use of DPP-4 inhibitors.

Cardiac Effects of GLP-1: Consequences of the Treatment with Incretin Mimetics and DPP-4 Inhibitors

The GLP-1 receptor is expressed in the heart. In GLP-1 receptor knock-out mice structural and functional cardiac abnormalities are typical. In animals, exposure to GLP-1 reduces the size of myocardial necroses in the case of induced infarction. In a pilot study with patients treated for acute myocardial infarction, a 48-h infusion of GLP-1 improved left-ventricular function and a wall-motility index. In a dog model of dilated cardiomyopathy, GLP-1 increased glucose uptake and left-ventricular function. These findings, together with the cardiovascular benefit expected from significant weight loss, make it appear possible, that incretin mimetics and/or DPP-4 inhibitors may be agents with the potential to reduce the incidence of cardiovascular events in patients with type 2 diabetes, thus targeting one of the main clinical problems of this metabolic disease. Such potential benefits should be studied in randomized controlled trials of appropriate size and duration.

With incretin mimetics and DPP-4 inhibitors, two novel classes of antidiabetic agents have been developed and are in the course of being approved for the treatment of patients with type 2 diabetes, which will certainly broaden the armamentarium of anti-hyperglycemic therapy. This is valid based on their properties that have already been characterized in clinical trials. Some additional properties need to be explored in future studies, but hold the promise to make a substantial contribution to changing the course of type 2 diabetes, from the prevention of the transition between the prediabetic state to manifest diabetes, to improved and more durable metabolic control with less unwanted side effects and the prevention of diabetic complications.

GLP-1 is an intestinal incretin hormone that stimulates insulin ("incretin") and suppresses glucagon secretion, inhibits gastric emptying, and reduces appetite and food intake. In contrast to the other incretin hormone, GIP, GLP-1 remains active in patients with type 2 diabetes. GLP-1 itself, however, cannot be used for therapeutic purposes because of its rapid proteolytic degradation and inactivation (DPP-4) and renal elimination, leading to a $t_{1/2}$ of 1–2 min. Therapeutic use of the antidiabetic properties of incretins, especially GLP-1, can be made using degradation-resistant GLP-1 receptor agonists ("*incretin mimetics*"), or inhibitors of DPP-4 activity ("*incretin enhancers*").

Clinical studies with exenatide (two injections per day or long-acting release form administered once-weekly) and liraglutide (one injection per day) have proven the antidiabetic efficacy with reductions in fasting and postprandial glucose concentrations and HbA_{1c} (~1–2%), associated with weight loss (2–5 kg). Treatment with incretin mimetics is associated with mild nausea, which occurs early, mostly transiently, after initiation. Orally administered DPP-4 inhibitors (e.g., sitagliptin, vildagliptin) reduce HbA_{1c} by approximately 0.6–1.0%. DPP-4 inhibitors are weight-neutral. There are no specific safety of tolerability concerns emerging from clinical trials. Both incretin mimetics and DPP-4 inhibitors have the potential to increase β-cell mass as shown in animal studies. However, long-term clinical studies are required to ascertain specific benefits of using novel antidiabetic agents derived from the enteroinsular axis, in particular incretin hormones like GLP- 1, in the treatment of type 2 diabetes.

14

PHARMACOGENETICS

The use of drugs to treat cardiac arrhythmias is characterized by highly variable efficacy and serious toxicity. Both of these are difficult to predict in an individual patient. Studies of the mechanisms underlying this variability and unpredictability in drug action have been important platforms for defining the role of genetics in drug action and have also pointed to general mechanisms in the initiation and maintenance of abnormal cardiac rhythms. In practical terms, the past decade has seen a decline in the use of antiarrhythmic drugs, in part because of their unpredictable efficacy and toxicity. As well, "*non-pharmacologic*" techniques, including ablation of abnormal tissues underlying arrhythmias and implantable defibrillators, have matured and are increasingly used.

A common feature of most antiarrhythmic drugs is that they were developed without a clear understanding of the cellular and molecular mechanisms underlying cardiac arrhythmias. As a result, the molecular targets with which they interact to suppress (or occasionally exacerbate) arrhythmias and cause other forms of toxicity are only now being defined. Virtually all antiarrhythmic drugs target membrane proteins, including adrenergic receptors and ion channels, structures that generate ion-specific permeation pathways (pores) in response to changes in their environment; common examples of such changes include alterations in transmembrane voltage (generated by other ion channels) or the presence of ligands such as acetylcholine. Studies defining the genetics of variable antiarrhythmic drug responses have not only pointed to new disease mechanisms, but also to strategies for development of new drugs lacking serious adverse effects and targeting underlying disease processes that culminate in arrhythmias. This review will first summarize the impact of variants in genes determining drug disposition on the effects of therapies used in the treatment of arrhythmias. The role of genetics in determining variable pharmacodynamics will then be considered.

GENETICS OF ANTIARRHYTHMIC DRUG DISPOSITION

CYP3A

Therapeutic drug monitoring was developed to optimize treatment with drugs that have a narrow margin between dosage required to produce efficacy and those producing adverse effects. Examples of such drug classes to which this approach has been applied include antibiotics, anticonvulsants, and antiarrhythmics. Initial descriptions of variable drug disposition as a consequence of disease or of drug interactions generally did not include a clear understanding of the specific molecular mechanisms underlying such variability. Thus, for example, anticonvulsants were recognized 30 years ago to strikingly lower concentrations of quinidine and to reduce its therapeutic efficacy. In contemporary terms, this interaction reflects induction of CYP3A4 by anticonvulsant drugs, likely acting through orphan nuclear hormone receptors. While functionally important polymorphisms in the coding region of CPY3A4 have not been identified, there are such variants in CYP3A5, a closely related enzyme with overlapping substrate specificity and a prominent role in drug disposition in intestine. Given this view, variability in CYP3A expression becomes a logical candidate mechanism for modulating antiarrhythmic drug concentrations and hence effects; such variability could arise from polymorphisms in the promoter region of the CYP3A complex or in the genes encoding nuclear hormone receptors that mediate enzyme and transporter expression. Specific studies addressing these possibilities have not, however, been conducted.

CYP2D6

CYP2D6 is responsible for the biotransformation of a number of drugs used to control cardiac arrhythmias, notably some beta-adrenergic receptor antagonists (metoprolol, timolol, and carvedilol) as well as the sodium channel blocking antiarrhythmics encainide (no longer marketed), propafenone, and flecainide. The CYP2D6 poor metabolizers (PMs) making up 7% of Caucasian and African-American populations (and rare in Asian populations) display higher plasma concentrations and greater pharmacologic effects during treatment with CYP2D6 substrate beta-blockers. The molecular basis of variable CYP2D6 activity is discussed in detail elsewhere in this volume. The "*third-generation*" beta-blocker carvedilol is increasingly used in the treatment of heart failure and may be especially effective because of some vasodilator activity, possibly attributable to alpha-blockade. The extent of alpha- and beta-blockade by this drug does appear to be at least in part CYP2D6-mediated, although clinical trial data demonstrating that variable outcomes during carvedilol therapy in heart failure can be related to this polymorphism have not yet been developed.

Propafenone is another example of a drug that exerts multiple actions, and displays genetically determined variability in its clinical effects. In vitro, propafenone not only blocks sodium channels but also exerts beta- blocking activity. Initial reports of clinically significant adverse effects (such as bradycardia or bronchospasm) due to beta-blockade during propafenone therapy emphasized the unpredictable nature of this adverse effect. However, when CYP2D6 phenotype is considered, it becomes clear that PM subjects are at greater risk than extensive metabolizers (EMs) for clinically significant beta-blockade during treatment with the drug since they develop much higher concentrations of the parent drug than do EMs. It is also possible that consistent incorporation of beta-blockade into an antiarrhythmic molecule might improve its efficacy. Indeed, combining propafenone with low-dose quinidine (a CYP2D6 inhibitor) can result in phenocopying to the PM phenotype, and small trials have been undertaken to test the antiarrhythmic effects of the combination.

The antiarrhythmic drug encainide is biotransformed by CYP2D6 to a potent active metabolite, O-desmethyl encainide. Interestingly, this active metabolite, in turn, also undergoes CYP2D6-mediated biotransformation to a second active metabolite, 3-methoxy O-desmethyl encainide. Thus, variable CYP2D6 activity is a likely contributor to variable levels of the parent drug and its two active metabolites, and this may underlie some of the variability observed when the drug was used clinically. Flecainide, a compound with similar electrophysiologic properties, is bio-transformed to inactive metabolites by CYP2D6 and also undergoes renal excretion of parent drug. Thus, CYP2D6 phenotype has much less impact on flecainide plasma concentrations and effect, except in the rare patient with coexisting renal dysfunction.

CYP2C9

The anticoagulant warfarin is increasingly used to prevent thromboembolic complications in patients with atrial fibrillation. The drug is administered as racemate, and bio-inactivation of the active S-enantiomer is accomplished by CYP2C9. Relatively common variants in CYP2C9 that reduce its function have been described, and homozygotes for reduction of function alleles appear to be at increased risk for bleeding complications with the drug.

N-Acetyltransferase

Plasma concentration monitoring of procainamide and its metabolite, N-acetylprocainamide (NAPA), led to the recognition that acetylator status is the major determinant of the development of anti-nuclear antibodies and the drug-induced lupus syndrome during procainamide therapy. This finding, in turn, pointed to the metabolism of procainamide by non-acetyl transferase pathways as an important modulator of this form of drug toxicity and also formed the rational for considering NAPA as a potentially less toxic antiarrhythmic entity. NAPA was found to exert electrophysiologic activity in vitro and to suppress some arrhythmias in patients; importantly, the clinical studies also showed that NAPA was not back-converted to procainamide and did not cause antinuclear antibodies. However, NAPA was not an especially potent antiarrhythmic, and it commonly caused non-cardiovascular adverse effects such as nausea. Interestingly, while both procainamide and NAPA prolong cardiac repolarization (manifest on the surface ECG as QT, interval prolongation, thought at the time to correlate with antiarrhythmic activity), only the parent drug blocked cardiac sodium channels. Thus, the NAPA structure did provide a starting point for the development of a series of new and highly potent QT-prolonging anti- arrhythmic drugs that saw some enthusiasm for their use in the 1980s and 1990s.

Importantly, these clinical studies were executed at a time when the molecular basis of the slow and fast acetylator phenotypes were not well understood. We now know that there are two isoforms of the *N*-acetyltransferase enzyme arising from two different genes, NAT1 and NAT2. Constitutive expression of NAT1 accounts for basal enzyme function, and functionally important polymorphisms in NAT2, are thought to contribute to variability in overall enzymatic activity and thus to define the slow- and fast-acetylators phenotypes.

P-Glycoprotein

Digoxin is the prototypical substrate for transport by P-glycoprotein, the product of expression of the MDR1 gene. Elevation of serum digoxin concentration and increased risk of serious toxicity result from co-administration of drugs that inhibit P-glycoprotein; these include quinidine, amiodarone, verapamil, itraconazole, erythromycin, and cyclosporine. MDR1 DNA polymorphisms that are linked to variability in serum digoxin concentrations have been described, although whether the polymorphisms are causative or in linkage disequilibrium to regulatory sites in the gene is not yet fully established.

Antiarrhythmic Drug Pharmacodynamics

Even at equivalent plasma concentrations of parent drug (and relevant active metabolites) the effect of antiarrhythmic therapies still vary considerably among individuals. There are a number of mechanisms that may underlie such variability. One is variable uptake or efflux transporter function, responsible for delivery to and removal from key intercellular sites of action. Drug effects may be different in normal vs. diseased (e.g., scarred or hypertrophied) hearts. Finally, a substantial body of knowledge has been accumulating over the past decade attesting to a prominent role of genetic factors in modulating normal and abnormal cardiac electrophysiology and, in turn, their responses to drug exposure.

An extraordinarily important starting point for this work has been identification of specific genes whose expression results in key proteins determining cardiac electrogenesis. Ion channels, pore-forming structures that respond to ligands or changes in voltage to permit transmembrane movement of specific ions, are the most important class of these proteins. One very important approach to identifying ion channel and related genes has been the study of rare monogenic (familial) arrhythmia syndromes.

Most currently available antiarrhythmic drugs were developed at a time when molecular mechanisms underlying arrhythmias were not appreciated. As a consequence, these drugs interact with a very limited number of molecular targets: the cardiac sodium channel, beta-1 adrenergic receptors, L-type calcium channels, and one specific potassium current (termed I_{Kr}). The genes whose expression results in these currents or receptors are now well understood. Many other genes have been identified whose expression generates or modulates ion currents in heart or otherwise prominently modulates overall cardiac electrical behavior. Indeed, this work has generated a lengthy list of potential "new" antiarrhythmic drug targets: these include potassium currents (I_{Ks} and I_{Kur}), pacemaker current (I_f), novel calcium currents (I_{Ca-T}; the A1D isoform of I_{Ca-L}), and cardiac connexins C×43.

Study of the rare congenital arrhythmia syndromes has been important for ion channel biologists because it identifies genes whose expression plays a crucial role in normal cardiac electrophysiology. It has also been interesting to demonstrate that mutations in these genes may result not only in manifest congenital arrhythmia syndromes, but also subclinical phenotypes that can then be uncovered by drug administration. These are discussed next, followed by a consideration of how more common DNA polymorphisms, in these and other genes, might modulate drug responses.

Pharmacogenetics of QT Prolongation

One important implication of this increasingly complex view of the molecular basis of cardiac electrophysiology is that variations in many genes may modulate not only basal cardiac electrophysiology but also its response to drugs. One interesting and important example relates to the occasional development of marked prolongation of the QT interval on the surface electrocardiogram, a finding that is associated with a high risk of morphologically distinctive, potentially fatal, polymorphic ventricular tachycardia termed "*torsades de pointes*." Torsades de pointes characteristically occurs in one of two clinical settings: in patients with a familial arrhythmia syndrome (the congenital Long QT Syndrome) and in patients exposed to drugs that have the potential to prolong the QT interval. The latter includes not only antiarrhythmic drugs, but a wide range of "*non-cardiovascular*" agents. Indeed, unexpected QT prolongation, torsades de pointes, and sudden death with the use of such drugs has been the single commonest reason for drug withdrawal in the United States over the past decade. Hence, evolving concepts with respect to the underlying molecular mechanisms of this distinctive arrhythmia syndrome have implications not only for management of patients with a relatively uncommon familial syndrome, but also have important implications for drug development in general.

The QT interval on the surface electrocardiogram represents the integrated behavior of a number of important ion currents active during the repolarization phase of a typical cardiac action potential. These include L-type calcium currents, a small contribution by sodium current, and several repolarizing potassium currents, notably the rapid component of the delayed rectifier (I_{Kr}), the slow component of the delayed rectifier (I_{Ks}), and the inward rectifier (I_{K1}). Studies of the congenital Long QT Syndrome in the mid-1990s identified mutations in the genes whose expression underlies I_{Kr}, I_{Ks}, and the cardiac sodium channel as the commonest causes of the syndrome. Importantly, cloning of the gene whose expression results in I_{Kr}, the Human Ether-a-go-go-Related Gene, or HERG (now known as KCNH2), was followed shortly thereafter by the recognition that virtually all drugs that prolong the QT interval do so by interacting with this particular ion channel protein. This work, then, provides an important link between a drug-induced syndrome and the congenital syndrome.

Another key observation made in the course of studying patients with the congenital syndrome was the identification of family members of pro-bands in whom mutations could be identified but the QT interval appeared normal. This "*incomplete penetrance*" then raises the question of whether some or all of patients developing "*idiosyncratic*" drug-induced QT prolongation and torsades de pointes represent individuals with a subclinical form of the congenital syndrome. Addressing this issue is not straight-forward, in part because several hundred mutations, in seven different genes, have now been identified in kindreds with this disease. Thus, unlike other common genetic diseases like cystic fibrosis or sickle cell anemia, there is a not a single predominant disease-associated mutation. As a result, any DNA variant identified in a patient with drug-associated torsades de pointes may be a disease-associated mutation, a predisposing polymorphism, or an irrelevant polymorphism, and distinguishing among these may be difficult. Nevertheless, case reports and one systematic survey of approximately 100 individuals with drug-induced torsades de pointes do support the concept of a genetic predisposition increasing susceptibility to this arrhythmia syndrome in approximately 10% of subjects. Some of these individuals do, indeed, have variants that alter channel function in vitro and that are absent in large numbers of ethnically matched controls; such patients can therefore be viewed as having the congenital syndrome, clinically inapparent in absence of drug challenge. In fact, in some instances, other family members may have manifest QT-interval prolongation in the absence of drugs, further confirming the diagnosis of the congenital syndrome. DNA polymorphisms may also predispose to drug-induced torsades de pointes, as discussed further below.

Clinical studies have identified a multitude of risk factors for drug-induced torsades de pointes, including female gender, congestive heart failure, left ventricular hypertrophy, hypokalemia, bradycardia, and subclinical ion channel dysfunction. A unifying framework to account for how these multiple factors may modulate risk is that of "*repolarization reserve*," which suggests that the normal expression and function of multiple gene products—with potentially redundant function—ordinarily acts to maintain a QT interval within the normal range. Subtle dysfunction of such gene products may be clinically inapparent and only be exposed by administration of a QT-prolonging drug. Thus, an individual harboring a subclinical loss of function mutation or polymorphism in the gene encoding I_{Ks} may not display any clinical phenotype at baseline, because of a robust I_{Kr}. Administration of an I_{Kr} blocker to such an individual might leave them with very little repolarizing current and hence would cause marked QT-interval prolongation. The concept of "*reduced repolarization reserve*," developed to provide a unified approach to thinking about torsades de pointes risk, can be readily adapted to many other biological systems; in general, highly variable clinical responses to drug challenge may reflect subtle dysfunction of genes whose products modulate a highly complex phenotype like the QT interval.

Altered Sodium Channel Function

Mutations that result in a "*gain of function*" in the cardiac sodium channel gene (SCN5A) cause the long QT Syndrome. By contrast, mutations in the same gene may result in loss of function and a different congenital syndrome, the "*Brugada syndrome*". Individuals with Brugada Syndrome have structurally normal hearts, a high risk of ventricular fibrillation, and a morphologically distinctive electrocardiogram. As in the Long QT Syndrome, mutation carriers who have a normal baseline electrocardiogram have been identified. In such cases, exposure to a sodium channel-blocking drug (e.g., flecainide or procainamide) is often used to unmask the Brugada Syndrome ECG phenotype. Indeed it was the observation that sodium channel block may unmask the ECG phenotype that led to consideration of SCN5A as a candidate in the Brugada Syndrome; in ~20% of pro-bands, mutations can be found in this gene. Occasional patients treated clinically with sodium channel-blocking drugs such as drugs such as flecainide, procainamide, or tricyclic depressants do develop the typical Brugada Syndrome ECG pattern; whether such individuals actually harbor subclinical Brugada Syndrome or are otherwise predisposed to sudden death during administration of these agents is a logical possibility.

From Rare Syndromes to Common Polymorphisms

Cases of subclinical congenital arrhythmia syndromes exposed by drug challenge are quite rare, but nevertheless constitute an important "*proof of concept*" of a genetic basis for variable drug responses. On the other hand, intensive study of monogenic arrhythmia syndrome disease genes, as well as other genes whose expression contributes to normal electrophysiology, has identified polymorphisms, some quite common, that may also modulate arrhythmia susceptibility. Population and association studies have identified such polymorphisms, with minor allele frequencies of 1.5–13% in control populations that appear to be over-represented among patients with drug-induced torsades de pointes. In such cases, in vitro studies have provided further support for the idea that the variant allele predisposes to the arrhythmia, especially in the presence of environmental triggers. The best-studied trigger for such arrhythmia susceptibility remains drug challenge, although other environmental stimuli, such as adrenergic activation or acute myocardial ischemia, could well play a role in other patients.

S1102Y in SCN5A is present in 13% of African Americans, but is absent or extremely rare in other ethnic groups. In vitro electrophysiologic studies showed that this variant does alter channel function, and clinical association studies suggest an overrepresentation of the Y allele in African-American subjects with a variety of arrhzythmia syndromes, including drug-induced arrhythmias, compared to African-American controls. Similarly, Q9E was initially identified as a mutation in KCNE2 (encoding a function-modulating potassium channel subunit). The proband was an elderly African-American woman who displayed torsades de pointes on exposure to an I_{Kr}-blocking antibiotic (clarithromycin), and further study revealed that Q9E does, in fact, alter I_{Kr} function in vitro. More recently, Q9E has been recognized as a relatively common polymorphism (5% minor allele frequency), again detected only in African-Americans. Other polymorphisms have been described that appear to modulate normal cardiac electrophysiology, although none have yet been linked convincingly to increased susceptibility to drug-induced arrhythmias. Thus, for example, K897T in HERG has been associated with longer QT intervals, particularly among women. H558R in SCN5A does not appear to alter baseline sodium channel function, but does modulate the clinical and in vitro phenotype of a disease-associated mutation in the same channel. A promoter polymorphism in the gene encoding the connexin C×40, whose normal function underlies cell–cell communication especially in atrium, appears to reduce gene expression. This polymorphism thus becomes a logical candidate gene for modulating the development of the very common arrhythmia atrial fibrillation and thus its response to drugs. Polymorphisms in the promoter region of cardiac sodium channel have been described that modulate expression of the channel in vitro; whether such polymorphisms underlie variable expression of the channel in patients and thus variable responses to challenges such as sodium channel-blocking drugs or acute myocardial ischemia is not yet known. Finally, recent clinical and mechanistic studies implicate activation of a number of key signaling pathways, such as the beta-adrenergic system, the renin-angiotensin-aldosterone system, oxidant stress, or inflammation, as potential arrhythmia triggers. Variants in these pathways then become new candidates for modulating arrhythmia susceptibility.

Currently available arrhythmic drugs were developed at a time when the molecular basis of cardiac arrhythmias was not understood. Thus, therapy has been largely empiric, efficacy has been unpredictable, and serious side effects have been common. Some of variability in clinical action of antiarrhythmic drugs can be attributed directly to variable drug disposition, through specific pathways whose activity is now well recognized to be modulated by common DNA polymorphisms. An in-depth understanding of the molecular basis or normal cardiac electrophysiology has come from a number of approaches, notably including the intensive study of families with rare monogenic arrhythmia syndromes. Variations in the complex physiologic signaling system that results in normal electrical activity now appears to be a proximate cause of most cardiac arrhythmias. DNA variants in genes encoding elements of this system may result in disease, or may more commonly modulate arrhythmia risk in the face of exogenous stressors, including drugs, in the susceptible patient. Further definition of these molecular mechanisms and the polymorphisms that underlie such susceptibility should lead to the development of drug therapies targeting underlying pathophysiologic mechanisms, and lacking common and serious adverse effects. As in many areas of pharmacogenetics, real advances require a partnership between clinical and basic investigators to precisely identify variable and important clinical phenotypes and then define mechanisms underlying that variability.

15

NEW ANTICANCER AGENTS

Development of new anticancer and cancer prevention agents presents significant challenges to clinical trialists. The correct design of all phases of clinical trials is essential to ensure as rapid and as successful a development as possible. One must have a plan that will give the new agent the best chance of matching its preclinical activity. Because there have been problems with this in the past, it is virtually certain that many promising new agents were dismissed as being inactive because of flaws in clinical trial design. This chapter provides information on multiple types of clinical trial designs that can and have been used for approval of new anticancer (and prevention) agents.

METHODS TO SELECT AGENTS THAT WILL BE ACTIVE IN THE CLINIC

Of course, if people knew for certain how to select agents that would definitely work in the clinic it is likely we would be much further along in our treatment of patients with cancer. However, there are some techniques that have been reported in the literature and that our drug development teams in San Antonio and in Tucson have used to increase the chances of bringing agents into clinical trials that will eventually be approved for clinical use. In the period of 1978–1983 our team just took the "next agent to come along" into the Phase I clinical trials. Unfortunately, only 3 of the 26 agents (12%) we took into Phase I trials during that time period were subsequently approved by the Food and Drug Administration (FDA). Clearly, we needed to do better than that.

In 1983, a significant publication by Staquet and colleagues reviewed the success of the various murine or human tumor cell lines that were being utilized as in vivo systems by the National Cancer Institute to evaluate all of the potential antineoplastic agents. In that study they noted that murine leukemias L1210 and P388, the murine B 16 melanoma, and the MX-1 mammary human tumor xenograft were the most predictive for antitumor activity in the clinic. These models were even more predictive if one used tumor regression or percent cure (≥ 45-d survivors) as an endpoint.

Models that were not predictive included the murine colon cancers Co26 and Co38, the CX-1 and LX-1, human tumor xenografts, and the Lewis lung model. When we utilized the Staquet suggested models to select agents for Phase I trials, the success rate for our program (as judged by the percent of new agents that were eventually approved by the FDA divided by all of the agents that we took into Phase I trials during that period) increased to 31%. In 1990 our team had the clinical impression that every time we took a new agent with a new mechanism of action into a Phase I clinical trial (e.g., tubulin inhibitors, such as docetaxel or paclitaxel, topoismerase I inhibitors such as topotecan or CPT11, or a chain terminator such as gemcitabine) it was very likely that the drug would eventually be approved. Using the additional parameter of a new mechanism of action, the success rate again appeared to improve.

The introduction of targeted monoclonal antibodies (MAbs) has also appeared to increase success rates. As is noted, by using the Staquet criteria plus the new mechanisms of action criteria, plus MAbs, it is estimated that nearly 67% of all new agents brought into Phase I trials will eventually demonstrate antitumor activity significant enough for approval by the FDA (provided that the appropriate pivotal trials are designed for the agent).

The point of MAbs is worth emphasizing. If one has a MAb specific to a particular cell surface antigen or receptor, it appears to be an excellent prognostic factor for activity and for approval. In summary, with some rather simplistic approaches, we believe some of the risk of development of new anticancer agents can be taken out of the process. In fact the likelihood of success can be very high.

Table 15.1. Example of new mechanism of action against specific targets: monoclonal antibodies against specific targets

Target	*Monoclonal antibody(s)*	*Clinical activity*
CD20	Rituximab (Rituxan)	Lymphoma
Her2/*neu*	Trastuzumab (Herceptin)	Breast, others
CD52	Alemtuzumab (CAMPATH)	CLL
CD20	Radiolabeled ibritumomab (Tiuxetan, Zevalin)	Lymphoma
EGFR	IMC-255; ABX-EGF	Colorectal
17-1A	Edrecolomab (Panorex)	Colorectal cancer
VEGF	Bevacizumab (Avastin)	Colorectal cancer renal cell, lung
Other	Many other	Other

General Aspects of Clinical Trial Design for Approval

It was stated above that agents with new mechanisms of action had a high probability of success—if the pivotal trials with the agent were designed correctly. To achieve that high probability of success some important aspects of clinical trial design include:

1. Try to select a clinical situation that closely mimics what was found in the preclinical data package. For example, if the new agent demonstrated only growth delays in an animal system, one should probably not design pivotal trials with response rate (e.g., tumor shrinkage) as a primary endpoint. Rather, one should utilize median survival or time to tumor progression (TTP) or time to treatment failure (TTF) as primary endpoints. The TTP or TTF endpoints are usually acceptable to regulatory agencies only if the trial is double-blinded. This is because clinicians caring for patients, and patients themselves, are most anxious to get off of a control arm and on to the new agent arm. This frequently will lead to a declaration that the control arm is not working so the patient can be crossed over to the new agent arm of the study. Thus, double-blinding is very helpful if it is at all possible. Another, more cumbersome method is to use an outside, independent, blinded review panel to assess tumor progression.
2. Make sure the sample size is large enough to give the new agent a real chance. For example, a sample size that allows one to detect only a 50% improvement in survival is too small of a sample size because that hurdle for any new agent is almost certainly too high (50% improvement). This is a setup for failure. Sample size must be large enough to give the new agent a chance e.g., a 25% improvement.
3. It is clear that if you are expecting an agent to be used to change the upfront treatment for patients with a specific type of tumor, two well controlled (and randomized) Phase III trials will need to

be performed. Normally two *well controlled* trials does not necessarily mean they have to be randomized trials. For example, well controlled could mean a well monitored study, or a study in which patients serve as their own controls. However, in the upfront situation, where the new agent is planned to change standard treatment, it is very likely that two *randomized* Phase III trials will be a necessity. There may be one exception to the two well controlled randomized Phase III trials requirement. It might be possible to obtain approval for the new agent to be used in an "upfront" situation if the level of significance for the primary endpoint of the Phase III trial is $p < 0.001$. As many experienced investigators can attest, a p value of that magnitude is indeed unusual in most Phase III trials.

4. It is frequently said that one must have an improvement in survival for a new agent to be approved. That is, of course, desirable. However, survival has not always been required. Table 3 details the new agents brought to the FDA Oncology Advisory Board for approval, the type of study(ies) that lead to approval, and the parameters used for that approval. As can be seen in that Table 3, there were 69 approvals and 16 disapprovals (note that some agents were brought multiple times for approval in different indications). As can be seen in that table there were 25 approvals based primarily on response, 16 on survival, 10 on TTP, and 18 based on other primary endpoints. There were 27 approvals based on Phase II trials and 42 approvals based on Phase III trials. One can also note that a variety of other endpoints have been used as primary parameters for approval (e.g., control of pleural effusion, reduction in dysplasia, etc.).

   It is this investigator's personal experience that regulatory agencies will entertain endpoints other than survival (see below) if that new endpoint is discussed prospectively with and in detail with the regulatory agencies. They, like us, like challenges.

5. As is noted above, the FDA and other world regulatory agencies have approved new agents based on response (as a surrogate for survival or for benefit for the patient). The landmark publication that really codified response rate as a surrogate was the article by O'Shaugnhessy and colleagues in which the general guidelines were put forth for approval based on Phase II results. There are many FDA observers who feel that response is no longer an approvable strategy, but it does document that it still can be a strategy for approval under the right circumstances, including:

   (a) a very high response rate or a substantial/complete response rate (where the responses are durable) which is something unexpected for a new agent. The best example of this is the high response rates noted with arsenic trioxide for patients with refractory acute promyelocytic leukemia.

   (b) a lower response rate but a low incidence of side effects. An excellent example of this is the Phase II experience with Herceptin for patients with refractory breast cancer (with response rates of 11% but with no significant side effects).

If you plan to use a Phase II strategy for approval, in general it is better to utilize a Phase II trial design with a reference arm. Otherwise there is a concern about patient selection (e.g., selection of long-term survivors regardless of treatment). Two possible strategies to give most reviewers confidence that it is indeed your new agent that is making a difference include trial designs such as:

(a) Patients with a refractory malignancy ↗ High dose of the new agent
↘ Lower dose of the new agent

Endpoints: response rate or time to tumor progression (if the arms are blinded).

(b) Patients with a refractory malignancy ↗ New agent
↘ Clinician's choice

Endpoint: response rate—as it is more difficult to blind the trial. (*Note*: this could be a 2:1 randomized of new agent vs clinician's choice.)

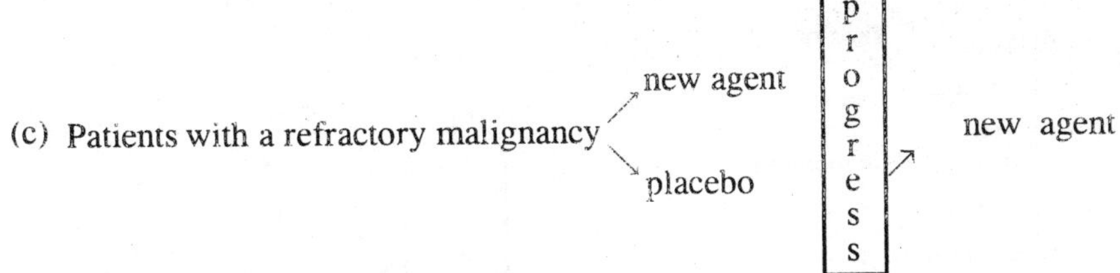

Endpoint: Time to tumor progression with a crossover allowed.

These types of randomized Phase II trials help (page 587) ensure everyone that there is no super-selection of your study population to select for patients who would have a favorable outcome irrespective of which treatment they were given.

Special Trial Designs, Particularly Suited for Cytostatic Agents

Patients as their Own Controls

This is a trial design that, until recently, was all but forgotten. There are at least two versions of this trial design. As can be seen, version 1, any patient who has a longer time on treatment on regimen B than on regimen A is considered a positive result (it is usually not an expected result for a patient to remain on treatment with a second- line regimen for a longer time than on a first-line regimen). This is certainly an inexact situation, as time on treatment is not the same as time to progression, but it is easier to measure when one does not have scans and X-ray films at regular intervals for the first regimen, as one usually has for the second regimen. Even though this is an inexact clinical trial situation, this trial design might offer some insight on whether or not the agent is having an effect on the natural history of the patient's disease. Based on past experience, if ≥30% of patients have a longer time on the new agent than on the regimen they received just prior to the new agent, that is a promising result that should be pursued.

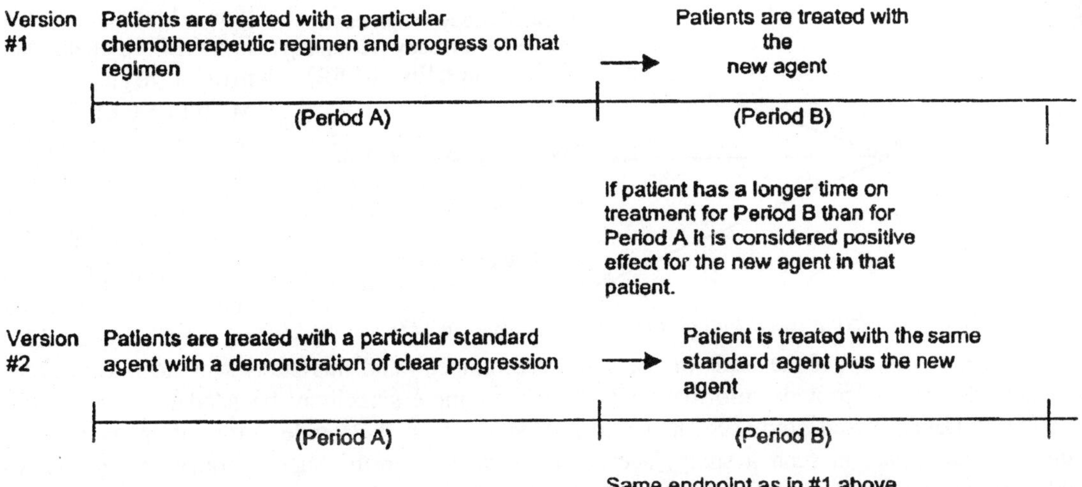

Fig. 15.1. Two versions of patients as their own control type of trial design.

To try version 2 of patients as their own controls one must have some preclinical information demonstrating that there is some synergy between the new cytostatic agent and the agent the patient is currently receiving. It is also critical in this design to make *very certain* that the patient is progressing on regimen A (best ascertained by an independent committee). It needs to be emphasized again that this type of trial is only an *exploratory trial*—but a trial that may again give hints of the agent changing the natural history of the disease. It is not a definitive trial design. This latter (version 2) design has already had a checkered start in that it was utilized for the design for the initial filing of the anti-epidermal growth factor receptor monoclonal antibody C225. The problem with that filing, however, was that it appears that there was unclear documentation as to whether or not the patient progressed on the initial regimen of CPT11 (period A) to which the C225 was added (during period B). That particular situation should not discourage the clinical investigator from trying version 2 of patients as their own controls *if* the new cytostatic agent demonstrates synergy with the standard cytotoxic agent (or other cytostatic agents for that matter).

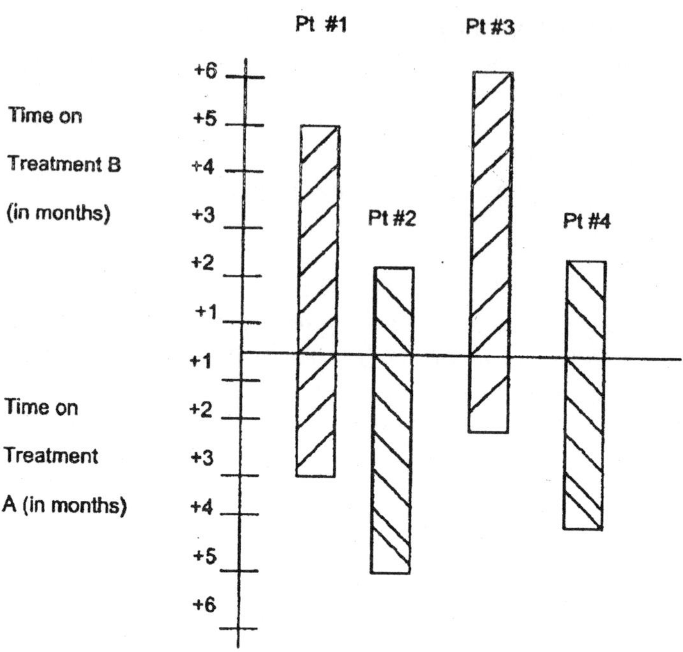

Fig. 15.2. Suggested manner for plotting time on treatment for period B vs time on treatment for period A.

Randomized Phase II Trial

This type of trial design was mentioned above. With some clever additional variations it can yield a great deal of information. As noted, the study was a three-arm study of chemotherapy vs chemotherapy plus a low dose of a MAb to VGEF vs chemotherapy plus a high dose of a MAb to VGEF. As can be seen, one of the endpoints for the study, in addition to toxicities, was the TTP. Once again, TTP can be a somewhat inexact endpoint and one that is not usually acceptable to a regulatory agency (except if the arms of the study are blinded—and this study was not). However, the above study design can provide information as to what sample sizes may be needed for an new drug application (NDA)-directed study. Such a study design can also provide information as to whether patients will participate in such a study, accrual rates, and so forth. Such a study design also yields valuable information on the safety of the various arms of the study.

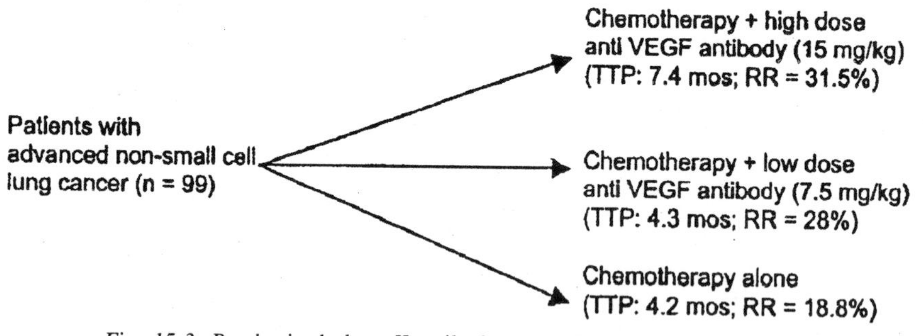

Fig. 15.3. Randomized phase II trail of a monoclonal antibody to VEGF.

An important option for the study is to continue with the study in a randomized fashion, selecting only one of the MAb-containing arms for comparison with the chemotherapy alone arm. This approach can save significant activation time for a new protocol (e.g., continue the randomized Phase II trial and power it up to be large enough for a Phase III trial rather than writing and activating a whole new Phase III trial). Another randomized Phase II trial that yielded very important information and which serves as an excellent model for solving drug development issues is a trial performed with the agent capecitabine (Xeloda). After results became available from the Phase I clinical trials with several different schedules of the agent, there was uncertainty as to just which schedule was the best. Therefore a randomized Phase II trial was conducted to determine which schedule (and dose) of capecitabine would be best to take into expanded Phase II and Phase III clinical trials. Patients were randomized to receive either: (a) 1331 mg/m^2/d continually; (b) 2510 mg/m^2/d intermittently, or (c) 1657 mg/m^2/d plus leucovorin 60 mg/d p.o. intermittently. The specific aims were to evaluate the safety and efficacy of each schedule. Cleverly, one of the efficacy endpoints utilized (in addition to response rate) was TTP. Utilizing TTP as a parameter of efficacy allowed a finer tuning because it allowed for a continuous assessment (in days) vs the dichotomous variable of response (response or no response). This clever randomized Phase II design showed that schedule "b" was the best schedule in terms of toxicities and efficacy. That schedule was then taken on into successful Phase II and Phase III trials, which led to the very rapid approval of capecitabine.

Randomized Discontinuation Trial Designs

This is a unique trial design for the development of cytostatic agents that has several very desirable features and yet seems as though it might be a very very difficult trial to complete. In reality, our team at the Arizona Cancer Center just participated in placing patients on a clinical trial utilizing this randomized discontinuation design and we have found excellent patient participation in the study. The design is particularly well suited for a new cytostatic agent that everyone wants to receive (just as the new agent endostatin was). All eligible patients initially received the new agent. Those who progress before 4 mo of treatment are completed are removed from the study. Those patients who do have a response or have stable disease for 4 mo are then randomized to continue the therapy or receive a placebo. The patients are carefully observed and if they have progressive disease (and are receiving placebo), they are placed back on the new agent. The endpoint for the study is the TTP for patients who continue on the therapy vs the TTP for patients who receive placebo.

The randomized discontinuation trial design has been used for testing new agents against the AIDS virus but it is just beginning to be used to evaluate new anticancer agents. Obviously when used in the situation with a new AIDs drug(s) one has viral titers to follow (vs computed axial tomography [CAT] scans and other imaging techniques for oncologists to follow a patient's tumor). The viral titers are more sensitive than our scans are. Also, some investigators question the ethics of randomizing patients who are responding to the new agent to continue, or discontinue that therapy. This problem can be addressed by randomizing only the patients with stable disease (and not the responders). Very carefully administered informed consent is obviously a necessity. One other potential problem with the randomized discontinuation design is that there is a theoretical problem in comparing the patients continued on

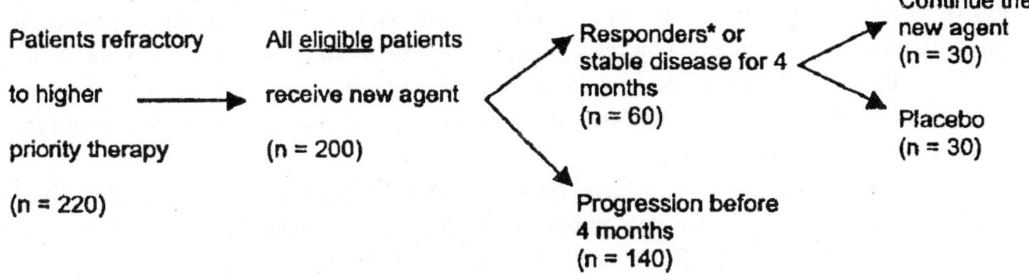

Fig. 15.4. Randomized discontinued design.

therapy vs those on placebo if there is a carryover effect of the agent (i.e., it could still be having an effect on the placebo group).

Regardless of its downsides, the randomized discontinuation trial design is one that should be considered for a new cytostatic agent. It does allow for a greater number of patients to have access to a potentially exciting new agent.

A Unique Endpoint for Approval

Clinical Benefit

In the early development of the chain terminator gemcitabine there were some patients with pancreatic cancer who demonstrated a decrease in their tumor-related pain and an increase in their appetite and weight. Gemcitabine had a new mechanism of action. It did not cause regression of pancreatic cancer growing in nude mice but rather it caused a slowing of growth of the pancreatic cancer xenografts growing in nude mice (MIA Pa Ca, PANC-1 and PAN C02). Therefore, it was likely that one would not see a complete or partial response in patients. In conversations with Dr. Bob Temple at the FDA and Dr. Gregory Burke our team was alerted to the fact that one endpoint they could accept in a trial was "fixing what bothers the patient." The term *clinical benefit* was derived from that conversation. Clinical benefit was not necessarily a quality of life parameter but it was an attempt to measure "fixing what bothers the patient." Because the three most common problems experienced by patients with pancreatic cancer included pain, weight loss, and a deterioration in performance status, Dr. John Anderson at Eli Lilly devised an algorithm to measure clinical benefit. This algorithm utilized pain performance status (measured by the Karnofsky scale because it had a broader range of 0–100 in increments of 10 rather than the ECOG or SWOG scales which have a range of only 0–5), and a direct measurement of weight (with clear cut definitions of what constituted weight gain or weight loss). The pivotal trial design for gemcitabine was as follows:

Patients with advanced, symptomatic pancreatic cancer ↗ Weekly gemcitabine
↘ Weekly 5 - FU

The primary endpoint for the study was an improvement in clinical benefit, with the secondary endpoints including response rate, median survival, and percentage of patients alive at 1 yr.

The study was positive for clinical benefit as well as for the other parameters. Gemcitabine was approved for use for treatment of patients with locally advanced or metastatic pancreatic cancer by the Oncology Drug Advisory Committee (ODAC) and by the FDA on the basis of this one study. In addition, there was a Phase II trial that was uncontrolled but demonstrated a similar survival (and response) to that found in the randomized phase III study. Gemcitabine was approved for treatment of patients with locally advanced or metastatic pancreatic cancer. Many observers who were present at the ODAC felt that gemcitabine would not have been approved if clinical benefit were the only parameter that was improved by gemcitabine. The other item of note is that gemcitabine was approved for frontline treatment of patients with advanced pancreatic cancer based on only one randomized trial. Observers at the ODAC felt that was because there were very few options for patients (and no prior controlled trials ever demonstrated an improvement in survival for any single agent) with advanced pancreatic cancer that gemcitabine was approved.

It is of note that no other attempts have been made to bring a new agent to the FDA using the clinical benefit parameter as the primary endpoint of the study. However, this investigator believes that with the proper algorithm it could be a solid primary endpoint for other pivotal trials with a new agent.

Special Challenges in Clinical Trial Designs for Approval

Analogs

Unfortunately in anticancer drug development we are still in the sulfonamide era—meaning that it is probably more productive to find agents with new mechanisms of action (for greater progress) than to work on analogs. However, there have been many commercial successes with analogs, largely based on less (or different) toxicities rather than on improved efficacy. The types of trials for approval for an analog program could be:

(a) Patients whose tumors are progressing on the parent compound (with very clear documentation of that progress) → Patient is treated with analog Endpoint: Response rate

Endpoint: Response rate

Issues with this design include a very refractory patient population. However, if the analog has activity in that setting, it will certainly have a substantial chance for approval.

(b) Treat patients with the new analog who have a tumor type that is not responsive to the parent compound → Patient is treated with the analog Endpoint: Response rate

Endpoint: Response rate

The issue here is that it is unlikely the analog will work in this situation. However, if it does work in this situation it also will have an excellent chance for eventual approval.

(c) Patient with a disease usually responsive to the parent compound ↗ New analog ↘ Parent compound

Endpoints: Survival, response rate, TTP toxicities

This is the best way to evaluate a new analog and the most likely way for an analog to be approved by regulatory agencies. Of course, superiority in one of the endpoints (not equivalence) is usually more convincing for approval.

Other Comments on Clinical Trials for Approval

Given the difficulty of treating patients with cancer, this author (as do many others in the field) believes that we should do everything we can to gain approval for new agents so patients have options. There are frequently numerous criticisms passing back and forth between investigators, regulators, educators, survivors, and others. At times their criticisms are valid—that perhaps we are asking for so much proof that an agent works (e.g., an improvement in survival) that it is discouraging to all involved and actually dampens any enthusiasm for development of new agents. It is this author's belief that the more these different constituencies communicate and work together (without assigning blame), the better chance we will have to develop innovative endpoints and trial designs for more rapid approval. Our job, together, is to obtain more options for clinical trial designs that allow development of new agents that work for our patients.

16

Antihypertensive Drugs

Recently, much attention has been focused on the interaction of small molecules with biological macromolecules. The search for selective enzyme inhibitors and receptor agonists or antagonists is one of the keys for target-oriented research in the pharmaceutical industry. Increased understanding of the mechanism of drug interaction on a molecular level has led to wide awareness of the importance of chirality as the key to the efficacy of many drug products. It is now known that in many cases only one enantiomer of a drug substance is required for efficacy and the other enantiomer is either inactive or exhibits considerably reduced activity. Pharmaceutical companies are aware that, where appropriate, new drugs for development should be homochiral to avoid the possibility of unnecessary side effects due to an undesirable enantiomer. In many cases where the switch from racemate drug substance to enantiomerically pure compound is feasible, there is the opportunity to extend the use of an industrial process. The physical characteristics of an enantiomer versus racemic compound may confer processing or formulation advantages.

Chiral drug intermediates can be prepared by different routes. One approach is to obtain them from naturally derived chiral synthons, produced mainly by fermentation processes. The chiral pool refers primarily to inexpensive, readily available, optically active natural products. A second approach is to carry out the resolution of racemic compounds. This approach can be achieved by preferential crystallization of enantiomers or diastereomers and by kinetic resolution of racemic compounds by chemical or biocatalytic methods. Finally, chiral synthons can also be prepared by asymmetric synthesis by either chemical or biocatalytic processes using microbial cells or enzymes derived therefrom. The advantages of microbial or enzyme-catalyzed reactions over chemical reactions are that they are stereoselective and can be carried out at ambient temperature and atmospheric pressure. The biocatalytic approach minimizes problems of isomerization, racemization, epimerization, and rearrangement that may occur during chemical processes. Biocatalytic processes are generally carried out in aqueous solution. These types of processes will avoid the use of environmentally harmful chemicals currently implemented in chemical processes and subsequent solvent waste disposal. Furthermore, microbial cells or enzymes derived therefrom can be immobilized and reused for many cycles. Recently, a number of review articles have been published on the use of enzymes in organic synthesis. This chapter provides some specific examples of preparation of chiral drug intermediates required for our antihypertensive agents.

Vasopeptidase Inhibitor

Enzymatic Synthesis of L-6-Hydroxynorleucine

L-6-Hydroxynorleucine is a chiral intermediate that is useful for the synthesis of a vasopeptidase inhibitor now in clinical trial and for the synthesis of C-7–substituted azepinones as potential intermediates

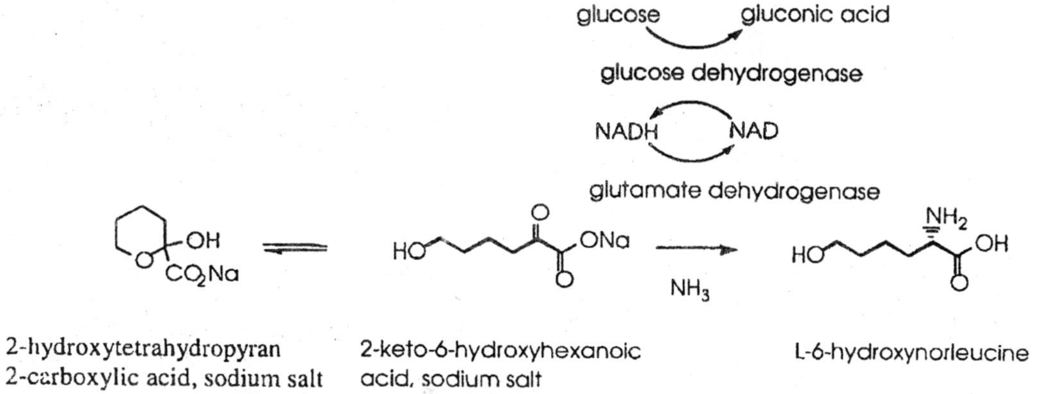

glucose → gluconic acid

glucose dehydrogenase

NADH ⇄ NAD

glutamate dehydrogenase

2-hydroxytetrahydropyran 2-carboxylic acid, sodium salt ⇌ 2-keto-6-hydroxyhexanoic acid, sodium salt —NH_3→ L-6-hydroxynorleucine

Fig. 16.1. Preparation of chiral synthon for vasopeptidase inhibitor.

for other antihypertensive metalloprotease inhibitors. It has also been used for the synthesis of siderophores, indospicines, and peptide hormone analogs. Previous synthetically useful methods for obtaining this intermediate have involved synthesis of the racemic compound followed by enzymatic resolution: D-Amino acid oxidase has been used to convert the D-amino acid to the ketoacid, leaving the L-enantiomer which was isolated by ion-exchange chromatography. In a second approach, racemic N-acetyl hydroxynorleucine has been treated with L-amino acid acylase to give the L-enantiomer. Both of these resolution methods give a maximum 50% yield and require separation of the desired product. Reductive amination of ketoacids using amino acid dehydrogenases has become a useful method for synthesis of natural and non-natural amino acids.

We have developed the synthesis and conversion of 2-keto-6-hydroxyhexanoic acid to L-6-hydroxynorleucine by a reductive amination process using beef liver glutamate dehydrogenase. 2-Keto-6-hydroxyhexanoic acid was converted completely to L-6-hydroxynorleucine by beef liver glutamate dehydrogenase. A nicotinamide adenine dinucleotide (NAD^+)-dependent formate dehydrogenase from *Candida boidinii* or glucose dehydrogenase from *Bacillus megaterium* was used for regeneration of reduced nicotinamide adenine dinucleotide (NADH) required for this reaction. The beef liver glutamate dehydrogenase was used for preparative reactions at 100 g/liter substrate concentration. 2-keto-6-hydroxyhexanoic acid, sodium salt, in equilibrium with 2-hydroxytetrahydropyran-2-carboxylic acid, sodium salt, is converted to L-6-hydroxynorleucine. The reaction requires ammonia and NADH. NAD^+ produced during the reaction was recycled to NADH by glucose dehydrogenase from *B. megaterium*. Reaction was completed in about 3 hr with reaction yields of 89–92%, and enantiomeric excess (e.e.) of >98% for L-6-hydroxynorleucine.

Chemical synthesis and isolation of 2-keto-6-hydroxyhexanoic acid required several steps. In a second, more convenient process, the ketoacid was prepared by treatment of racemic 6-hydroxynorleucine [produced by hydrolysis of 5-(4-hydroxybutyl)hydantoin] with D-amino acid oxidase and catalase. After the e.e. of the remaining L-6-hydroxynorleucine had risen to >99%, the reductive amination procedure was used to convert the mixture containing 2-keto-6-hydroxyhexanoic acid and L-6-hydroxynorleucine entirely to L-6-hydroxynorleucine with yields of 91–97% and e.e. of >98%. Sigma porcine kidney D-amino acid oxidase and beef liver catalase or *Trigonopsis variabilis* whole cells (source of oxidase and catalase) were used successfully for this transformation.

Enzymatic Synthesis of Allysine Ethylene Acetal

(*S*)-2-Amino-5-(1,3-dioxolan-2-yl)-pentanoic acid [allysine ethylene acetal] is one of three building blocks used for an alternative synthesis of omapatrilat, a vasopeptidase inhibitor. It has previously

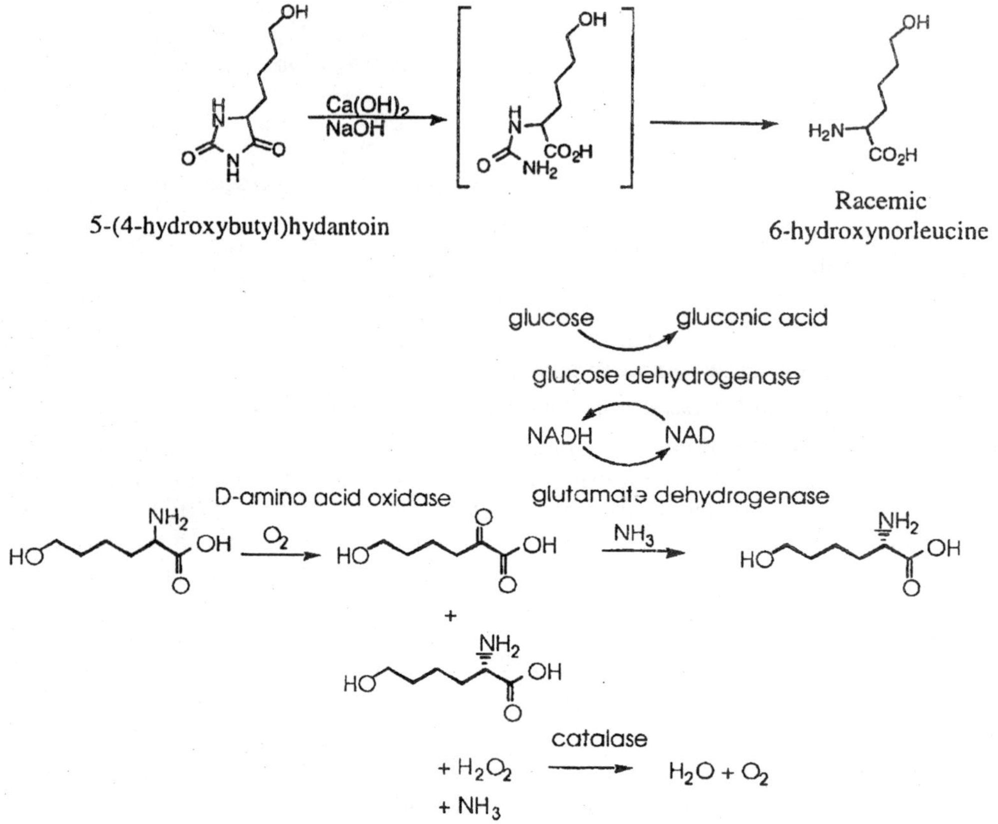

Fig. 16.2. Chemical conversion of 5-(4-hydroxybutyl)hydantoin to racemic 6-hydroxynorleucine.

been prepared in an eight- step synthesis from 3,4-dihydro-2H-pyran. The reductive amination of ketoacid acetal to acetal amino acid was demonstrated using phenylalanine dehydrogenase from *Thermoactinomyces intermedius*. The reaction requires ammonia and NADH. NAD^+ produced during the reaction was recycled to NADH by the oxidation of formate to CO_2 using formate dehydrogenase from *C. boidinii*. An initial process was developed using heat-dried cells of*T. intermedius* ATCC 33205 as a source of phenylalanine dehydrogenase, and heat-dried cells of methanol-grown *C. boidinii* as a source of formate dehydrogenase.

An improved process was also developed using phenylalanine dehydrogenase from *T. intermedius* expressed in *Escherichia coli BL21 (DE3)* (pPDH155K) [SC16144] in combination with *C. boidinii* as a source of formate dehydrogenase. A third-generation process using methanol-grown *Pichia pastoris* as a source of endogenous formate dehydrogenase and *E. coli* SC16144 expressing *T. intermedius* phenylalanine dehydrogenase was also developed.

Glutamate, alanine, leucine, and phenylalanine dehydrogenases converted to the desired amino acid. Using an extract of *T. intermedius* ATCC 33205 as a source of phenylalanine dehydrogenase and formate dehydrogenase from *C. boidinii* for NADH regeneration, the reaction yield of 80% was obtained, and the process was developed using this enzyme combination. Heat-dried cells of*T. intermedius* and *C. boidinii* SC13822 grown on methanol were used for the reaction.

Phenylalanine dehydrogenase activities in cells recovered from fermentations. *T. intermedius* gave useful activity on a small scale (15 liters), but lysed soon after the end of the growth period, making

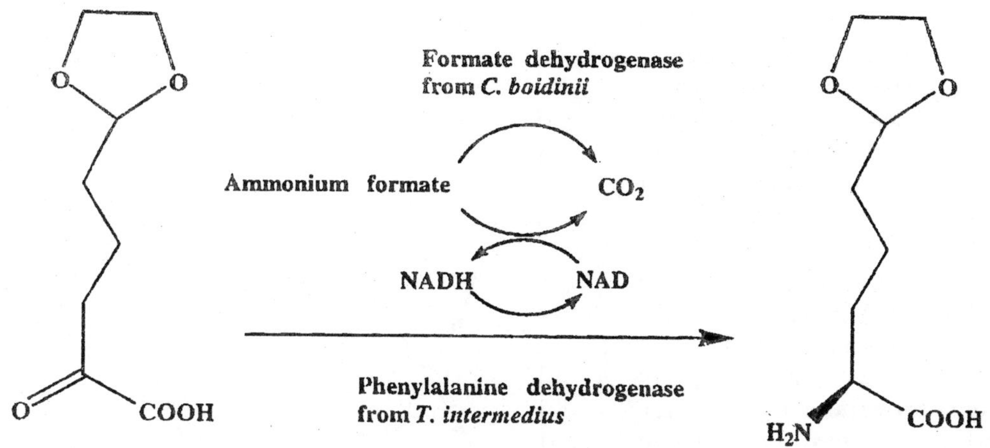

Fig. 16.3. Preparation of chiral synthon for vasopeptidase inhibitor.

recovery of activity difficult or impossible on a large scale (4000 liters). The problem was solved by cloning and expressing the *T. intermedius* phenylalanine dehydrogenase in *E. coli*, inducible by isopropyl thiogalactoside. Fermentation of *T. intermedius* yielded 184 units of phenylalanine dehydrogenase activity per liter of whole broth in 6 hr. At harvest, because the activity was unstable, the fermentor needed to be cooled rapidly. In contrast, the recombinant *E. coli* produced over 19,000 units per liter of whole broth in about 14 hr, and the activity was stable at harvest. *C. boidinii* grown on methanol was a useful source of formate dehydrogenase as described previously. In order to recover the cells on a large scale, 0.5% methanol was added to stabilize the cells.

P. pastoris grown on methanol was also a useful source of formate dehydrogenase. Expression of *T. intermedius* phenylalanine dehydrogenase in *P. pastoris*, inducible by methanol, allowed both enzymes to be obtained from a single fermentation. Formate dehydrogenase activity per gram of wet cells was 2.7-fold greater than for *C. boidinii*, and fermentor productivity was increased by 8.7-fold compared to *C. boidinii*. Fermentor productivity for phenylalanine dehydrogenase in *P. pastoris* was about 28% of the recombinant *E. coli* productivity.

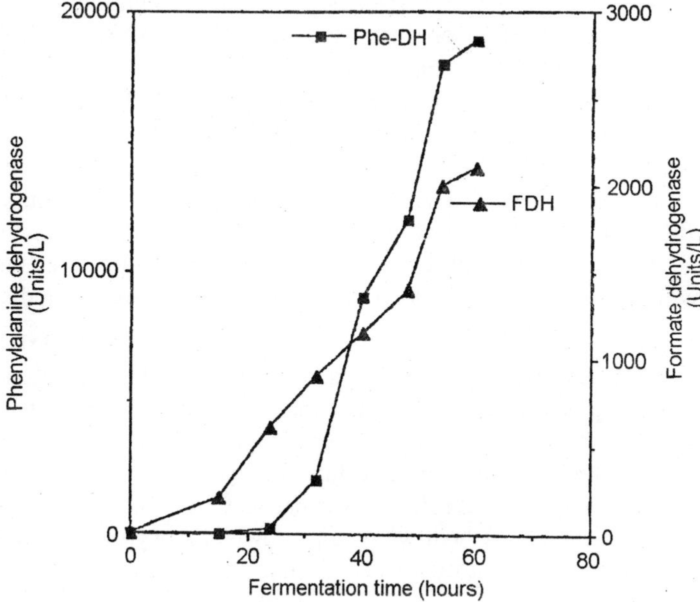

Fig. 16.4. Production of phenylalanine dehydrogenase and formate dehydrogenase in P. pastoris.

Formate dehydrogenase has been reported to have a pH optimum of 7.5–8.5. The pH optimum for the reductive amination of by an extract of *T. intermedius* was found to be about 8.7. Reductive amination reactions were carried out at pH 8.0. The time course for a representative batch showing conversion of ketoacid to amino acid using *E. coli/C. boidinii* heat-dried cells.

The procedure using heat-dried cells of *E. coli* containing cloned phenylalanine dehydrogenase and heat-dried *C. boidinii* was scaled up. A total of 197 kg of was produced in three 1600-liter batches using a 5% concentration of substrate with an average yield of 91 M% and e.e. of >98%.

Third-generation procedure, using dried recombinant *P. pastoris* expressing *T. intermedius* phenylalanine dehydrogenase inducible with methanol, and endogenous formate dehydrogenase induced when *P. pastoris* was grown in medium containing methanol, allowed both enzymes to be produced during a single fermentation. The two enzymes were conveniently produced in about the right ratio that was used for the reaction. The *Pichia* reaction procedure had the following modifications of the *E. coli*/ *C. boidinii* procedure: concentration of substrate was increased to 100 g/liter, one-fourth the amount of NAD was used, and dithiothreitol was omitted. The procedure with *P. pastoris* was also scaled up to produce 15.5 kg of with 97 M% yield and e.e. >98% in a 180 liter batch using 10% ketoacid concentration.

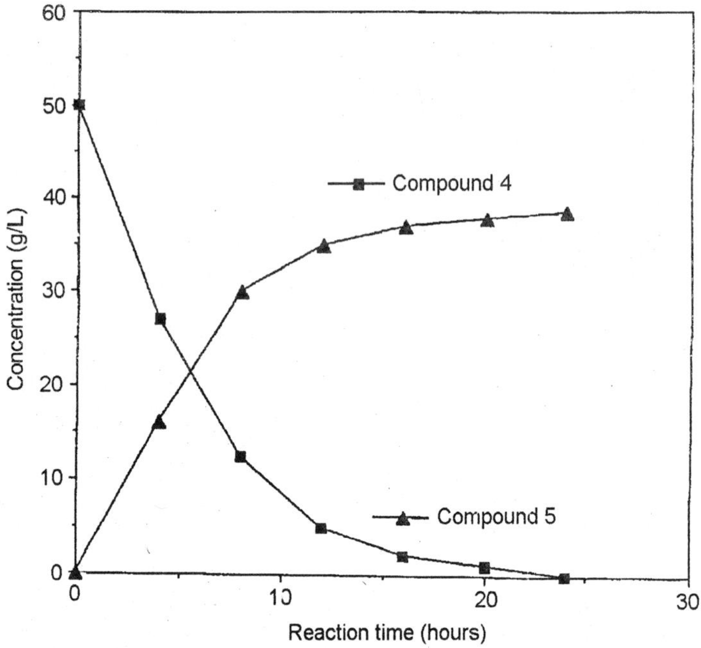

Fig. 16.5. Kinetics of enzymatic conversion of ketoacid acetal to amino acid acetal by phenylalanine dehydrogenase from recombinant E. coli and formate dehydrogenase from C. boidinii.

For reusability, formate dehydrogenase could be immobilized on Eupergit C and phenylalanine dehydrogenase on Eupergit C250L. The immobilized enzymes were tested for reusability in a jacketed reactor maintained at 40° C, and were used five times for the conversion without much loss of any activity and productivity. At the end of each reaction, the solution was drained from the reactor through a 80/400-mesh stainless steel sieve, which retained the immobilized enzymes, then the reactor was recharged with fresh substrate solution. After the fifth reuse, the reaction rate was decreased; however, the original reaction rate was restored in the seventh-reuse studies by addition of formate dehydrogenase.

β-3-Receptor Agonist

β-Adrenoceptors have been classified as β1 and β2. Increased heart rate is the primary consequence of β1-receptor stimulation, while bronchodilation and smooth muscle relaxation are mediated from β-2 receptor stimulation. Rat adipocyte lipolysis was initially thought to be a β-1-mediated process. However, recent results indicate that this type of lipolysis is neither β1 nor β2 receptor-mediated, but is due to "atypical" receptors, later called β3-adrenergic receptors. β3-Adrenergic receptors are found on the cell surface of both white and brown adipocytes and are responsible for lipolysis, thermogenesis, and relaxation of intestinal smooth muscle. Consequently, several research groups are engaged in developing selective β-3 agonists for the treatment of gastrointestinal disorders, type II diabetes, and obesity. Efficient biocatalytic syntheses of chiral intermediates required for the total chemical syntheses of β-3 receptor agonists have been reported by us.

The biocatalytic approaches include (1) the microbial reduction of 4-benzyloxy-3-methanesulfonylamino-2'-bromoacetophenone to the corresponding (*R*)-alcohol by *Sphingomonas paucimobilis*

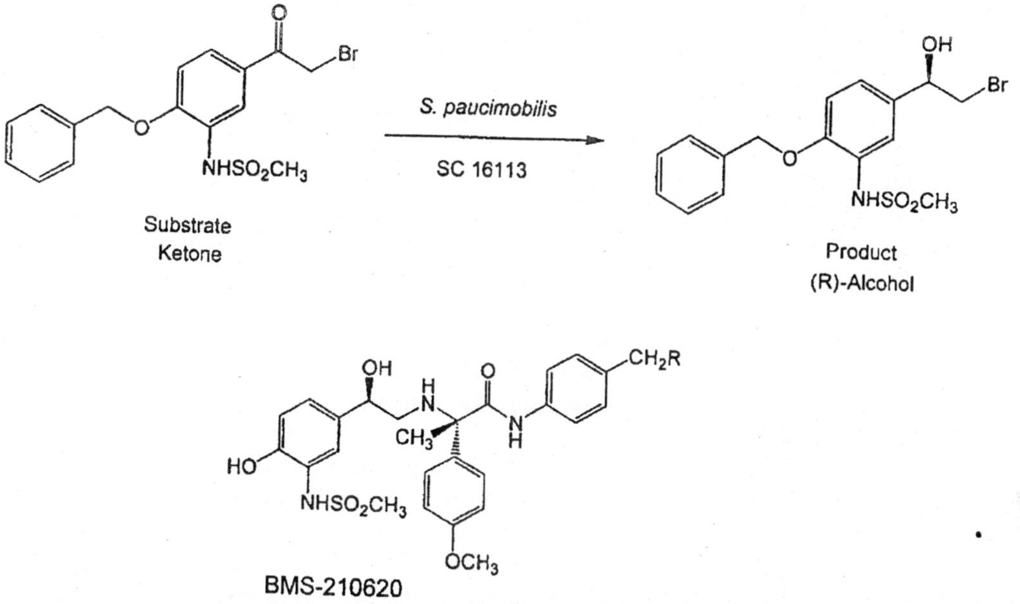

S. paucimobilis
SC 16113
NHSO2CH3
Substrate
Ketone
OH
Br
Product
(R)-Alcohol
OH
CH2R
HO
NHSO2CH3
CH3
OCH3
BMS-210620

Fig. 16.6. Preparation of chiral synthon for β-3-receptor agonist.

SC 16113; (2) the enzymatic resolution of racemic (α-methyl)phenylalanine amide and α-(4-methoxyphenyl) alanine amide by amidase from *Mycobacterium neoaurum* ATCC 25795 to prepare the corresponding (*S*)-amino acids, the asymmetric hydrolysis of methyl-(4-methoxyphenyl)-propanedioic acid, diethyl ester, to the corresponding (*S*)-monoester by pig liver esterase.

(A)
M. neoaurum
ATCC 25795
Substrate
Product
(B)
M. neoaurum
ATCC 25795
Substrate
Product
(C)
Pig Liver Esterase
Diester
S-(-)-Monoester

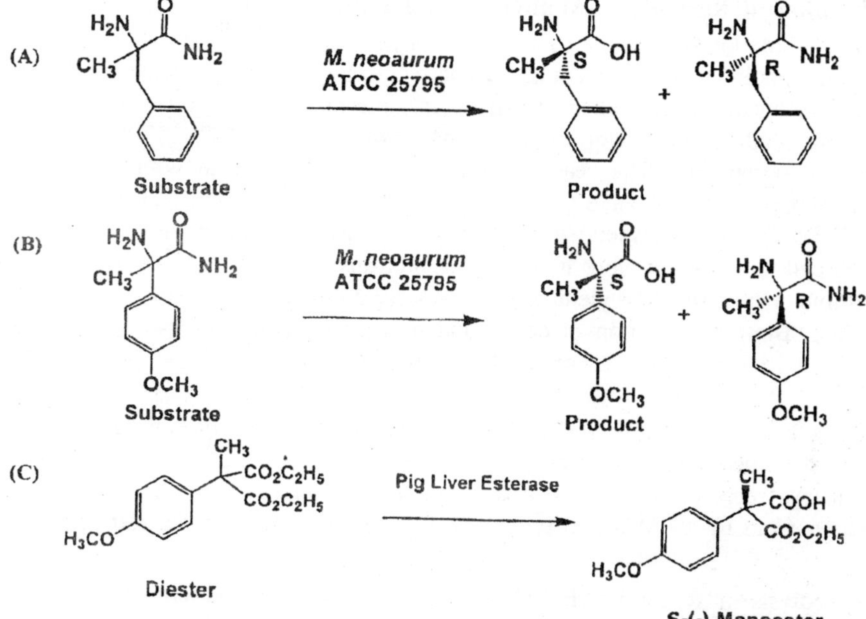

Fig. 16.7. Preparation of chiral synthon for β-3-receptor: (A) enzymatic resolution of racemic amino acid amide by amidase from M. neoaurum ATCC 25795; (B) enzymatic resolution of racemic amino acid amide by amidase from M. neoaurum ATCC 25795; (C) enzymatic asymmetric hydrolysis of diester to the corresponding (S)-monoester by pig liver esterase.

Microbial Reduction of 4-Benzyloxy-3-Methanesulfonylamino-2'-Bromoacetophenone

The microbial reduction of 4-benzyloxy-3-methanesulfonylamino-2'-bromoacetophenone to the corresponding (*R*)-alcohol was demonstrated by *S. paucimobilis* SC 16113. Among cultures evaluated, *Hansenula anamola* SC 13833, *H. anamola* SC 16142, *Rhodococcus rhodochrous* ATCC 14347, and *S. paucimobilis* SC 16113, gave desired alcohol in >96% e.e. and >15% reaction yield. *S. paucimobilis* SC 16113, in the initial screening, catalyzed the efficient conversion of ketone to the desired chiral alcohol in 58% reaction yield and >99.5% e.e.

The fermentation of *S. paucimobilis* SC 16113 culture was carried out in a 750-liter fermentor. From each fermentation batch, about 60 kg of wet cell paste was collected. Cells harvested from the fermentor were used to conduct the biotransformation in 1-, 10-, and 210-liter preparative batches under aerobic or anaerobic conditions. The cells were suspended in 80 mM potassium phosphate buffer (pH 6.0) to 20% (w/v, wet cells) concentration. Compound (1–2 g/liter) and glucose (25 g/liter) were added to the fermentor and the reduction reaction was carried out at 37°C. In some batches, at the end of the fermentation cycle, the cells were concentrated sevenfold by ceramic crossflow microfiltration using a 0.2-μm filter, diafiltered using 10 mM potassium phosphate buffer (pH 7.0), and used directly in the bioreduction process. In all batches of biotransformation, the reaction yield of >85% and the e.e. of >98% were obtained. The isolation of compound from the 210-liter preparative batch was carried out to obtain 100 g of product. The isolated gave 83% chemical purity and an e.e. of 99.5%.

In an alternative process, frozen cells of *S. paucimobilis* SC 16113 were used with resin adsorbed (XAD-16 resin) substrate at 5- and 10-g/liter substrate concentrations. In this process, an average reaction yield of 85% and an e.e. of >99% were obtained for product. At the end of the biotransformation, the reaction mixture was filtered on a 100-mesh (150-m) stainless steel screen, and the resin retained by the screen was washed with 2 liters of water. The product was then desorbed from the resin and crystallized in an overall 75 M% yield with 91% homogeneity and 99.8% e.e.

Enzymatic Resolution of Racemic (α-Methyl)phenylalanine Amides

The enzymatic resolution of racemic (α-methyl)phenylalanine amide and α-(4-methoxyphenyl)alanine amide to the corresponding (*S*)-amino acids, respectively, by an amidase from *M. neoaurum* ATCC 25795 has been developed. The chiral amino acids are intermediates for the syntheses of β-3-receptor agonists. The cells (10%, w/v, wet cells) of *M. neoaurum* ATCC 25795 were evaluated for biotransformation of compound. The reaction was completed in 75 min with a reaction yield of 48 M% (theoretical max. 50%) and an e.e. of 95% for the desired product. Freeze-dried cells of *M. neoaurum* ATCC 25795 were suspended in 100 mM potassium phosphate buffer (pH 7.0) at 1% concentration and cell suspensions were used for the biotransformation of compound. The reaction was completed in 60 min with a reaction yield of 49.5 M% (theoretical max. 50%) and an e.e. of 99% for the desired product. Biotransformation of compound was also carried out using a purified amidase. A reaction yield of 49 M% and an e.e. of 99.8% were obtained for desired product after 60 min of reaction time.

Freeze-dried cells of *M. neoaurum*ATCC 25795 and partially purified amidase were used for the biotransformation of compound. A reaction yield of 49 M% and an e.e. of 78% were obtained for the desired product using freeze-dried cells. The reaction was completed in 50 hr. Using partially purified amidase, a reaction yield of 49 M% and e.e. of 94% were obtained for desired product after a 70-hr reaction time.

Asymmetric Hydrolysis of Racemic Methyl-(4-Methoxyphenyl)-Propanedioic Acid, Diethyl Ester

The enzymatic asymmetric hydrolysis of methyl-(4-methoxyphenyl)-propanedioic acid, diethyl ester to the corresponding (*S*)-monoester by pig liver esterase (PLE) has been demonstrated. Chiral (*S*)-monoester is a key intermediate for the syntheses of β-3-receptor agonists.

Various organic solvents were tested for the PLE-catalyzed asymmetric hydrolysis of diester in a biphasic system. The results indicate that the reaction yields and e.e. of monoester were dependent on the solvent used in the asymmetric hydrolysis. Tetrahydrofuran (THF), methyl isobutyl ketone (MIBK), hexane, and dichloromethane inhibited PLE. Lower reaction yields (28–56 M%) and lower e.e. (59–72%) were obtained using *t*-butyl methyl ether, dimethylformamide (DMF), and dimethylsulfoxide (DMSO) as cosolvent. Higher e.e. (>91%) was obtained using methanol, ethanol, and toluene as cosolvent. Ethanol gave highest reaction yield (96.7%) and e.e. (96%) for monoester.

The effect of temperature and pH were evaluated for the PLE-catalyzed hydrolysis of diester in a biphasic system using ethanol as cosolvent. It was observed that the e.e. of desired monoester was increased with decreasing temperature from 25°C to 10°C. The optimum pH for asymmetric hydrolysis of diester in a biphasic system using ethanol as a cosolvent was 7.2 at 10°C. A semipreparative-scale asymmetric hydrolysis of diester was carried out in a biphasic system using 10% ethanol as cosolvent. Substrate (3 g) was used in a 300-ml reaction mixture. The reaction was carried out at 10°C, 125 rpm agitation, and at pH 7.2 for 11 hr. Reaction yield of 96 M% and an e.e. of 96.9% were obtained. From the reaction mixture, 2.6 g of monoester were isolated in 86.3 M% overall yield. The e.e. of isolated *S*-(–)-monoester was 96.9%.

Angiotensin Converting Enzyme (ACE) and Neutral Endopeptidase Inhibitors

Captopril is designated chemically as 1-[(2*S*)-3-mercapto-2-methylpropionyl]-L-proline. It is used as an antihypertensive agent through suppression of the renin–angiotensin–aldosterone system. Captopril and other compounds such as enalapril and lisinopril prevent the conversion of angiotensin I to angiotensin II by inhibition of ACE. The potency of captopril as an inhibitor of ACE depends critically on the configuration of the mercaptoalkanoyl moiety; the compound with the S-configuration is about

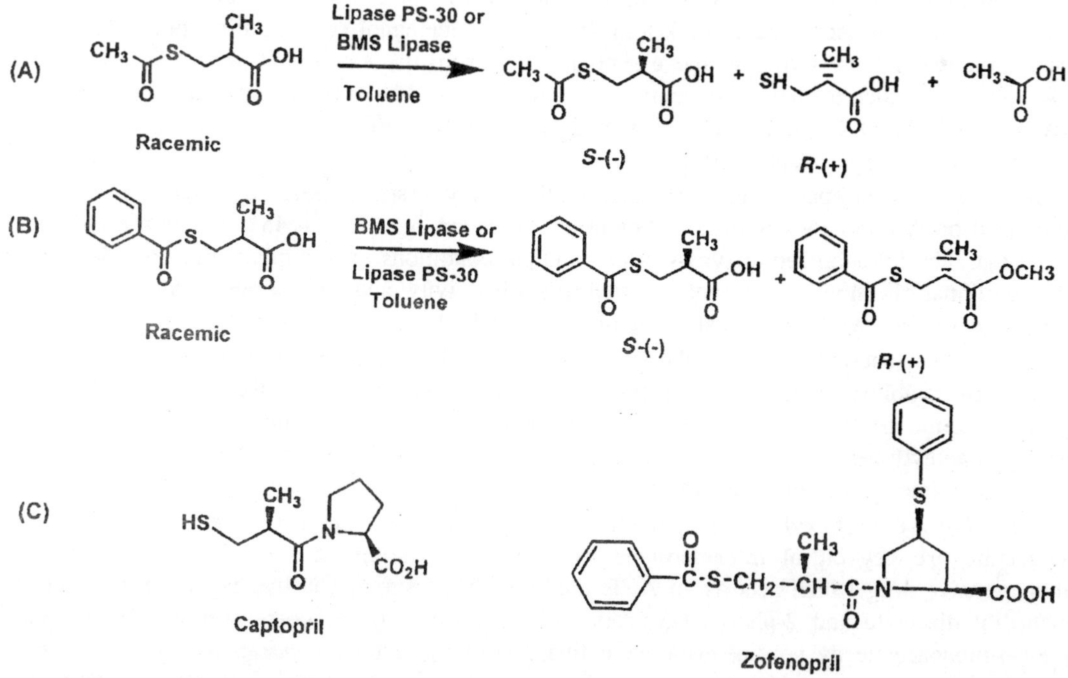

(A) Racemic — Lipase PS-30 or BMS Lipase, Toluene → *S*-(-) + *R*-(+) + CH_3COOH

(B) Racemic — BMS Lipase or Lipase PS-30, Toluene → *S*-(-) + *R*-(+)

(C) Captopril; Zofenopril

Fig. 16.8. (A) Synthesis of captopril side-chain S-(–): stereoselective enzymatic hydrolysis of racemic 3-acylthio-2-methylpropionoic acid. (B) Synthesis of zofenopril side-chain S-(–); stereoselective enzymatic esterification of racemic 3-behzylthio-2-methylpropionic acid. (C) Structures of captopril and zofenopril.

100 times more active than its corresponding *R*-enantiomer. The required 3-mercapto-(2*S*)-methylpropionic acid moiety has been prepared from microbially derived chiral 3-hydroxy-(2*R*)-methylpropionic acid, which is obtained by the hydroxylation of isobutyric acid.

The use of extracellular lipases of microbial origin to catalyze the stereo- selective hydrolysis of esters of 3-acylthio-2-methylpropionic acid in an aqueous system has been demonstrated to produce optically active 3-acylthio-2-methylpropionic acid. The synthesis of the chiral side chain of captopril by the lipase-catalyzed enantioselective hydrolysis of the thioester bond of racemic 3-acetylthio-2-methylpropionic acid to yield *S*-(–) has been demonstrated. Among various lipases evaluated, lipase from *Rhizopus oryzae* ATCC 24563 (heat-dried cells), BMS lipase (extracellular lipase derived from the fermentation of *Pseudomonas* sp. SC 13856), and lipase PS-30 from *Pseudomonas cepacia* in an organic solvent system (1,1,2-trichloro-1,2,2-trifluoroethane or toluene) catalyzed the hydrolysis of thioester bond of undesired enantiomer of racemic to yield desired *S*-(–), *R*-(+)-3-mercapto-2-methylpropionic acid and acetic acid. The reaction yield of >24% (theoretical max. 50%) and e.e. of >95% were obtained for *S*-(–) using each lipase in an independent experiment.

In an alternative approach to prepare the chiral side chain of captopril and zofenopril, the lipase-catalyzed stereoselective esterification of racemic 3-benzoylthio-2-methylpropionic acid in an organic solvent system was demonstrated to yield *R*-(+)-methyl ester and unreacted acid enriched in the desired *S*-(–)-enantiomer. Using lipase PS-30 with toluene as solvent and methanol as nucleophile, the desired *S*-(–) was obtained in 37% reaction yield (theoretical max. 50%) and 97% e.e. Substrate was used at 22-g/ liter concentration. The amount of water and the concentration of methanol supplied in the reaction mixture was very critical. Water was used at 0.1% concentration in the reaction mixture. More than 1% water led to the aggregation of enzyme in the organic solvent, with a decrease in the rate of reaction which was due to mass transfer limitation. The rate of esterification decreased as the methanol to substrate ratio was increased from 1:1 to 4:1. Higher methanol concentration probably inhibited the esterification reaction by stripping the essential water from the enzyme. Lower e.e. of product S-(–) was obtained at higher methanol concentration. Crude lipase PS-30 was immobilized on three different resins, XAD-7, XAD-2 and Accurel polypropylene (Accurel PP) in absorption efficiencies of about 68%, 71%, and 98.5%, respectively.

These immobilized lipases were evaluated for the ability to stereoselectively esterify racemic. Enzyme immobilized on Accurel PP catalyzed efficient esterification, giving 36– 45% reaction yield and 97.7% e.e. of *S*(–). The immobilized enzyme under identical conditions gave similar e.e. and yield of product in 23 additional reaction cycles without any loss of activity and productivity. *S*-(–) is a key chiral intermediate for the synthesis of captopril or zofenopril.

The *S*-(–)-α-[(acetylthio)methyl]phenylpropionic acid is a key chiral intermediate for the neutral endopeptidase inhibitor. We have demonstrated the lipase-catalyzed stereoselective hydrolysis of thioester bond of racemic α-[(acetylthio)methyl]phenylpropionic acid in organic solvent to yield *R*-(+)-α-[(mercapto)methyl]phenylpropionic acid and *S*-(–). Using lipase PS-30, the *S*-(–) was obtained in 40% reaction yield (theoretical max. 50%) and 98% e.e.

The *S*-(–)-2-cyclohexyl-1,3-propanediol monoacetate and the *S*-(–)-2-phenyl-1,3-propanediol monoacetate are key chiral intermediates for the chemoenzymatic synthesis of Monopril, a new antihypertensive drug which acts as an ACE inhibitor. The asymmetric hydrolysis of 2-cyclohexyl-1,3-propanediol diacetate and 2-phenyl-1,3-propanediol diacetate to the corresponding *S*-(–)-monoacetate and *S*-(–)-monoacetate by porcine pancreatic lipase (PPL) and *Chromobacterium viscosum* lipase have been demonstrated by Patel et al. In a biphasic system using 10% toluene, the reaction yield of >65% and e.e. of 99% were obtained for *S*-(–) using each enzyme. *S*-(–) was obtained in 90% reaction yield and 99.8% e.e. using *C. viscosum* lipase under similar conditions.

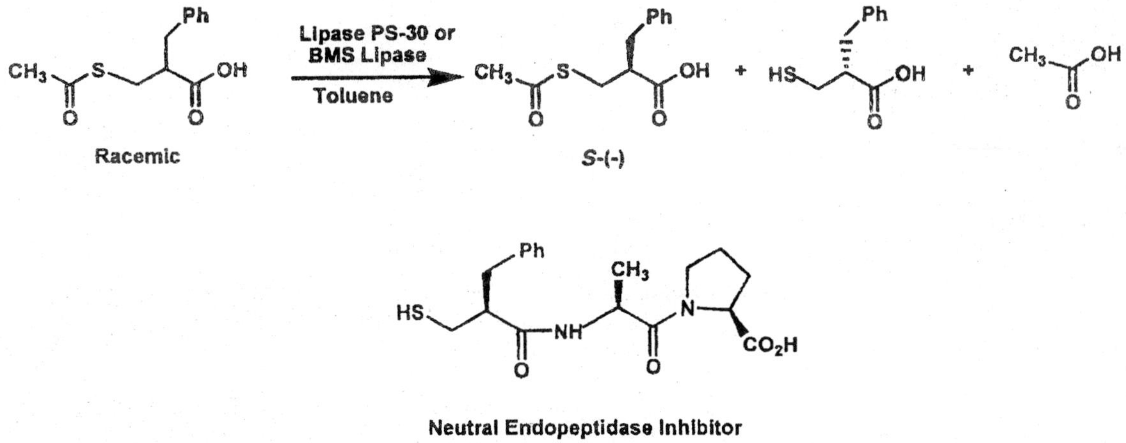

Fig. 16.9. Preparation of chiral synthon for neutral endopeptidase inhibitor: stereoselective enzymatic hydrolysis of racemic α-[(acetylthio)methyl]phenylpropionic acid.

Ceranopril is another ACE inhibitor which requires chiral intermediate 2-(*S*)-hydroxy-6-(carbobenzyloxyamino)-hexanoic acid. A biotransformation process was developed by Hanson et al. to prepare the 2-(*S*)-hydroxy-6-(carbobenzyloxyamino)-hexanoic acid. N-ε-carbobenzoxy(CBZ)-L-lysine was first converted to the corresponding keto acid by oxidative deamination using cells of *Providencia alcalifaciens* SC 9036 which contained L-amino acid oxidase and catalase. The keto acid was subsequently converted to 2-(*S*)-hydroxy-6-(carbobenzyloxyamino)-hexanoic acid using L-2-hydroxyisocaproate (HIC) dehydrogenase from *Lactobacillus confusus*. The NADH required for this reaction was regenerated using formate dehydrogenase from *C. boidinii*. The reaction yield of 95% with 98.5% e.e. was obtained in the overall process.

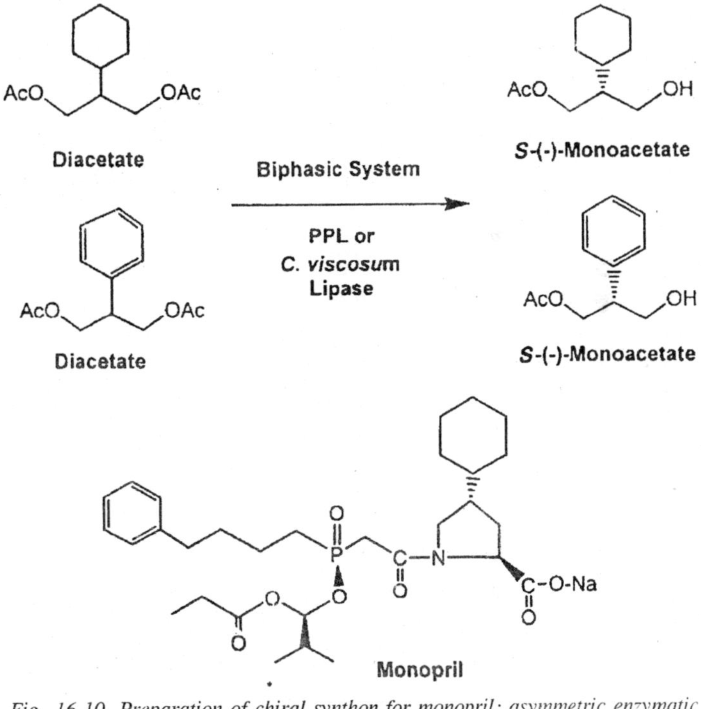

Fig. 16.10. Preparation of chiral synthon for monopril: asymmetric enzymatic hydrolysis of 2-cyclohexyl- and 2-phenyl-1,3-propanediol diacetate and the corresponding S-(–)-monoacetates.

Thromboxane A2 Antagonists

Thromboxane A2 (TxA2) is an exceptionally potent pro-aggregatory and vasoconstrictor substance produced by the metabolism of arachidonic acid in blood platelets and other tissues. Together with potent anti-aggregatory and vasodilator compounds, TxA2 plays an important role in the maintenance of vascular homeostasis and contributes to the pathogenesis of a variety of vascular disorders. Approaches toward limiting the effect of TxA2 have focused on either inhibiting its synthesis or blocking its action at its receptor sites by means of an antagonist. The lactol or lactone are key chiral intermediates for the total synthesis of

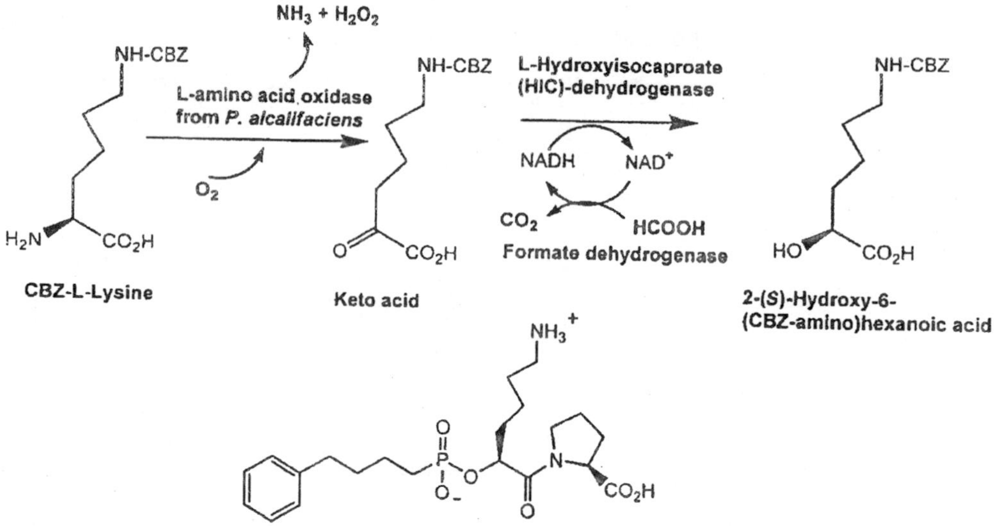

$NH_3 + H_2O_2$

NH-CBZ L-amino acid oxidase from *P. alcalifaciens* O_2 H_2N CO_2H **CBZ-L-Lysine**

NH-CBZ O CO_2H **Keto acid**

L-Hydroxyisocaproate (HIC)-dehydrogenase NADH NAD^+ CO_2 HCOOH **Formate dehydrogenase**

NH-CBZ HO CO_2H **2-(*S*)-Hydroxy-6-(CBZ-amino)hexanoic acid**

NH_3^+ O P O O N CO_2H O

Ceranopril

Fig. 16.11. Synthesis of chiral synthon for ceranopril: enzymatic conversion of CBZ-L-lysine to (S)-hydroxy-6-(carbobenzyloxyamino)-hexanoic acid.

compound, a new cardiovascular agent useful in the treatment of thrombolic disease. Horse liver alcohol dehydrogenase (HLADH) catalyzes the oxidoreduction of a variety of compounds. It has been demonstrated that HLADH catalyzes the stereospecific oxidation of only one of the enantiotopic hydroxyl groups of acyclic and monocyclic meso-diols. The authors demonstrated the oxidation of meso exo- and endo-7-oxabicyclo [2.2.1]heptane-2,3-dimethanol to the corresponding enantiomerically pure γ-lactones by HLADH. NAD and flavin adenine dinucleotide (FAD) at concentrations of 1 and 20 mmol, respectively, were required for the stereoselective oxidation of 12.7 mmol of substrate. Due to the high cost of enzyme and required cofactors, this process for preparing chiral lactones was economically not feasible for scale-up. Patel et al. described the stereoselective oxidation of (exo,exo)-7-oxabicyclo[2.2.1]heptane-2,3-dimethanol to the corresponding chiral lactol and lactone by cell suspension (10% w/v, wet cells) of *Nocardia globerula* ATCC 21505 or *Rhodococcus* sp. ATCC 15592. The reaction yield of 70 M% and e.e. of 96% were for chiral lactone after a 96-hr biotransformation process at 5-g/liter substrate concentration using cell suspensions of *N. globerula* ATCC 21505. An overall reaction yield of 46 M% (lactol and lactone combined) and e.e. of 96.7% and 98.4% were obtained for lactol and lactone, respectively, using cell suspensions of *Rhodococcus* sp. ATCC 15592. Substrate was used at 5-g/ liter concentration.

The asymmetric hydrolysis of (exo,exo)-7-oxabicyclo[2.2.1]heptane-2,3-dimethanol, diacetate ester to the corresponding chiral monoacetate ester has been demonstrated with lipases. Lipase PS-30 from *P. cepacia* was most effective in asymmetric hydrolysis to obtain the desired enantiomer of monoacetate ester. The reaction yield of 75 M% and e.e. of >99% were obtained when the reaction was conducted in a biphasic system with 10% toluene at 5 g/liter of the substrate. Lipase PS-30 was immobilized on Accurel PP and the immobilized enzyme was reused (5 cycles) without loss of enzyme activity, productivity, or e.e. of product. The reaction process was scaled up to 80 liters (400 g of substrate) and monoacetate ester was isolated in 80 M% yield with 99.3% e.e. The product was isolated in 99.5% chemical purity. The chiral monoacetate ester was oxidized to its corresponding aldehyde and subsequently hydrolyzed to give chiral lactol. The chiral lactol obtained by this enzymatic process was used in chemoenzymatic synthesis of thromboxane A2 antagonist.

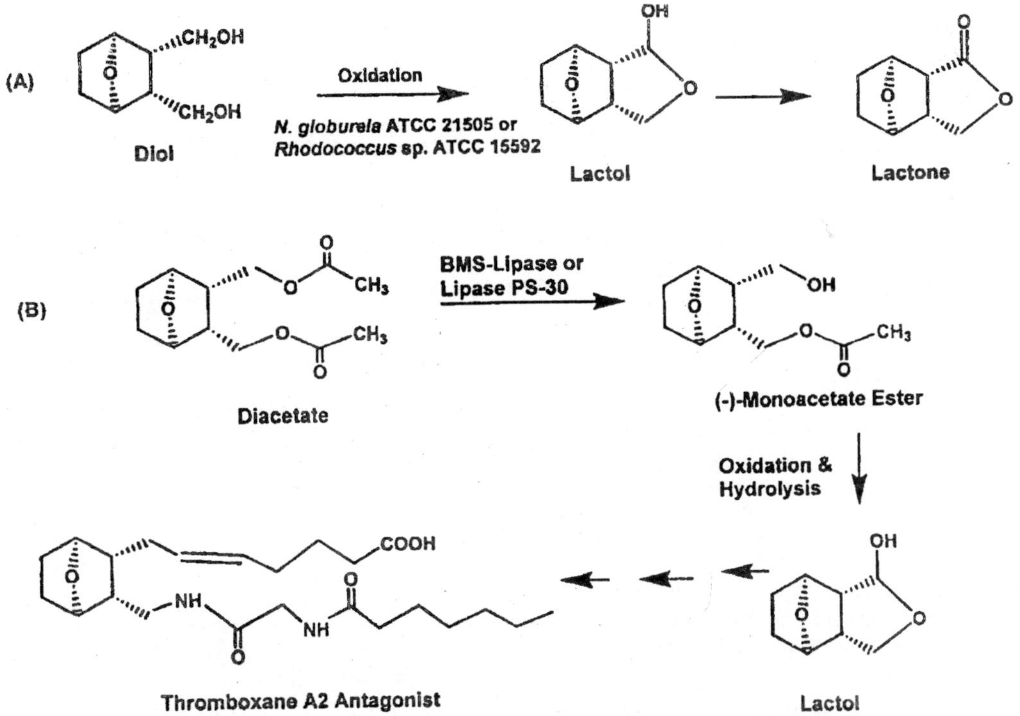

Fig. 16.12. Synthesis of chiral synthon for thromboxane A2 antagonist: (A) stereoselective microbial oxidation of (exo,exo)-7-oxabicyclo[2.2.1]hepatane-2,3-dimethanol to the corresponding lactol and lactone; (B) asymmetric enzymatic hydrolysis of (exo,exo)-7-oxabicyclo[2.2.1]heptane-2,3-dimethanol, diacetate to the corresponding S-(–)-monoacetate ester.

ANTICHOLESTEROL DRUGS

Chiral β-hydroxy esters are versatile synthons in organic synthesis, specifically in the preparation of natural products. Recently, we have described the reduction of the methyl ester of 4-chloro-3-oxobutanoic acid to the methyl ester of *S*-(–)-4-chloro-3-hydroxybutanoic acid by cell suspensions of *Geotrichum candidum* SC 5469. *S*(–) is a key chiral intermediate in the total chemical synthesis of a cholesterol antagonist (SQ 33600), which acts by inhibiting hydroxymethylglutaryl CoA (HMG CoA) reductase. In the biotransformation process, a reaction yield of 95% and e.e. of 96% were obtained for *S*-(–) by glucose, acetate-, or glycerol-grown cells (10% w/v) of *G. candidum* SC 5469. Substrate was used at 10-g/liter concentration. The e.e. of *S*-(–) was increased to 98% by heat treatment of cell suspensions (55°C for 30 min) prior to conducting the bioreduction.

Glucose-grown cells of *G. candidum* SC 5469 have also catalyzed the stereoselective reduction of ethyl-, isopropyl-, and tertiary-butyl esters of 4- chloro-3-oxobutanoic acid and methyl and ethyl esters of 4-bromo-3-oxobutanoic acid. A reaction yield of >85% and e.e. of >94% were obtained. NAD^+-dependent oxido-reductase responsible for the stereoselective reduction of â-keto esters of 4-chloro- and 4-bromo-3-oxobutanoic acid was purified 100-fold. The molecular weight of purified enzyme is 950,000. The purified oxido-reductase was immobilized on Eupergit C and used to catalyze the reduction. The cofactor NAD^+ required for the reduction reaction was regenerated by glucose dehydrogenase.

So far, most microorganisms and enzymes derived therefrom have been used in the reduction of a single keto group of β-keto or α-keto compounds. Recently, Patel et al. have demonstrated the stereoselective reduction of 3,5-dioxo-6-(benzyloxy)hexanoic acid, ethyl ester, to (3*S*,5*R*)-dihydroxy-6-(benzyloxy)hexanoic acid, ethyl ester. The compound is a key chiral intermediate required for the

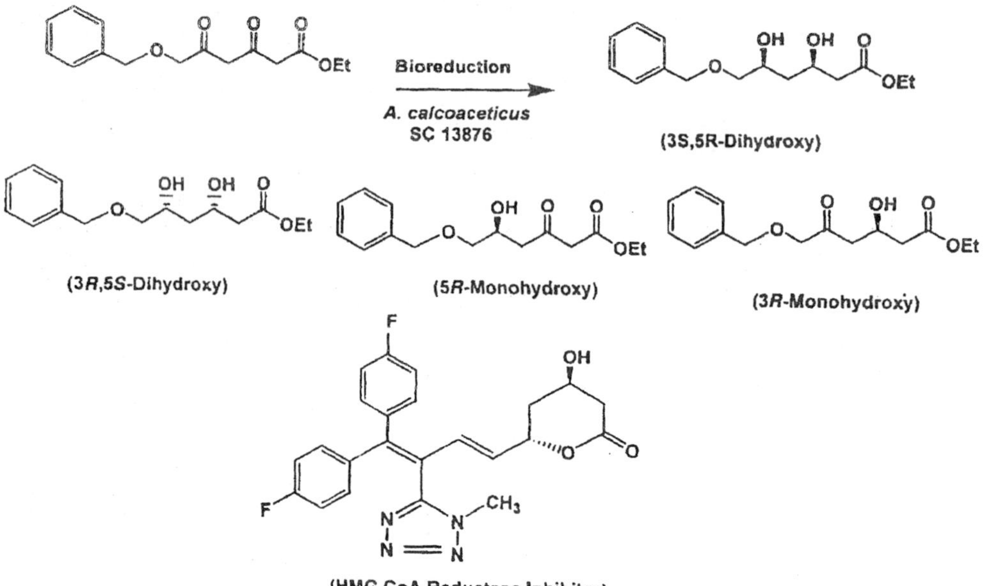

Fig. 16.13. Synthesis of chiral synthon for anticholesterol drug R-(+): stereoselective microbial reduction of 3,5-dioxo-6-(benzyloxy)hexanoic acid, ethyl ester.

chemical synthesis of [4-[4α,6β(E)]]-6-[4,4-bis(4-fluorophenyl)-3-(1-methyl-1H-tetrazol-5-yl)-1,3-butadienyl]-tetrahydro-4-hydroxy-2H-pyran-2-one, compound *R*-(+), a new anticholesterol drug that acts by inhibition of HMG CoA reductase. Among various microbial cultures evaluated for the stereoselective reduction of diketone, cell suspensions of *Acinetobacter calcoaceticus* SC 13876 reduced. The reaction yield of 85% and e.e. of 97% were obtained using glycerol-grown cells. The substrate was used at 2 g/liter and cells were used at 20% (w/v, wet cells) concentration.

Cell extracts of *A. calcoaceticus* SC 13876 in the presence of NAD^+, glucose, and glucose dehydrogenase reduced to the corresponding monohydroxy compounds and [3-hydroxy-5-oxo-6-(benzyloxy)hexanoic acid ethyl ester and 5-hydroxy-3-oxo-6-(benzyloxy)hexanoic acid ethyl ester]. Both were further reduced to (3*S*,4*R*)-dihydroxy compound using the cell extracts. The reaction yield of 92% and the e.e. of 98% were obtained when the reaction was carried out in a 1-liter batch using cell extracts. The substrate was used at 10 g/liter. Product was isolated from the reaction mixture in 72% overall yield. The HPLC area percent purity of the isolated product was 99% and the e.e. was 98.5%. The reductase which converted was purified about 200-fold from cell extracts of *A. calcoaceticus* SC 13876. The purified enzyme gave a single protein band on SDS-PAGE corresponding to 33,000 Da.

Using an enzymatic resolution process, chiral alcohol *R*-(+) was also prepared by the lipase-catalyzed stereoselective acetylation of racemic in organic solvent. We evaluated various lipases, among which lipase PS-30 and BMS lipase (produced by fermentation of *Pseudomonas* strain SC 13856) efficiently catalyzed the acetylation of the undesired enantiomer of racemic to yield *S*-(–)-acetylated product and unreacted desired *R*-(+). A reaction yield of 49 M% (theoretical max. 50 M%) and e.e. of 98.5% were obtained for *R*-(+) when the reaction was conducted in toluene as solvent in the presence of isopropenyl acetate as acyl donor. Substrate was used at 4 g/ liter concentration. In methyl ethyl ketone at 50-g/liter substrate concentration, a reaction yield of 46 M% and e.e. of 96% were obtained for *R*-(+).

Lipase PS-30 was immobilized on Accurel PP and the immobilized enzyme was reused five times without any loss of activity or productivity in the resolution process to prepare *R*-(+). The enzymatic

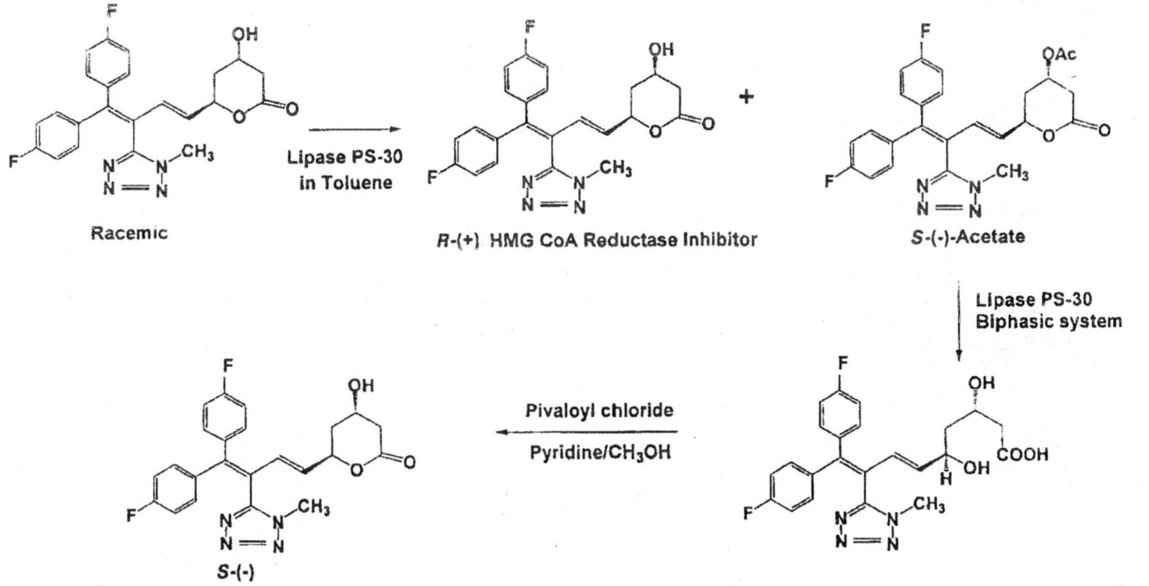

Fig. 16.14. Synthesis of chiral anticholesterol drug R-(+)-racemic: stereoselective enzymatic acetylation of racemic.

process was scaled up to a 640- liter preparative batch using immobilized lipase PS-30 at 4 g/liter racemic substrate in toluene as a solvent. From the reaction mixture, *R*-(+) was isolated in 35 M% overall yield with 98.5% e.e. and 99.5% chemical purity. The undesired *S*-(–)-acetate produced by this process was enzymatically hydrolyzed by lipase PS-30 in a biphasic system to prepare the corresponding *S*-(–)-alcohol. Thus both enantiomers of alcohol were produced by the enzymatic process.

Pravastatin and Mevastatin are anticholesterol drugs which act by competitively inhibiting HMG CoA reductase. Pravastatin sodium is produced by two fermentation steps. The first step is the production of compound ML-236B by *Penicillium citrinum*. The purified compound was converted to its sodium salt with sodium hydroxide and in the second step was hydroxylated to Pravastatin sodium by *Streptomyces carbophilus*. A cytochrome P-450–containing enzyme system has been demonstrated from *S. carbophilus* which catalyzed the hydroxylation reaction.

Squalene synthase is the first pathway-specific enzyme in the biosynthesis of cholesterol and catalyzes the head-to-head condensation of two molecules of farnesyl pyrophosphate (FPP) to form squalene. It has been implicated in the transformation of

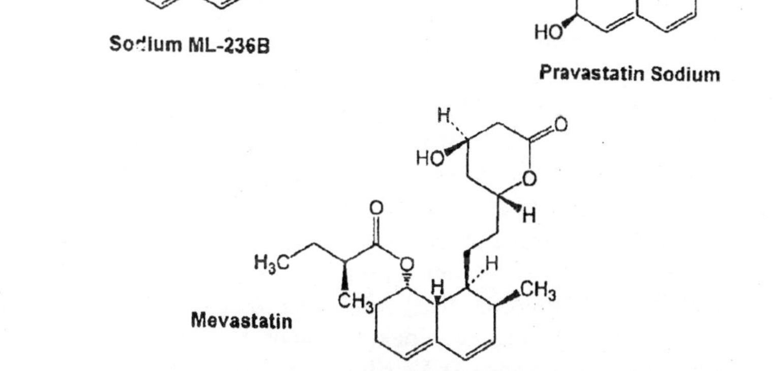

Fig. 16.15. Stereoselective microbial hydroxylation of ML-236B to Pravastain.

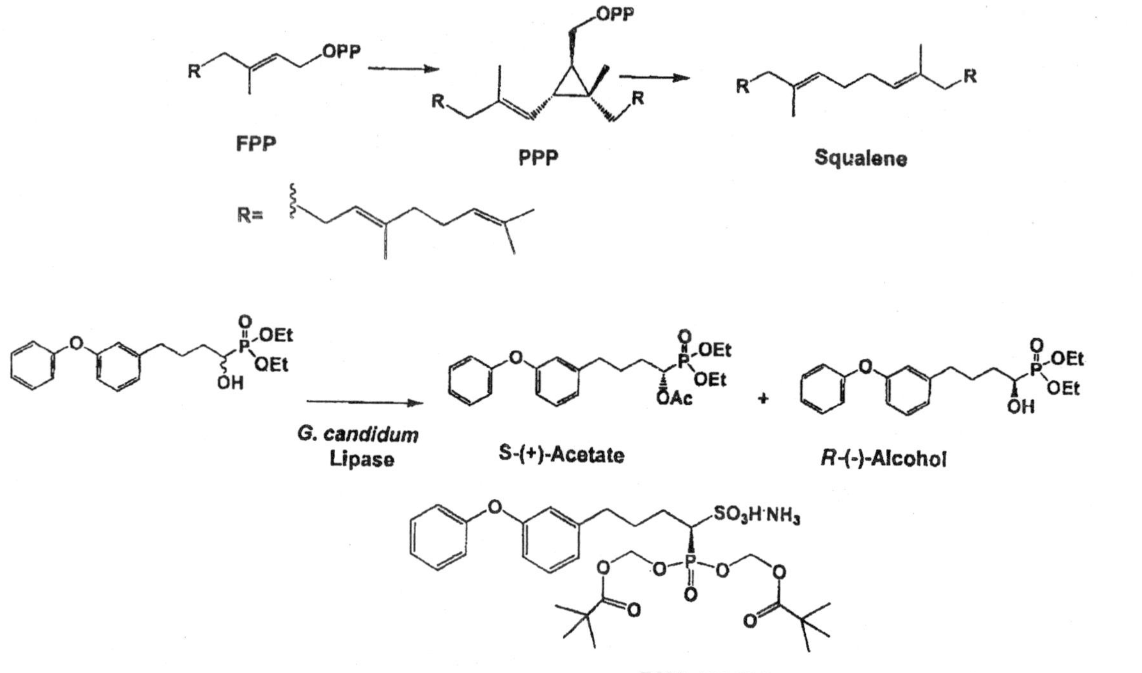

Fig. 16.16. Enzymatic synthesis of chiral synthon for BMS-188494, a squalene synthase inhibitor: stereoselective acetylation of racemic.

FPP into presqualene pyrophosphate (PPP). FPP analogs are a major class of inhibitors of squalene synthase. However, this class of compounds lacks specificity and are potential inhibitors of other FPP consuming transferases such as geranyl-geranyl pyrophosphate synthase. To increase enzyme specificity, analogs of PPP and other mechanism-based enzyme inhibitors have been synthesized. BMS-188494 is a potent squalene synthase inhibitor that is effective as an anticholesterol drug. (*S*)[1-(acetoxy)-4-(3-phenoxyphenyl)butyl]phosphonic acid, diethyl ester is a key chiral intermediate required for the total chemical synthesis of BMS-188494. The stereoselective acetylation of racemic [1-(hydroxy)-4-(3-phenoxyphenyl)butyl]phosphonic acid, diethyl ester, was carried out using *G. candidum* lipase in toluene as solvent and isopropenyl acetate as acyl donor. A reaction yield of 38% (theoretical max. 50%) and an e.e. of 95% were obtained for chiral.

Calcium Channel Blocking Agents

Dilthiazem, a benzothiazepinone calcium channel blocking agent that inhibits influx of extracellular calcium through L-type voltage-operated calcium channels, has been widely used clinically in the treatment of hypertension and angina. Since dilthiazem has a relatively short duration of action, recently an 8-chloro derivative has been introduced in the clinic as a more potent analog of dilthiazem. Lack of extended duration of action and little information on structure–activity relationships in this class of compounds led Floyd et al. and Das et al. to prepare isosteric 1-benzazepin-2-ones which resulted in the identification of a 6-trifluoromethyl-1-benzazepin-2-one derivative as a longer-lasting and more potent antihypertensive agent. A key chiral intermediate [(3*R*-*cis*)-1,3,4,5-tetrahydro-3-hydroxy-4-(4-methoxyphenyl)-6-(trifluoromethyl)-2H-1-benzazepin-2-one] was required for the total chemical synthesis of the new calcium channel blocking agent [(*cis*)-3-(acetoxy)-1-[2-(dimethylamino)ethyl]-1,3,4,5-tetrahydro-4-(4-methoxyphenyl)-6-(trifluoromethyl)-2H-1-benzazepin-2-one]. A stereoselective microbial process was developed for the reduction of 4,5-dihydro-4-(4-methoxyphenyl)-6-(trifluoromethyl)-1H-1

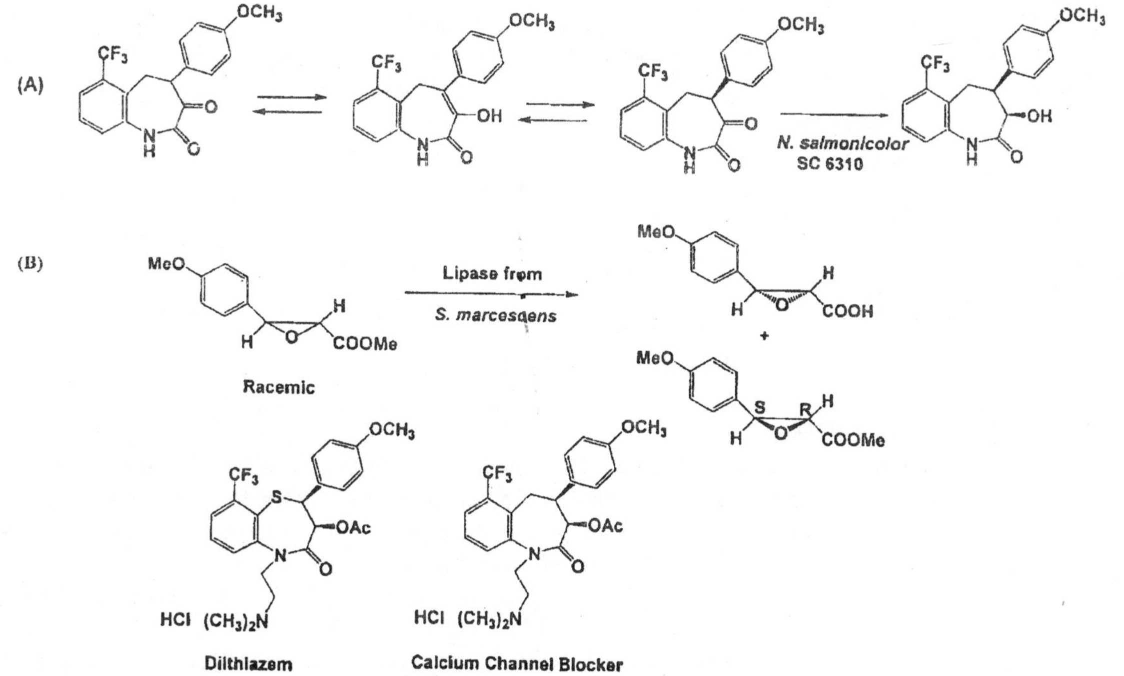

Fig. 16.17. Synthesis of chiral synthon for calcium channel blocker.

-benzazepin-2,3-dione to chiral. Compound exists predominantly in the achiral enol form, which is in rapid equilibrium with the two keto-form enantiomers. Reduction of could give rise to formation of four possible alcohol stereoisomers. Remarkably, conditions were found under which only the single alcohol isomer was obtained by microbial reduction. Among various cultures evaluated, microorganisms from the genera *Nocardia*, *Rhodococcus*, *Corynebacterium*, and *Arthrobacter* reduced compound to compound with 60–70% conversion yield at 1-g/liter substrate concentration. The most effective culture, *Nocardia salmonicolor* SC 6310, catalyzed the bioconversion in 96% reaction yield with 99.8% e.e. at 2-g/liter substrate concentration. Product was isolated and identified by NMR and MS. A preparative-scale fermentation process for growth of *N. salmonicolor* and a bioreduction process using cell suspensions of the organism were demonstrated.

A chiral intermediate (2*R*,3*S*)-3-(4-methoxyphenyl)glycidic acid methyl ester [(–)-MPGM] is required for the synthesis of dilthiazem. Matsumae et al. screened over 700 microorganisms and identified a lipase from *Serratia marcescens* which catalyzed the enantioselective hydrolysis of racemic MPGM in a biphasic system using toluene as organic phase. The reaction yield of 48% and the e.e. of 99.8% were obtained for (–)-MPGM.

Potassium Channel Openers

The study of potassium K-channel biochemistry, physiology, and medicinal chemistry has flourished, and numerous papers and reviews have been published in recent years. It has long been known that K-channels play a major role in neuronal excitability and a critical role in the basic electrical and mechanical functions of a wide variety of tissues, including smooth muscle, cardiac muscle, and glands. A new class of highly specific pharmacological compounds has been developed which either open or block K-channels. K-channel openers are powerful smooth muscle relaxants with in vivo antihypertensive and bronchodilator activities. Recently, the synthesis and antihypertensive activity of a series of novel K-

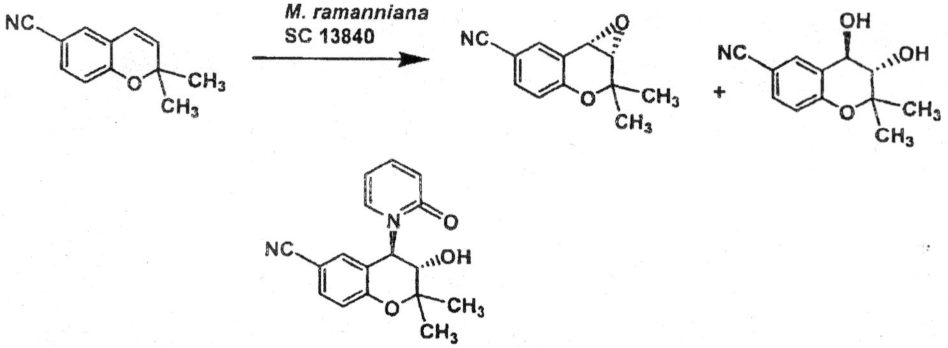

Potassium Channel Opener

Fig. 16.18. Oxygenation of 2,2-dimethyl-2H-1-benzopyran-6-carbonitrile to the corresponding chiral expoxide and (+)-trans-diol by M. ramanniana SC 13840.

channel openers based on monosubstituted *trans*-4-amino-3,4-dihydro-2,2-dimethyl-2H-l-benzopyran-3-ol have been demonstrated. Chiral epoxide and diol are potential intermediates for the synthesis of K-channel activators that are important as antihypertensive and bronchodilator agents. The stereoselective microbial oxygenation of 2,2-dimethyl-2H-1-benzopyran-6-carbonitrile to the corresponding chiral epoxide and chiral diol has been demonstrated. Among microbial cultures evaluated, the best culture, *Mortierella ramanniana* SC 13840, gave reaction yields of 67.5 M% and e.e. of 96% for the (+)-*trans*-diol. A single-stage process (fermentation/epoxidation) for the biotransformation was developed using *M. ramanniana* SC 13840. In a 25-liter fermentor, the (+)-*trans*-diol was obtained in the reaction yield of 60.7 M% and e.e. of 92.5%.

Using a 3-liter cell suspension (10% w/v, wet cells) of *M. ramanniana* SC 13840, the (+)-*trans*-diol was obtained in 76 M% yield with an e.e. of 96%. The reaction was carried out in a 5-liter Bioflo fermentor with 2-g/liter substrate and 1 0-g/liter glucose concentrations. Glucose was supplied to regenerate NADH required for this reaction. From the reaction mixture, (+)-*trans*-diol was isolated in 65 M% (4.6 g) overall yield. An enantiomeric excess of 97% and a chemical purity of 98% were obtained for the isolated (+)-*trans*-diol. In an enzymatic resolution approach, chiral (+)-*trans*-diol was prepared by the stereoselective acetylation of racemic diol with lipases from *Candida cylindraceae* and *P. cepacia*. Both enzymes catalyzed the acetylation of the undesired enantiomer of racemic diol to yield monoacetylated product and unreacted desired (+)-*trans*-diol. A reaction yield of 40% and an e.e. of >90% were obtained using each lipase.

Antiarrhythmic Agents

Larsen and Lish reported the biological activity of a series of phenethanolamine-bearing alkyl sulfonamido groups on the benzene ring. Within this series, some compounds possessed adrenergic and antiadrenergic actions. D-(+)-sotalol is a β-blocker that, unlike other β-blockers, has antiarrhythmic properties and has no other peripheral actions. The β-adrenergic blocking drugs such as propranolol and sotalol have been separated chemically into the dextrorotatory and levorotatory optical isomers, and it has been demonstrated that the activity of the levo isomer is 50 times that of the corresponding dextro isomer. Chiral alcohol is a key intermediate for the chemical synthesis of D-(+)-sotalol. The stereoselective microbial reduction of N-(4-(2-chloro-acetyl)phenyl)methanesulfonamide to the corresponding (+)-alcohol has been demonstrated. Among numbers of microorganisms screened for the transformation of ketone to (+)-alcohol, *Rhodo coccus* sp. ATCC 29675, *Rhodococcus rhodochrous* ATCC 21243, *N. salmonicolor* SC 6310, and *Hansenula polymorpha* ATCC 26012 gave the desired (+)-alcohol in >90% e.e. *H. polymorpha* ATCC 26012 catalyzed the efficient conversion of ketone to (+)-alcohol in 95% reaction yield and >99% e.e. Growth of *H. polymorpha* ATCC 26012 culture was carried out in a 380-liter fermentor and cells harvested from the fermentor were used to conduct transformation in a 3-liter preparative batch. Cell suspensions (20% wet cells in 1 liter of 10 mM potassium phosphate buffer, pH 7.0) were supplemented with 12 g of ketone and 225 g of glucose and the reduction reaction was carried out at 25°C, 200 rpm, and pH 7. Complete conversion of ketone to (+)-alcohol was obtained in a 20-hr reaction. Using preparative HPLC, 8.2 g of (+)-alcohol were isolated from the reaction mixture in overall 68% yield with >99% e.e.

The production of optically active chiral intermediates is a subject of increasing importance in the pharmaceutical industry. Increasing regulatory pressure by the Food and Drug Administration to market homochiral drugs has led to the use of alternative approaches, including biocatalysis for the synthesis of chiral compounds. Organic synthesis has been one of the most successful scientific disciplines and has enormous practical utility. One can ask the question, then, why biocatalysis? What does biocatalysis have to offer to synthetic organic chemists? Biocatalysis gives an added dimension and enormous opportunity to prepare industrially useful chiral compounds. The advantages of biocatalysis over chemical catalysis are that enzyme-catalyzed reactions are stereoselective and regioselective and can be carried out at ambient temperature and atmospheric pressure. In biocatalytic processes, microbial cells and enzymes can be immobilized and an immobilized biocatalyst can be reused for many cycles. In addition, enzymes can be overexpressed to make biocatalytic processes economically efficient. The use of different classes of enzymes in catalysis of different types of chemical reactions is essential to generate a variety of chiral compounds for chemoenzymatic synthesis of pharmaceutical products. This includes the use of hydrolytic enzymes such as lipases, esterases, proteases, dehalogenases, acylases, amidases, nitrilases, lyases, epoxide hydrolases, decarboxylases, and hydantoinases in resolution of racemic compounds and in asymmetric synthesis of optically active compounds. Oxidoreductases and aminotransferases have been used in synthesis of chiral alcohols, aminoalcohols, amino acids, and amines. Aldolases and decarboxylases have been effectively used in asymmetric synthesis by aldol condensation and acyloin condensation reactions. Oxygenases such as monooxygenases have been used in stereoselective and regioselective hydroxylation and epoxidation reactions and dioxygenases in the chemoenzymatic synthesis of chiral diols.

The idea of designing biocatalysts that act specifically in desired reactions of interest can change the face of synthesis. Tailored enzymes made by random and site-directed mutagenesis with modified activity and preparation of thermostable and pH stable enzymes can lead to the production of novel stereoselective biocatalysts. The use of enzymes inorganic solvents has led to hundreds of publications on enzyme-catalyzed asymmetric synthesis and resolution processes. Molecular recognition and selective catalysis are key chemical processes in life which are embodied in enzymes. In the course of the last decades, the progress in biochemistry, protein chemistry, molecular cloning, random and site-directed mutagenesis, and fermentation technology has opened up unlimited access to a variety of enzymes and microbial cultures as valuable tools in organic synthesis.

17

Pharmacology of Central Nervous System

The central nervous system (CNS) is responsible for controlling bodily functions as well as being the center for behavioral and intellectual abilities. Neurons within the CNS are organized into highly complex patterns that mediate information through synaptic interactions. CNS drugs often attempt to modify the activity of these neurons in order to treat specific disorders or to alter the general level of arousal of the CNS. This chapter presents a simplified introduction to the organization of the CNS and the general strategies that can be used with drugs to alter activity within the brain and spinal cord.

CNS Organization

The CNS can be grossly divided into the brain and spinal cord. The brain is subdivided according to anatomic or functional criteria. The following is a brief overview of the general organization of the brain and spinal cord, with some indication of where particular CNS drugs tend to exert their effects. This chapter is not intended to be an extensive review of neuroanatomy—a more elaborate discussion of CNS structure and function can be found in several excellent sources.

Cerebrum

The largest and most rostral aspect of the brain is the *cerebrum*. The cerebrum consists of bilateral hemispheres, with each hemisphere anatomically divided into several lobes (frontal, temporal, parietal, and occipital). The outer cerebrum, or cerebral cortex, is the highest order of conscious function and integration in the CNS. Specific cortical areas are responsible for sensory and motor functions as well as intellectual and cognitive abilities. Other cortical areas are involved in short-term memory and speech. The cortex also operates in a somewhat supervisory capacity regarding lower brain functioning and may influence the control of other activities such as the autonomic nervous system. With regard to CNS drugs, most therapeutic medications tend to affect cortical function indirectly by first altering the function of lower brain and spinal cord structures. An exception is the group of drugs used to treat epilepsy; these drugs are often targeted directly for hyperexcitable neurons in the cerebral cortex. In addition, drugs that attempt to enhance cognitive function in conditions such as Alzheimer disease (cholinergic stimulants) might also exert their primary effects in the cerebrum.

Basal Ganglia

A group of specific areas located deep within the cerebral hemispheres is collectively termed the *basal ganglia*. Components of the basal ganglia include the caudate nucleus, putamen, globus pallidus, lentiform nucleus, and substantia nigra. The basal ganglia are primarily involved in the control of motor activities; deficits in this area are significant in movement disorders such as Parkinson disease and Huntington chorea. Certain medications used to treat these movement disorders exert their effects by interacting with basal ganglia structures.

Diencephalon

The area of the brain enclosing the third ventricle is the *diencephalon*. This area consists of several important structures, including the thalamus and hypothalamus. The thalamus contains distinct nuclei that are crucial in the integration of certain types of sensations and their relay to other areas of the brain (such as the somatosensory cortex). The hypothalamus is involved in the control of diverse body functions including temperature control, appetite, water balance, and certain emotional reactions. The hypothalamus is also significant in its control over the function of hormonal release from the pituitary gland. Several CNS drugs affecting sensation and control of the body functions listed, manifest their effects by interacting with the thalamus and hypothalamus.

Mesencephalon and Brainstem

The *mesencephalon*, or *midbrain*, serves as a bridge between the higher areas of the brain (cerebrum and diencephalon) and the *brainstem*. The brainstem consists of the pons and the medulla oblongata. In addition to serving as a pathway between the higher brain and spinal cord, the midbrain and brainstem are the locations of centers responsible for controlling respiration and cardiovascular function (vasomotor center).

The reticular formation is also located in the midbrain and brainstem. The reticular formation is comprised of a collection of neurons that extend from the reticular substance of the upper spinal cord through the midbrain and the thalamus. The reticular formation monitors and controls consciousness and is also important in regulating the amount of arousal or alertness in the cerebral cortex. Consequently, CNS drugs that affect the arousal state of the individual tend to exert their effects on the reticular formation. Sedative-hypnotics and general anesthetics tend to decrease activity in the reticular formation, whereas certain CNS stimulants (caffeine, amphetamines) may increase arousal through a stimulatory effect on reticular formation neurons.

Cerebellum

The *cerebellum* lies posterior to the brainstem and is separated from it by the fourth ventricle. Anatomically it is divided into two hemispheres, each consisting of three lobes (anterior, posterior, and flocculonodular). The function of the cerebellum is to help plan and coordinate motor activity and to assume responsibility for comparing the actual movement with the intended motor pattern. The cerebellum interprets various sensory input and helps modulate motor output so that the actual movement closely resembles the intended motor program. The cerebellum is also concerned with the vestibular mechanisms responsible for maintaining balance and posture. Therapeutic medications are not usually targeted directly for the cerebellum, but incoordination and other movement disorders may result if a drug exerts a toxic side effect on the cerebellum.

Limbic System

So far, all of the structures described have been grouped primarily by their anatomic relationships with the brain. The *limbic system* is comprised of several structures that are dispersed throughout the brain but are often considered as a functional unit or system within the CNS. Major components of the limbic system include cortical structures (such as the amygdala, hippocampus, and cingulate gyrus), the hypothalamus, certain thalamic nuclei, mamillary bodies, septum pellucidum, and several other structures and tracts. These structures are involved in the control of emotional and behavioral activity. Certain aspects of motivation, aggression, sexual activity, and instinctive responses may be influenced by activity within the limbic system. CNS drugs affecting these aspects of behavior, including some antianxiety and antipsychotic medications, are believed to exert their beneficial effects primarily by altering activity in the limbic structures.

Spinal Cord

At the caudal end of the brainstem, the CNS continues distally as the *spinal cord*. The spinal cord is cylindrically shaped and consists of centrally located gray matter that is surrounded by white matter. The gray matter serves as an area for synaptic connections between various neurons. The white matter consists of the myelinated axons of neurons, which are grouped into tracts ascending or descending between the brain and specific levels of the cord. Certain CNS drugs exert some or all of their effects by modifying synaptic transmission in specific areas of gray matter, while other CNS drugs, such as narcotic analgesics, may exert an effect on synaptic transmission in the gray matter of the cord as well as on synapses in other areas of the brain. Some drugs may be specifically directed toward the white matter of the cord. Drugs such as local anesthetics can be used to block action potential propagation in the white matter so that ascending or descending information is interrupted (i.e., a spinal block).

Blood-Brain Barrier

The *blood-brain barrier* refers to the unique structure and function of CNS capillaries. Certain substances are not able to pass from the bloodstream into the CNS, despite the fact that these substances are able to pass from the systemic circulation into other peripheral tissues. This fact suggests the existence of some sort of unique structure and function of the CNS capillaries that prevents many substances from entering the brain and spinal cord—hence, the term *blood-brain barrier*. This barrier effect is caused primarily by the tight junctions that occur between capillary endothelial cells; in fact, CNS capillaries lack the gaps and fenestrations that are seen in peripheral capillaries. Also, nonneuronal cells in the CNS (e.g., astrocytes) and the capillary basement membrane seem to contribute to the relative impermeability of this barrier. Functionally, the blood-brain barrier acts as a selective filter and seems to protect the CNS by limiting the harmful substances that enter into the brain and spinal cord.

The blood-brain barrier obviously plays an important role in clinical pharmacotherapeutics. To exert their effects, drugs targeted for the CNS must be able to pass from the bloodstream into the brain and spinal cord. In general, nonpolar, lipid-soluble drugs are able to cross the blood-brain barrier by passive diffusion. Polar and lipophobic compounds are usually unable to enter the brain. Some exceptions occur because of the presence of carrier-mediated transport systems in the blood-brain barrier. Some substances (such as glucose) are transported via facilitated diffusion, while other compounds (including some drugs) may be able to enter the brain by active transport. However, the transport processes that carry drugs into the brain are limited to certain specific compounds, and the typical manner by which most drugs enter the brain is by passive lipid diffusion.

Several active transport systems also exist on the blood-brain barrier that are responsible for *removing* drugs and toxins from the brain. That is, certain drugs can enter the brain easily via diffusion or another process, but these drugs are then rapidly and efficiently transported out of the brain and back into the systemic circulation. This effect creates an obvious problem because these drugs will not reach therapeutic levels within the CNS, and won't be beneficial. Hence, the blood-brain barrier has many structural and functional characteristics that influence CNS drugs, and researchers continue to explore ways that these characteristics can be modified to ensure adequate drug delivery to the brain and spinal cord.

CNS Neurotransmitters

The majority of neural connections in the human brain and spinal cord are characterized as chemical synapses. The term *chemical synapse* indicates that a chemical neurotransmitter is used to propagate the nervous impulse across the gap that exists between two neurons. Several distinct chemicals have been identified as neurotransmitters within the brain and spinal cord. Groups of neurons within the CNS tend to use one of these neurotransmitters to produce either excitation or inhibition of the other neurons. Although each neurotransmitter can be generally described as either excitatory or inhibitory within the CNS, some transmitters may have different effects depending on the nature of the postsynaptic receptor involved. The interaction of the transmitter and the receptor dictates the effect on the postsynaptic neuron. The fact that several distinct neurotransmitters exist and that neurons using specific transmitters are organized functionally within the CNS has important pharmacologic implications. Certain drugs may alter the transmission in pathways using a specific neurotransmitter while having little or no effect on other transmitter pathways. This allows the drug to exert a rather specific effect on the CNS, so many disorders may be rectified without radically altering other CNS functions. Other drugs may have a much more general effect and may alter transmission in many CNS regions. To provide an indication of neurotransmitter function, the major categories of CNS neurotransmitters and their general locations and effects are discussed subsequently.

Acetylcholine

Acetylcholine is the neurotransmitter found in many areas of the brain as well as in the periphery (skeletal neuromuscular junction, some autonomic synapses). In the brain, acetylcholine is abundant in the cerebral cortex, and seems to play a critical role in cognition and memory. Neurons originating in the large pyramidal cells of the motor cortex and many neurons originating in the basal ganglia also secrete acetylcholine from their terminal axons. In general, acetylcholine synapses in the CNS are excitatory in nature.

Monoamines

Monoamines are a group of structurally similar CNS neurotransmitters that include the *catecholamines* (dopamine, norepinephrine) and 5-hydroxytryptamine (serotonin). *Dopamine* exerts different effects at various locations within the brain. Within the basal ganglia, dopamine is secreted by neurons that originate in the substantia nigra and project to the corpus striatum. As such, it is important in regulating motor control, and the loss of these dopaminergic neurons results in symptoms commonly associated with Parkinson disease. Dopamine also influences mood and emotions, primarily via its presence in the hypothalamus and other structures within the limbic system. Although its effects within the brain are very complex, dopamine generally inhibits the neurons onto which it is released.

Norepinephrine is secreted by neurons that originate in the locus caeruleus of the pons and projects throughout the reticular formation. Norepinephrine is generally regarded as an inhibitory transmitter within the CNS, but the overall effect following activity of norepinephrine synapses is often general excitation of the brain, probably because norepinephrine directly inhibits other neurons that produce inhibition. This phenomenon of *disinhibition* causes excitation by removing the influence of inhibitory neurons.

Serotonin (also known as 5-hydroxytryptamine) is released by cells originating in the midline of the pons and brainstem and is projected to many different areas, including the dorsal horns of the spinal cord and the hypothalamus. Serotonin is considered to be a strong inhibitor in most areas of the CNS and is believed to be important in mediating the inhibition of painful stimuli. It is also involved in controlling many aspects of mood and behavior, and problems with serotonergic activity have been implicated in several psychiatric disorders, including depression and anxiety.

Amino Acids

Several amino acids, such as glycine and gamma-aminobutyric acid (GABA), are important inhibitory transmitters in the brain and spinal cord. Glycine seems to be the inhibitory transmitter used by certain interneurons located throughout the spinal cord, and this amino acid also causes inhibition in certain areas of the brain. Likewise, GABA is found throughout the CNS, and is believed to be the primary neurotransmitter used to cause inhibition at presynaptic and postsynaptic neurons in the brain and spinal cord. Other amino acids such as aspartate and glutamate have been found in high concentrations throughout the brain and spinal cord; these substances cause excitation of CNS neurons. These excitatory amino acids have received a great deal of attention lately because they may also produce neurotoxic effects when released in large amounts during CNS injury and certain neurologic disorders (epilepsy, amyotrophic lateral sclerosis, and so forth).

Peptides

Many peptides have already been established as CNS neurotransmitters. One peptide that is important from a pharmacologic standpoint is substance P, which is an excitatory transmitter that is involved in spinal cord pathways transmitting pain impulses. Increased activity at substance P synapses in the cord serves to mediate the transmission of painful sensations, and certain drugs such as the opioid analgesics may decrease activity at these synapses. Other peptides that have important pharmacologic implications include three families of compounds: the endorphins, enkephalins, and dynorphins. These peptides, also known as the endogenous opioids, are excitatory transmitters in certain brain synapses that inhibit painful sensations. Hence, endogenous opioids in the brain are able to decrease the central perception of pain. Finally, peptides such as galanin, leptin, neuropeptide Y, vasoactive intestinal polypeptide (VIP), and pituitary adenylate cyclase–activating polypeptide (PACAP) have been identified in various areas of the CNS. These and other peptides may affect various CNS functions, either by acting directly as neurotransmitters or by acting as cotransmitters moderating the effects of other neurotransmitters.

Other Transmitters

In addition to the well-known substances, other chemicals are continually being identified as potential CNS neurotransmitters. Recent evidence has implicated substances such as adenosine and adenosine triphosphate (ATP) as transmitters or modulators of neural transmission in specific areas of the brain and in the autonomic nervous system. Many other chemicals that are traditionally associated with functions outside the CNS are being identified as possible CNS transmitters, including histamine, nitric oxide, and certain hormones (vasopressin, oxytocin). As the function of these chemicals and other new transmitters becomes clearer, the pharmacologic significance of drugs that affect these synapses will undoubtedly be considered.

CNS Drugs: General Mechanisms

The majority of CNS drugs work by modifying synaptic transmission in some way. Most drugs that attempt to rectify CNS-related disorders do so by either increasing or decreasing transmission at specific synapses. For instance, psychotic behavior has been associated with overactivity in central synapses that use dopamine as a neurotransmitter. Drug therapy in this situation consists of agents that decrease activity at central dopamine synapses. Conversely, Parkinson disease results from a decrease in activity at specific dopamine synapses. Antiparkinsonian drugs attempt to increase dopaminergic transmission at these synapses and bring synaptic activity back to normal levels. A drug that modifies synaptic transmission must somehow alter the quantity of the neurotransmitter that is released from the presynaptic terminal or affect the stimulation of postsynaptic receptors, or both. When considering a typical synapse, there are several distinct sites at which a drug may alter activity in the synapse. Specific ways a drug may modify synaptic transmission are presented here.

Presynaptic Action Potential

The arrival of an action potential at the presynaptic terminal initiates neurotransmitter release. Certain drugs, such as local anesthetics, block propagation along neural axons so that the action potential

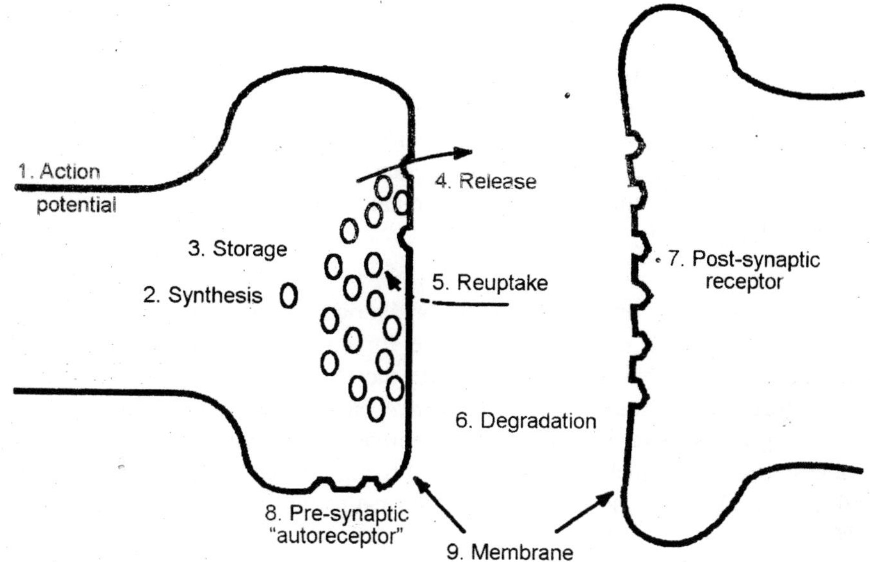

Fig. 17.1. Sites at which drugs can alter transmission at a CNS synapse.

fails to reach the presynaptic terminal, which effectively eliminates activity at that particular synapse. Also, the amount of depolarization or the height of the action potential arriving at the presynaptic terminal is directly related to the amount of transmitter released.

Any drug or endogenous chemical that limits the amount of depolarization occurring in the presynaptic terminal will inhibit the synapse because less neurotransmitter is released. In certain situations, this is referred to as *presynaptic inhibition*, because the site of this effect is at the presynaptic terminal. The endogenous neurotransmitter GABA is believed to exert some of its inhibitory effects via this mechanism.

Synthesis of Neurotransmitter

Drugs that block the synthesis of neurotransmitter will eventually deplete the presynaptic terminal and impair transmission. For example, metyrosine (Demser) inhibits an enzyme that is essential for catecholamine biosynthesis in the presynaptic terminal. Treatment with metyrosine results in decreased synthesis of transmitters such as dopamine and norepinephrine.

Storage of Neurotransmitter

A certain amount of chemical transmitter is stored in presynaptic vesicles. Drugs that impair this storage will decrease the ability of the synapse to continue to transmit information for extended periods. An example of this is the antihypertensive drug reserpine (Serpalan, Serpasil), which impairs the ability of adrenergic terminals to sequester and store norepinephrine in presynaptic vesicles.

Release

Certain drugs will increase synaptic activity by directly increasing the release of neurotransmitter from the presynaptic terminal. Amphetamines appear to exert their effects on the CNS primarily by increasing the presynaptic release of catecholamine neurotransmitters (e.g., norepinephrine). Conversely, other compounds may inhibit the synapse by directly decreasing the amount of transmitter released during each action potential. An example is botulinum toxin (Botox), which can be used as a skeletal muscle relaxant because of its ability to impair the release of acetylcholine from the skeletal neuromuscular junction.

Reuptake

After the neurotransmitter is released, some chemical synapses terminate activity primarily by transmitter reuptake. Reuptake involves the movement of the transmitter molecule back into the presynaptic terminal. A drug that impairs the reuptake of transmitter allows more of it to remain in the synaptic cleft and continue to exert an effect. Consequently, blocking reuptake actually increases activity at the synapse. For instance, tricyclic antidepressants impair the reuptake mechanism that pumps amine neurotransmitters back into the presynaptic terminal, which allows the transmitter to continue to exert its effect and prolong activity at the synapse.

Degradation

Some synapses rely primarily on the enzymatic breakdown of the released transmitter to terminate synaptic activity. Inhibition of the enzyme responsible for terminating the transmitter allows more of the active transmitter to remain in the synaptic cleft, thereby increasing activity at the synapse. An example is using a drug that inhibits the *cholinesterase* enzyme as a method of treating myasthenia gravis. In myasthenia gravis, there is a functional decrease in activity at the skeletal neuromuscular junction. Anticholinesterase drugs such as neostigmine (Prostigmin) and pyridostigmine (Mestinon) inhibit acetylcholine breakdown, allowing more of the released neurotransmitter to continue to exert an effect at the neuromuscular synapse.

Postsynaptic Receptor

Chemical antagonists can be used to block the postsynaptic receptor, thus decreasing synaptic transmission. The best-known example of this is the use of beta blockers. These agents are antagonists that are specific for the beta-adrenergic receptors on the myocardium, and they are frequently used to treat hypertension, cardiac arrhythmias, and angina pectoris. Other drugs may improve synaptic transmission by affecting the receptor directly so there is a tendency for increased neurotransmitter binding or improved receptor–effector coupling, or both. For instance, benzodiazepines (e.g., diazepam [Valium], chlordiazepoxide [Librium, others]) appear to enhance the postsynaptic effects of the inhibitory neurotransmitter GABA.

Presynaptic Autoreceptors

In addition to postsynaptic receptors, there are also receptors on the presynaptic terminal of some types of chemical synapses. These presynaptic receptors seem to serve as a method of negative feedback in controlling neurotransmitter release. During high levels of synaptic activity, the accumulation of neurotransmitter in the synaptic cleft may allow binding to the presynaptic receptors and limit further release of chemical transmitter. Certain drugs may also be able to attenuate synaptic activity through presynaptic autoreceptors. For instance, clonidine (Catapres), may exert some of its antihypertensive effects by binding to presynaptic receptors on sympathetic postganglionic neurons and impairing the release of norepinephrine onto the peripheral vasculature. The use of drugs that alter synaptic activity by binding to these autoreceptors is still somewhat new, however, and the full potential for this area of pharmacology remains to be determined.

Membrane Effects

Drugs may alter synaptic transmission by affecting membrane organization and fluidity. Membrane fluidity is basically the amount of flexibility or mobility of the lipid bilayer. Drugs that alter the fluidity of the presynaptic membrane could affect the way that presynaptic vesicles fuse with and release their neurotransmitter. Drug-induced changes in the postsynaptic membrane would affect the receptor environment and thereby alter receptor function. Membrane modification will result in either increased or decreased synaptic transmission, depending on the drug in question and the type and magnitude of membrane change. Alcohol (ethanol) and general anesthetics were originally thought to exert their effects by producing reversible changes in the fluidity and organization of the cell membranes of central neurons. Although this idea has been challenged somewhat, these drugs may still exert some of their effects via neuronal membranes. A CNS drug does not have to adhere specifically to only one of these methods of synaptic modification. Some drugs may affect the synapse in two or more ways. For example, the antihypertensive agent guanethidine (Ismelin) impairs both presynaptic storage and release of norepinephrine. Other drugs such as barbiturates may affect both the presynaptic terminal and the postsynaptic receptor in CNS synapses.

Sedative-Hypnotic and Antianxiety Agents

Drugs that are classified as sedative-hypnotics are used both to relax the patient and to promote sleep. As the name "*sedative*" implies, these drugs exert a calming effect and serve to pacify the patient. At higher doses, the same drug can produce drowsiness and initiate a relatively normal state of sleep (hypnosis). At still higher doses, some sedative-hypnotics (especially barbiturates) will eventually bring on a state of general anesthesia. Because of their general central nervous system (CNS)-depressant effects, some sedative- hypnotic drugs are also used for other functions such as treating epilepsy or producing muscle relaxation. However, the sleep-enhancing effects will be of concern here.

By producing sedation, many drugs will also decrease the level of anxiety in a patient. Of course, these anxiolytic properties often cause a decrease in the level of alertness in the individual. However, certain agents are available that can reduce anxiety without an overt sedative effect.

Sedative-hypnotic and antianxiety drugs are among the most commonly used drugs worldwide. For example, it is estimated that insomnia affects between 10 to 15 percent of the general population, and that pharmacological management can be helpful in promoting normal sleep. Moreover, people who are ill, or who have recently been relocated to a new environment (hospital, nursing home), will often have difficulty sleeping and might need some form of sedative-hypnotic agent. Likewise, a person who sustains an injury or illness will certainly have some apprehension concerning his or her welfare. If necessary, this apprehension can be controlled to some extent by using antianxiety drugs during the course of rehabilitation. Consequently, many patients receiving physical therapy and occupational therapy take sedative-hypnotic and antianxiety agents to help promote sleep and decrease anxiety; rehabilitation specialists should understand the basic pharmacology of these agents.

Sedative-Hypnotic Agents

Sedative-hypnotics fall into two general categories: benzodiazepines and nonbenzodiazepines. At present, benzodiazepines are typically used to promote normal sedation and sleep, especially in relatively acute or short-term situations. These agents will be addressed first, followed by a description of the nonbenzodiazepine hypnotics.

Benzodiazepines

Benzodiazepines are a family of compounds that share the same basic chemical structure and pharmacological effects. Although the more famous members of this family are associated with treating anxiety (e.g., diazepam), several benzodiazepines are indicated specifically to promote sleep. These agents exert hypnotic effects similar to those of nonbenzodiazepines—such as the barbiturates—but benzodiazepines are generally regarded as safer because there is less of a chance for lethal overdose. Benzodiazepines, however, are not without their drawbacks, and they can cause residual effects the day after they are administered; prolonged use can also cause tolerance and physical dependence.

Mechanism of benzodiazepine effects

The benzodiazepines exert their effects by increasing the inhibitory effects at CNS synapses that use the neurotransmitter gamma-aminobutyric acid (GABA). These inhibitory synapses are associated with a membrane protein complex containing three primary components: (1) a binding site for GABA, (2) a binding site for benzodiazepines, and (3) an ion channel that is specific for chloride ions. GABA typically exerts its inhibitory effects by binding to its receptor site on this complex and by initiating an increase in chloride conductance through the channel. Increased chloride conductance facilitates chloride entry into the neuron and results in hyperpolarization, or a decreased ability to raise the neuron to its firing threshold. By binding to their own respective site on the complex, benzodiazepines potentiate the effects of GABA and increase the inhibition at these synapses.

Consequently, the presence of the GABA-benzodiazepine–chloride ion channel complex accounts for the specific mechanism of action of this class of sedative-hypnotics. By increasing the inhibitory effects at GABAergic synapses located in the reticular formation, benzodiazepines can decrease the level of arousal in the individual. In other words, the general excitation level in the reticular activating system decreases, and relaxation and sleep are enhanced.

Research has also indicated that there are at least three primary types of GABA receptors, and these receptors are classified as GABA A, B, and C according to their structural and functional characteristics. $GABA_A$ and $GABA_C$ receptors, for example, cause inhibition by increasing chloride entry, whereas $GABA_B$ receptors may cause inhibition by increasing potassium *exit* (efflux) from CNS neurons. At the present time, it appears that benzodiazepines act primarily on the $GABA_A$ subtype and that the therapeutic effects of these drugs (sedation, hypnosis, decreased anxiety) are mediated through the $GABA_A$ receptor, which is found in the brain. Hence, clinically used benzodiazepines are basically $GABA_A$ receptor agonists.

Furthermore, the $GABA_A$ receptor is composed of several subunits (alpha, beta, gamma); it appears that individual subunits on this receptor mediate specific effects. Sedation, for example, seems to be mediated by the alpha 1 subunit, whereas other beneficial effects such as decreased anxiety might be mediated by the alpha 2 and alpha 3 subunits. Benzodiazepines seem to affect all of these subunits, hence their ability to produce sedative and antianxiety effects.

These drugs, however, might also exert certain side effects (tolerance, dependence) by affecting other subunits on the $GABA_A$ receptor. A drug that is selective for only the alpha 1 subunit might exert sedative effects without producing as many side effects. Some of the newer nonbenzodiazepine drugs such as zolpidem (Ambien) and zaleplon (Sonata) appear to be more specific for the alpha 1 subunit, and might therefore produce sedative effects with fewer side effects.

Because of these new advances, scientists continue to study the molecular biology of the $GABA_A$ receptor, and clarify how benzodiazepines affect these receptors. Likewise, differences between the principal GABA receptors (A, B, C) has encouraged the development of drugs that are more selective to GABA receptors located in certain areas of the CNS. The muscle relaxant baclofen (Lioresal), for example, may be somewhat more selective for $GABA_B$ receptors in the spinal cord than for other $GABA_A$ or $GABA_C$ receptors that are found in the brain. Future drug development will continue to exploit the differences between the GABA receptor subtypes so that drugs are more selective and can produce more specific beneficial effects with fewer side effects.

Finally, the discovery of a CNS receptor that is specific for benzodiazepines has led to some interesting speculation as to the possible existence of some type of endogenous sedative-like agent. The presence of a certain type of receptor to indicate that the body produces an appropriate agonist for that receptor makes sense. For instance, the discovery of opiate receptors initiated the search for endogenous opiate-like substances, which culminated in the discovery of the enkephalins. It has been surmised that certain endogenous steroids such as allopregnanolone (a metabolic byproduct of progesterone) can bind to the GABA receptors in the CNS and produce sedative-hypnotic effects. Continued research in this area may someday reveal the exact role of steroids and other endogenous substances, and the focus of pharmacologic treatment can then be directed toward stimulating the release of endogenous sedative-hypnotic agents

Nonbenzodiazepines

Barbiturates

The barbiturates are a group of CNS depressants that share a common chemical origin: barbituric acid. The potent sedative-hypnotic properties of these drugs have been recognized for some time, and their status as the premier medication used to promote sleep went unchallenged for many years. However, barbiturates are associated with a relatively small therapeutic index; approximately 10 times the therapeutic dose can often be fatal. These drugs are also very addictive, and their prolonged use is often a problem in terms of drug abuse. Consequently, the lack of safety of the barbiturates and their strong potential for addiction and abuse necessitated the development of alternative nonbarbiturate drugs such as the benzodiazepines.

Despite their extensive use in the past, the exact mechanism of the barbiturates remains somewhat unclear. When used in sedative-hypnotic doses, barbiturates may function in a similar fashion to the benzodiazepines in that they also potentiate the inhibitory effects of GABA. This idea suggests that barbiturates may affect the GABA-benzodiazepine–chloride ion channel complex described above. Indeed, considerable evidence exists that barbiturates bind directly to the $GABA_A$ receptor at a site that is different from the binding site for GABA or benzodiazepines. Barbiturates may, however, also exert effects that are not mediated through an effect on the GABA-benzodiazepine–chloride ion channel. At higher doses, for instance, barbiturates may also directly increase the release of inhibitory transmitters such as glycine, and increase the release of excitatory transmitters such as glutamate. Regardless of their exact mechanism, barbiturates are effective sedative-hypnotics because of their specificity for neurons in the midbrain portion of the reticular formation as well as some limbic system structures. At higher doses, barbiturates also depress neuronal excitability in other areas of the brain and spinal cord.

Newer, nonbenzodiazepine sedative-hypnotics

Several drugs including zolpidem (Ambien) and zaleplon (Sonata) were developed recently as sedative-hypnotics. These drugs are chemically different from the benzodiazepines, but still seem to affect the $GABA_A$ receptors in the brain. That is, these newer drugs bind to the $GABA_A$ receptor, which then causes GABA to bind more effectively, thus increasing chloride conductance and the level of inhibition in the neuron. Increased inhibition in certain areas of the brain results in less arousal and the promotion of sleep. These newer drugs appear to be as effective as the benzodiazepines in promoting sleep. The drugs also seem to have a lower risk of producing certain side effects and causing problems when discontinued. This difference might be explained by the fact that newer, nonbenzodiazepine drugs bind preferentially to the alpha 1 subunit of the $GABA_A$ receptor. As discussed earlier, stimulation of this particular subunit seems to mediate sedation without producing other side effects. Hence, drugs like zolpidem and zaleplon are gaining acceptance for the treatment of sleep disorders, and efforts continue to develop other nonbenzodiazepine drugs that selectively affect this receptor.

Other Nonbenzodiazepines

Several other nonbenzodiazepine compounds can be prescribed for their sedative-hypnotic properties. These compounds are chemically dissimilar from one another, but share the ability to promote relaxation and sleep via depressing the CNS. Cyclic ethers and alcohols (including ethanol) can be included in this category, but their use specifically as sedative-hypnotics is fairly limited at present. The recreational use of ethanol in alcoholic beverages is an important topic in terms of abuse and long-term effects. However, since this area is much too extensive to be addressed here, only their effects as sedative-hypnotics is considered.

Alcohol (ethanol) and other sedative-hypnotics— neither benzodiazepine nor barbiturate in nature— work through mechanisms that are poorly understood. In the past, it was thought that alcohols exerted their CNS-depressant effects directly on neuronal membrane composition and fluidity. These and other highly lipid-soluble substances could simply dissolve in the lipid bilayer and inhibit neuronal excitability by temporarily disrupting membrane structures in the presynaptic and postsynaptic regions of CNS neurons. Recent evidence, however, suggests that alcohol may act on protein receptors much in the same way as the benzodiazepines and barbiturates. That is, alcohol may exert most of its effects by activating $GABA_A$ receptors and increasing GABA-mediated inhibition in the CNS. In any event, alcohol and similar agents bring about a decrease in neuronal transmission, which causes fairly widespread CNS depression which accounts for the subsequent sedative effects of such compounds.

Pharmacokinetics

Benzodiazepine and nonbenzodiazepine sedative-hypnotics are usually highly lipid soluble. They are typically administered orally and are absorbed easily and completely from the gastrointestinal tract. Distribution is fairly uniform throughout the body, and these drugs reach the CNS readily because of their high degree of lipid solubility. Sedative-hypnotics are metabolized primarily by the oxidative enzymes of the drug-metabolizing system in liver cells. Termination of their activity is accomplished either by hepatic enzymes or by storage of these drugs in non-CNS tissues; that is, by sequestering the drugs in adipose and other peripheral tissues, their CNS-depressant effects are not exhibited. However, when the drugs slowly leak out of their peripheral storage sites, they can be redistributed to the brain and can cause low levels of sedation. This occurrence may help explain the "hangoverlike" feelings that are frequently reported the day after taking sedative-hypnotic drugs. Finally, excretion of these drugs takes place through the kidney after their metabolism in the liver. As with most drug biotransformations, metabolism of sedative-hypnotics is essential in creating a polar metabolite that is readily excreted by the kidney.

Problems and Adverse Effects

Residual Effects

The primary problem associated with sedative- hypnotic use is the residual effects that can occur the day after administration. Individuals who take a sedative-hypnotic to sleep at night sometimes complain of drowsiness and decreased motor performance the next day. These hangoverlike effects may be caused by the drug being redistributed to the CNS from peripheral storage sites or may simply occur because the drug has not been fully metabolized.

Anterograde amnesia is another problem sometimes associated with sedative-hypnotic use. The patient may have trouble recalling details of events that occurred for a certain period of time before the drug was taken. Although usually a minor problem, this can become serious if the drug-induced amnesia exacerbates an already existing memory problem, as might occur in some elderly patients.

These residual problems can be resolved somewhat by taking a smaller dose or by using a drug with a shorter half-life. Also, newer nonbenzodiazepine agents such as zolpidem and zaleplon appear to have milder effects, perhaps because of their relatively short half-life and the limited duration of action. These newer drugs have therefore been advocated in people who are prone to residual effects (e.g., older adults), and people who need to use these drugs for an extended period of time.

Tolerance and Physical Dependence

Another potential problem with long-term sedative- hypnotic drug use is that prolonged administration may cause tolerance and physical dependence. *Drug tolerance* is the need to take more of a drug to exert the same effect. *Dependence* is described as the onset of withdrawal symptoms if drug administration is ceased. Although these problems were originally thought to be limited to barbiturates, benzodiazepines and other sedative-hypnotics are now recognized as also causing tolerance and dependence when taken continually for several weeks.

The manner and severity of withdrawal symptoms varies according to the type of drug and the extent of physical dependence. Withdrawal after short-term benzodiazepine use may be associated with problems such as sleep disturbances (i.e., so-called rebound insomnia). As discussed earlier, withdrawal effects seem to be milder with the newer nonbenzodiazepine agents (zolpidem and zaleplon). Newer agents, however, are not devoid of these problems and care should be taken with prolonged use, especially in people with psychiatric disorders or a history of substance abuse.

Consequently, the long-term use of these drugs should be avoided, and other nonpharmacologic methods of reducing stress and promoting relaxation (e.g., mental imagery, biofeedback) should be instituted before tolerance and physical dependence. If the sedative-hypnotic drug has been used for an extended period, tapering off the dosage rather than abruptly stopping it has been recommended as a safer way to terminate administration.

Other Side Effects

Other *side effects* such as gastrointestinal discomfort (nausea and vomiting), dry mouth, sore throat, and muscular incoordination have been reported, but these occur fairly infrequently and vary according to the exact drug used. Cardiovascular and respiratory depression may also occur, but these problems are dose-related and are usually not significant, except in cases of overdose.

ANTIANXIETY DRUGS

Anxiety can be described as a fear or apprehension over a situation or event that an individual feels is threatening. These events can range from a change in employment or family life to somewhat irrational phobias concerning everyday occurrences. Anxiety disorders can also be classified in several clinical categories including generalized anxiety disorder, social anxiety disorder, panic disorder, obsessive-compulsive disorder, and posttraumatic stress syndrome. Antianxiety drugs can help decrease the tension and nervousness associated with many of these syndromes until the situation is resolved or until the individual is counseled effectively in other methods of dealing with his or her anxiety. Many drugs—including sedative-hypnotics—have the ability to decrease anxiety levels, but this is usually at the expense of an increase in sedation. Frequently, alleviating anxiety without producing excessive sedation is desirable so that the individual can function at home, on the job, and so on. Consequently, certain drugs are available that have significant anxiolytic properties at doses that produce minimal sedation. Benzodiazepine drugs and other nonbenzodiazepine strategies for dealing with anxiety are discussed here.

Benzodiazepines

As discussed previously, because of their relative safety, the benzodiazepines are typically the front-line drugs used to treat many forms of anxiety. In terms of anxiolytic properties, diazepam (Valium) is the prototypical antianxiety benzodiazepine. The extensive use of this drug in treating nervousness and apprehension has made the trade name of this compound virtually synonymous with a decrease in tension and anxiety. When prescribed in anxiolytic dosages, diazepam and certain other benzodiazepines will decrease anxiety without major sedative effects. Some sedation, however, may occur even at anxiolytic dosages; these drugs can be used as sedative-hypnotics simply by increasing the dosage.

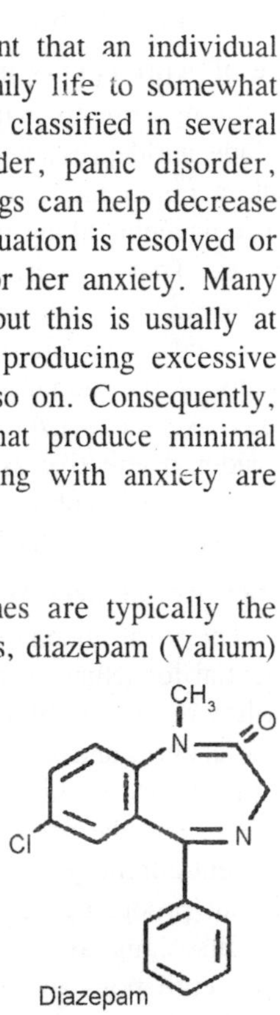

Diazepam

Fig. 17.2. Dizepam.

The mechanism of action of the benzodiazepines was discussed previously in this chapter. The antianxiety properties of these drugs involve a mechanism similar or identical to their sedative-hypnotic effects (i.e., potentiating GABAergic transmission). Benzodiazepines also seem to increase inhibition in the spinal cord, which produces some degree of skeletal muscle relaxation, which may contribute to their antianxiety effects by making the individual feel more relaxed.

Buspirone

Buspirone (BuSpar) is an antianxiety agent that was approved in 1986 for treating general anxiety disorder. This agent is not a benzodiazepine. It belongs instead to a drug class known as the azapirones. Therefore, buspirone does not act on the GABA receptor, but exerts its antianxiety effects by increasing the effects of 5-hydroxytryptamine (serotonin) in certain areas of the brain. Buspirone is basically a serotonin agonist that stimulates certain serotonin receptors, especially the 5-HT1A serotonin receptor subtype. This increase in serotonergic influence is beneficial in treating general anxiety disorder and possibly in panic disorder, obsessive-compulsive disorder, posttraumatic stress syndrome, and various other disorders that are influenced by CNS serotonin levels. More importantly, buspirone has a much better side-effect profile than traditional antianxiety drugs. Buspirone seems to produce less sedation and psychomotor impairment than benzodiazepine agents. There is a much smaller risk of developing tolerance and dependence to buspirone and the potential for abuse is much lower than with other anxiolytics. Buspirone has only moderate efficacy, however, and this drug may not take effect as quickly in patients with severe anxiety. Nonetheless, buspirone offers a safer alternative to traditional antianxiety drugs such as benzodiazepines, especially if patients need to receive treatment for an extended period of time. Development of additional azapirones and other drugs that influence serotonin activity may continue to provide better and safer antianxiety agents in the future.

Use of Antidepressants in Anxiety

Many patients with anxiety also have symptoms of depression. It therefore seems reasonable to include antidepressant drugs as part of the pharmacological regimen in these patients. Hence, patients with a combination of anxiety and depression often take a traditional antianxiety agent such as a benzodiazepine along with an antidepressant. Antidepressant drugs, however, might have direct anxiolytic effects. That is, certain antidepressants such as paroxetine (Paxil) or venlafaxine (Effexor) can help reduce anxiety independent of their effects on depression. These antidepressants have therefore been advocated as an alternative treatment for anxiety, especially for people who cannot tolerate the side effects of traditional anxiolytics, or who might be especially susceptible to the addictive properties of drugs like the benzodiazepines. Moreover, antidepressants such as paroxetine or venlafaxine are now considered effective as the primary treatment for several forms of anxiety, including generalized anxiety disorder, social phobia, and panic disorder. Antidepressants, either used alone or in combination with antianxiety drugs, have become an important component in the treatment of anxiety.

Other Antianxiety Drugs

The ideal antianxiety agent is nonaddictive, safe (i.e., relatively free from harmful side effects and potential for lethal overdose), and not associated with any sedative properties. Drugs such as meprobamate (Miltown) and barbiturates are not currently used to any great extent because they do not meet any of these criteria and are no more effective in reducing anxiety than benzodiazepines. As indicated earlier, buspirone and certain antidepressants currently offer an effective and somewhat safer method of treating anxiety, and the use of these agents has increased dramatically in recent years. Another option includes the beta-adrenergic antagonists (beta blockers) because these drugs can decrease situational anxiety without producing sedation. In particular, beta blockers such as propranolol (Inderal) have been used by musicians and other performing artists to decrease cardiac palpitations, muscle tremors, hyperventilation, and other manifestations of anxiety that tend to occur before an important performance. Beta blockers probably exert their antianxiety effects through their ability to decrease activity in the sympathetic nervous system, that is, through their sympatholytic effects. These drugs may exert both peripheral sympatholytic effects (e.g., blockade of myocardial beta-1 receptors) as well as decreasing central sympathetic tone. In any event, beta blockers may offer a suitable alternative to decrease the effects of nervousness without a concomitant decrease in levels of alertness or motivation. Again, these drugs have gained popularity with performing artists as a way to blunt the symptoms of performance anxiety without actually diminishing the anticipation and excitement that is requisite for a strong performance.

Problems and Adverse Effects

Most of the problems that occur with benzodiazepine anxiolytic drugs are similar to those mentioned regarding the use of these agents as sedative-hypnotics. Sedation is still the most common side effect of anxiolytic benzodiazepines, even though this effect is not as pronounced as with their sedative-hypnotic counterparts. Still, even short-term use of these drugs can produce psychomotor impairment, especially during activities that require people to remain especially alert, such as driving a car. Addiction and abuse are problems with chronic benzodiazepine use, and withdrawal from these drugs can be a serious problem. Also, anxiety can return to, or exceed, pretreatment levels when benzodiazepines are suddenly discontinued, a problem known as rebound anxiety. The fact that chronic benzodiazepine use can cause these problems reinforces the idea that these drugs are not curative and should be used only for limited periods of time as an adjunct to other nonpharmacologic procedures such as psychologic counseling. Problems and side effects associated with buspirone include dizziness, headache, nausea, and restlessness. Antidepressants such as paroxetine and venlafaxine also produce a number of side effects depending on the specific agent. Nonetheless, these newer, nonbenzodiazepine anxiolytics tend to produce less sedation, and their potential for addiction is lower compared to benzodiazepines. Hence, nonbenzodiazepine drugs might be an attractive alternative, especially in patients who are prone to sedation (e.g., older adults), patients with a history of substance abuse, or people who need chronic anxiolytic treatment.

Special Consideration of Sedative-Hypnotic and Antianxiety Agents in Rehabilitation

Although these drugs are not used to directly influence the rehabilitation of musculoskeletal or other somatic disorders, the prevalence of their use in patient populations is high. Any time a patient is hospitalized for treatment of a disorder, a substantial amount of apprehension and concern exists. The foreign environment of the institution as well as a change in the individual's daily routine can understandably result in sleep disturbances. Likewise, older adults often have trouble sleeping, and the use of sedative- hypnotic agents is common, especially in patients living in nursing homes or other facilities. Individuals who are involved in rehabilitation programs, both as inpatients and as outpatients, may also have a fairly high level of anxiety because of concern about their health and ability to resume normal functioning. Acute and chronic illnesses can create uncertainty about a patient's future family and job obligations as well as doubts about his or her self- image. The tension and anxiety produced may necessitate pharmacologic management.

The administration of sedative-hypnotic and antianxiety drugs has several direct implications for the rehabilitation session. Obviously the patient will be much calmer and more relaxed after taking an antianxiety drug, thus offering the potential benefit of gaining the patient's full cooperation during a physical or occupational therapy treatment. Anxiolytic benzodiazepines, for example, reach peak blood levels 2 to 4 hours after oral administration, so scheduling the rehabilitation session during that time may improve the patient's participation in treatment. Of course, this rationale will backfire if the drug produces significant hypnotic effects. Therapy sessions that require the patient to actively participate in activities such as gait training or therapeutic exercise will be essentially useless and even hazardous if the patient is extremely drowsy. Consequently, scheduling patients for certain types of rehabilitation within several hours after administration of sedative-hypnotics or sedative-like anxiolytics is counterproductive and should be avoided.

Finally, benzodiazepines and other drugs used to treat sleep disorders and anxiety are often associated with falls and subsequent trauma including hip fractures, especially in older adults. The risk of falls is greater in people who have a history of doing so or who have other problems that would predispose them to falling (vestibular disorders, impaired vision, and so forth). Therapists can identify such people and intervene to help prevent this through balance training, environmental modifications (removing cluttered furniture, throw rugs, and so forth), and similar activities. Therapists can help plan and implement nonpharmacological interventions to help decrease anxiety and improve sleep. Interventions such as regular physical activity, massage, and various relaxation techniques may be very helpful in reducing stress levels and promoting normal sleep. Therapists can therefore help substitute nonpharmacological methods for traditional sedative-hypnotic and antianxiety drugs, thus improving the patient's quality of life by avoiding drug-related side effects.

Sedative-hypnotic and antianxiety drugs play a prominent role in today's society. The normal pressures of daily life often result in tension and stress, which affects an individual's ability to relax or cope with stress. These problems are compounded when there is some type of illness or injury present. As would be expected, a number of patients seen in a rehabilitation setting are taking these drugs. Benzodiazepines have long been the premier agents used to treat sleep disorders and anxiety; they all share a common mechanism of action, and they potentiate the inhibitory effects of GABA in the CNS. With regard to their sedative-hypnotic effects, benzodiazepines such as flurazepam and triazolam are commonly used to promote sleep. Although these drugs are generally safer than their forerunners, they are not without their problems. Newer nonbenzodiazepine sedative-hypnotics such as zolpidem and zaleplon may also be effective in treating sleep disorders, and these newer agents may be somewhat safer than their benzodiazepine counterparts. Benzodiazepines such as diazepam (Valium) leave as are also used frequently to reduce anxiety, but the introduction of newer drugs such as buspirone and specific antidepressants (paroxetine, venlafaxine) have provided an effective but somewhat safer alternative for treating anxiety. Because of the potential for physical and psychologic dependence, sedative-hypnotic and antianxiety drugs should not be used indefinitely. These drugs should be prescribed judiciously as an adjunct to helping patients deal with the source of their problems.

18

SKELETAL MUSCLE RELAXANTS

Skeletal muscle relaxants are used to treat conditions associated with hyperexcitable skeletal muscle—specifically, spasticity and muscle spasms. Although these two terms are often used interchangeably, spasticity and muscle spasms represent two distinct abnormalities. The use of relaxant drugs, however, is similar in each condition because the ultimate goal is to normalize muscle excitability without a profound decrease in muscle function. Considering the number of rehabilitation patients with muscle hyperexcitability that is associated with either spasm or spasticity, skeletal muscle relaxants represent an important class of drugs to the rehabilitation specialist.

Drugs discussed in this chapter are used to decrease muscle excitability and contraction via an effect at the spinal cord level, at the neuromuscular junction, or within the muscle cell itself. Some texts also classify neuromuscular junction blockers such as curare and succinylcholine as skeletal muscle relaxants. However, these drugs are more appropriately classified as skeletal muscle *paralytics* because they eliminate muscle contraction by blocking transmission at the myoneural synapse. This type of skeletal muscle paralysis is used primarily during general anesthesia. Skeletal muscle relaxants do not typically prevent muscle contraction; they only attempt to normalize muscle excitability to decrease pain and improve motor function.

INCREASED MUSCLE TONE: SPASTICITY VERSUS MUSCLE SPASMS

Much confusion and consternation often arise from the erroneous use of the terms "spasticity" and "spasm." For the purpose of this text, these terms will be used to describe two different types of increased excitability, which result from different underlying pathologies. *Spasticity* occurs in many patients following an injury to the central nervous system (CNS), including cord-related problems (multiple sclerosis, spinal cord transection) and injuries to the brain (CVA, cerebral palsy, acquired brain injury). Although there is considerable controversy about the exact changes in motor control, most clinicians agree that spasticity is characterized primarily by an exaggerated muscle stretch reflex. This abnormal reflex activity is velocity-dependent, with a rapid lengthening of the muscle invoking a strong contraction in the stretched muscle.

The neurophysiologic mechanisms underlying spasticity are complex, but this phenomenon occurs when supraspinal inhibition or control is lost because of a lesion in the spinal cord or brain. Presumably, specific upper motor neuron lesions interrupt the cortical control of stretch reflex and alpha motor neuron excitability. Spasticity, therefore, is not in itself a disease but rather the motor sequela to pathologies such as cerebral vascular accident (CVA), cerebral palsy, multiple sclerosis (MS), and traumatic lesions to the brain and spinal cord (including quadriplegia and paraplegia).

Skeletal muscle *spasms* are used to describe the increased tension often seen in skeletal muscle after certain musculoskeletal injuries and inflammation (muscle strains, nerve root impingements, etc.) occur. This tension is involuntary, so the patient is unable to relax the muscle. Spasms differ from spasticity because spasms typically arise from an orthopedic injury to a musculoskeletal structure or peripheral nerve root rather than an injury to the CNS. Likewise, muscle spasms are often a continuous, tonic contraction of specific muscles rather than the velocity-dependent increase in stretch reflex activity commonly associated with spasticity. The exact reasons for muscle spasms are poorly understood. According to some authorities, muscle spasms occur because a vicious cycle is created when the initial injury causes muscular pain and spasm, which increases afferent nociceptive input to the spinal cord, further exciting the alpha motor neuron to cause more spasms, and so on. Other experts believe that muscle spasms occur because of a complex protective mechanism, whereby muscular contractions are intended to support an injured vertebral structure or peripheral joint. Regardless of the exact reason, tonic contraction of the affected muscle is often quite painful because of the buildup of pain-mediating metabolites (e.g., lactate). Consequently, various skeletal muscle relaxants attempt to decrease skeletal muscle excitation and contraction in cases of spasticity and spasm. Specific drugs and their mechanisms of action are discussed here.

Specific Agents Used to Produce Skeletal Muscle Relaxation

Skeletal muscle relaxants are categorized in this chapter according to their primary clinical application: agents used to decrease spasms and agents used to decrease spasticity. One agent, diazepam (Valium), is indicated for both conditions and will appear in both categories. Finally, the use of botulinum toxin (Botox) as an alternative strategy for reducing focal spasms or spasticity will be addressed.

Agents Used to Treat Muscle Spasms

Diazepam

The effects of diazepam (Valium) on the CNS and its use as an antianxiety drug are discussed in Chapter 6. Basically, diazepam and other benzodiazepines work by increasing the central inhibitory effects of gamma-aminobutyric acid (GABA); that is, diazepam binds to receptors located at GABAergic synapses and increases the GABA-induced inhibition at that synapse. Diazepam appears to work as a muscle relaxant through this mechanism, potentiating the inhibitory effect of GABA on alpha motor neuron activity in the spinal cord. The drug also exerts some supraspinal sedative effects; in fact, some of its muscle relaxant properties may derive from the drug's ability to produce a more generalized state of sedation.

Uses

Diazepam is one of the oldest medications for treating muscle spasms, and has been used extensively in treating spasms associated with musculoskeletal injuries such as acute low-back strains. Diazepam has also been used to control muscle spasms associated with tetanus toxin; the use of valium in this situation can be life-saving as well by inhibiting spasms of the larynx and other muscles.

Adverse effects

The primary side effect with diazepam is that dosages successful in relaxing skeletal muscle also produce sedation and a general reduction in psychomotor ability. However, this effect may not be a problem and may actually be advantageous for the patient recovering from an acute musculoskeletal injury. For example, a patient with an acute lumbosacral strain may benefit from the sedative properties because he or she will remain fairly inactive, thereby allowing better healing during the first few days after the injury. Continued use, however, may be problematic because of diazepam's sedative effects. The drug can also produce tolerance and physical dependence, and sudden withdrawal after prolonged use can cause seizures, anxiety, agitation, tachycardia, and even death. Likewise, an overdose with diazepam can result in coma or death as well. Hence, this drug might be beneficial for the short-term management of acute muscle spasms, but long-term use should be discouraged.

Polysynaptic Inhibitors

A variety of centrally acting compounds have been used in an attempt to enhance muscle relaxation and decrease muscle spasms. Some examples are carisoprodol (Soma, Vanadom), chlorphenesin carbamate (Maolate), chlorzoxazone (Paraflex, Parafon Forte, others), cyclobenzaprine (Flexeril), metaxalone (Skelaxin), methocarbamol (Carbacot, Robaxin, Skelex), and orphenadrine citrate (Antiflex, Norflex, others). The mechanism of action of these drugs is not well defined. Research in animals has suggested that these drugs may decrease polysynaptic reflex activity in the spinal cord, hence the term "*polysynaptic inhibitors.*" A polysynaptic reflex arc in the spinal cord is comprised of several small interneurons that link incoming (afferent) input into the dorsal horn with outgoing (efferent) outflow onto the alpha motor neuron. By inhibiting the neurons in the polysynaptic pathways, these drugs could decrease alpha motor neuron excitability and therefore cause relaxation of skeletal muscle.

It is not clear, however, exactly how these drugs inhibit neurons involved in the polysynaptic pathways. There is preliminary evidence that one of these compounds (cyclobenzaprine) might block serotonin receptors on spinal interneurons, thereby decreasing the excitatory influence of serotonin on alpha motor neuron activity. Although this effect has been attributed to cyclobenzaprine in animals (rats), the effect of this drug and other muscle relaxants in humans remains to be determined.

On the other hand, these compounds have a general depressant effect on the CNS; that is, they cause a global decrease in CNS excitability that results in generalized sedation. It therefore seems possible that some of their muscle relaxant effects are caused by their sedative powers rather than a selective effect on specific neuronal reflex pathways. This observation is not to say that they are ineffective, because clinical research has shown that these drugs can be superior to a placebo in producing subjective muscle relaxation. However, the specific ability of these drugs to relax skeletal muscle remains doubtful, and it is generally believed that their muscle relaxant properties are secondary to a nonspecific CNS sedation.

Uses

These drugs are typically used as adjuncts to rest and physical therapy for the short-term relief of muscle spasms associated with acute, painful musculoskeletal injuries. When used to treat spasms, these compounds are often given with a nonsteroidal anti-inflammatory agent (NSAIDs), or sometimes incorporated into the same tablet with an analgesic such as acetaminophen or aspirin. For instance, Norgesic is one of the brand names for orphenadrine combined with aspirin (and caffeine). Such combinations have been reported to be more effective than the individual components given separately.

Adverse effects

Because of their sedative properties, the primary side effects of these drugs are drowsiness and dizziness. A variety of additional adverse effects, including nausea, light-headedness, vertigo, ataxia, and headache, may occur depending on the patient and the specific drug administered. Cases of fatal overdose have also been documented for several of these drugs, including cyclobenzaprine and metaxolone. Long term or excessive use of these medications may also cause tolerance and physical dependence. In particular, carisoprodol should be used cautiously because this drug is metabolized in the body to form meprobamate, which is a controlled substance that has sedative/anxiolytic properties but is not used extensively because it has strong potential for abuse. Hence, use of carisoprodol represents a rather unique situation where the drug itself or its metabolic byproduct (meprobamate) can produce effects and side effects that lead to addiction and abuse, especially in people with a history of substance abuse. Likewise, discontinuing carisoprodol suddenly after long term use can lead to withdrawal symptoms such as anxiety, tremors, muscle twitching, and hallucinations. Consequently, polysynaptic inhibitors can help provide short-term relief for muscle spasms associated with certain musculoskeletal conditions, and they may work synergistically with physical therapy and other interventions during acute episodes of back pain, neck pain, and so forth. Nonetheless, they have some rather serious side effects and potential for abuse, and the long-term use of these drugs should be discouraged.

Agents Used to Treat Spasticity

The three agents traditionally used in the treatment of spasticity are baclofen, diazepam, and dantrolene sodium. Two newer agents, gabapentin and tizanidine, are also available for treating spasticity in various conditions. All of these agents are addressed below.

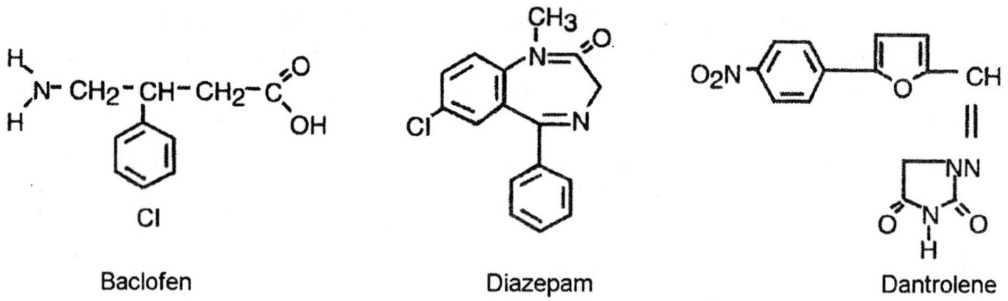

Baclofen Diazepam Dantrolene

Fig. 18.1. Structure of three primary antispasticity drugs.

Baclofen

The chemical name of baclofen is beta (*p*-chlorophenyl)-GABA. As this name suggests, baclofen is a derivative of the central inhibitory neurotransmitter GABA. However, there appear to be some differences between baclofen and GABA. Baclofen seems to bind preferentially to certain GABA receptors, which have been classified as $GABA_b$ receptors (as opposed to $GABA_a$ receptors). Preferential binding to $GABA_b$ receptors enables baclofen to act as a GABA agonist, inhibiting transmission within the spinal cord at specific synapses. To put this in the context of its use as a muscle relaxant, baclofen appears to have an inhibitory effect on alpha motor neuron activity within the spinal cord. This inhibition apparently occurs via inhibiting excitatory neurons that synapse with the alpha motor neuron (presynaptic inhibition), as well as directly affecting the alpha motor neuron itself (postsynaptic inhibition). The result is decreased firing of the aipha motor neuron, with a subsequent relaxation of the skeletal muscle.

Uses

Baclofen is administered orally to treat spasticity associated with lesions of the spinal cord, including traumatic injuries resulting in paraplegia or quadriplegia and spinal cord demyelination resulting in MS. Baclofen is often the drug of choice in reducing the muscle spasticity associated with MS because it produces beneficial effects with a remarkable lack of adverse side effects when used in patients with MS. The drug also does not cause as much generalized muscle weakness as direct-acting relaxants such as dantrolene, which can be a major advantage of baclofen treatment in many patients with MS. Baclofen also appears to produce fewer side effects when used appropriately to reduce spasticity secondary to traumatic spinal cord lesions, thus providing a relatively safe and effective form of treatment. When administered systemically, baclofen is less effective in treating spasticity associated with supraspinal lesions (stroke, cerebral palsy), because these patients are more prone to the adverse side effects of this drug and beoause baclofen does not readily penetrate the blood-brain barrier.

Oral baclofen has also been used to reduce alcohol consumption in people who are chronic alcohol abusers. Apparently, relatively low doses of baclofen can reduce the cravings and desire for alcohol consumption via the effects of this drug on CNS GABA receptors. Future studies will help clarify the role of this drug in treating chronic alcoholism.

Adverse effects

When initiating baclofen therapy, the most common side effect is transient drowsiness, which usually disappears within a few days. When given to patients with spinal cord lesions, there are usually few other adverse effects. When given to patients who have had a CVA or to elderly individuals, there is sometimes a problem with confusion and hallucinations. Other side effects, occurring on an individual basis, include fatigue, nausea, dizziness, muscle weakness, and headache.

Abrupt discontinuation of baclofen may also cause withdrawal symptoms such as hyperthermia, hallucinations, and seizures. Increased seizure activity has also been reported following baclofen overdose, and in selected patient populations such as certain children with cerebral palsy and certain adults with multiple sclerosis.

Intrathecal Baclofen

Although baclofen is administered orally in most patients it can also be administered intrathecally in patients with severe, intractable spasticity. Intrathecal administration is the delivery of a drug directly into the subarachnoid space surrounding a specific level of the spinal cord. This places the drug very close to the spinal cord, thus allowing increased drug effectiveness with much smaller drug doses. Likewise, fewer systemic side effects occur because the drug tends to remain in the area of the cord rather than circulating in the bloodstream and causing adverse effects on other tissues.

When baclofen is administered intrathecally for the long-term treatment of spasticity, a small catheter is usually implanted surgically so that the open end of the catheter is located in the subarachnoid space and the other end is attached to some type of programmable pump. The pump is implanted subcutaneously in the abdominal wall and is adjusted to deliver the drug at a slow, continuous rate. The rate of infusion is adjusted over time to achieve the best clinical reduction in spasticity.

Intrathecal baclofen delivery using implantable pumps has been used in patients with spasticity of spinal origin (spinal cord injury, multiple sclerosis), and in patients with spasticity resulting from supraspinal (cerebral) injury, including cerebral palsy, CVA, and traumatic brain injury. Studies involving these patients have typically noted a substantial decrease in rigidity (as indicated by decreased Ashworth scores, decreased reflex activity, and so forth). Patient satisfaction is generally favorable, and caregivers for younger children report ease of care following implantation of intrathecal baclofen pumps. There is growing evidence that intrathecal baclofen can also reduce pain of central origin in people with spasticity; that is, continuous baclofen administration to the subarachnoid space may inhibit the neural circuitry that induces chronic pain in people with stroke and other CNS injuries.

Uses

Intrathecal baclofen can result in decreased spasticity and increased comfort in many people with severe spasticity. This intervention can also result in functional improvements, especially in cases where voluntary motor control was being masked by spasticity. Ambulatory patients with spasticity resulting from a CVA, for example, may be able to increase their walking speed and increase their functional mobility after intrathecal baclofen therapy.

These functional improvements, however, may not occur in all types of spasticity. Patients with severe spasticity of spinal origin, for example, may not experience improvements in mobility or decreased disability. If these patients do not have adequate voluntary motor function there is simply not enough residual motor ability to perform functional tasks after spasticity is reduced. Nonetheless, these patients may still benefit from intrathecal baclofen because of decreased rigidity and pain, which can result in improved self-care and the ability to perform daily living activities.

Adverse effects

Despite these benefits, intrathecal baclofen is associated with a number of potential complications. Primary among these is the possibility of a disruption in the delivery system; that is, a pump malfunction or a problem with the delivery catheter can occur. In particular, the catheter can become obstructed, or the tip of the catheter can become displaced so that baclofen is not delivered into the correct area of the subarachnoid space. Increased drug delivery due to a pump malfunction could cause overdose and lead to respiratory depression, decreased cardiac function, and coma. Conversely, abruptly stopping the drug due to pump failure, pump removal, or delivery catheter displacement/blockage may cause a withdrawal syndrome that includes fever, confusion, delirium, and seizures.

A second major concern is the possibility that tolerance could develop with long-term, continuous baclofen administration. Tolerance is the need for more of a drug to achieve its beneficial effects when used for prolonged periods. Several studies have reported that dosage must indeed be increased progressively when intrathecal baclofen systems are used for periods of several months to several years. Tolerance to intrathecal baclofen, however, can usually be dealt with by periodic adjustments in dosage, and tolerance does not usually develop to such an extent that intrathecal baclofen must be discontinued.

Hence, intrathecal baclofen offers a means of treating certain patients with severe spasticity who have not responded to more conventional means of treatment including oral baclofen. Additional research will help determine optimal ways that this intervention can be used to decrease spasticity. Further improvements in the technologic and mechanical aspects of intrathecal delivery, including better pumps and catheter systems, will also make this a safer and more practical method of treating these patients.

Dantrolene Sodium

The only muscle relaxant available that exerts its effect directly on the skeletal muscle cell is dantrolene sodium (Dantrium). This drug works by impairing the release of calcium from the sarcoplasmic reticulum within the muscle cell during excitation. In response to an action potential, the release of calcium from sarcoplasmic storage sites initiates myofilament cross-bridging and subsequent muscle contraction. By inhibiting this release, dantrolene attenuates muscle contraction and therefore enhances relaxation.

Uses

Dantrolene is often effective in treating severe spasticity, regardless of the underlying pathology. Patients with traumatic cord lesions, advanced MS, cerebral palsy, or CVAs will probably experience a reduction in spasticity with this drug. This drug is also invaluable in treating malignant hyperthermia, which is a potentially life-threatening reaction occurring in susceptible individuals following exposure to general anesthesia, muscle paralytics used during surgery, or certain antipsychotic medications (a condition also called neuroleptic malignant syndrome). In this situation, dantrolene inhibits skeletal muscle contraction throughout the body, thereby limiting the rise in body temperature generated by strong, repetitive skeletal muscle contractions. Dantrolene is not prescribed to treat muscle spasms caused by musculoskeletal injury.

Adverse effects

The most common side effect of dantrolene is generalized muscle weakness; this makes sense considering that dantrolene impairs sarcoplasmic calcium release in skeletal muscles throughout the body, not just in the hyperexcitable tissues. Thus, the use of dantrolene is sometimes counterproductive because the increased motor function that occurs when spasticity is reduced may be offset by generalized motor weakness. This drug may also cause severe hepatotoxicity, and cases of fatal hepatitis have been reported. The risk of toxic effects on the liver seems to be greater in women over 40 years of age, and in individuals receiving higher doses of this drug (over 300 mg). Other, less serious side effects that sometimes occur during the first few days of therapy include drowsiness, dizziness, nausea, and diarrhea, but these problems are usually transient.

Diazepam

As indicated earlier, diazepam is effective in reducing spasticity as well as muscle spasms because this drug increases the inhibitory effects of GABA in the CNS.

Uses

Diazepam is used in patients with spasticity resulting from cord lesions and is sometimes effective in patients with cerebral palsy.

Adverse effects

Use of diazepam as an antispasticity agent is limited by the sedative effects of this medication; that is, patients with spasticity who do not want a decrease in mental alertness will not tolerate diazepam therapy very well. Extended use of the drug can cause tolerance and physical dependence, and use of diazepam for the long-term treatment of spasticity should be avoided whenever possible.

Gabapentin

Developed originally as an antiseizure drug, gabapentin (Neurontin) has also shown some promise in treating spasticity. This drug appears to cause inhibition in the spinal cord in a manner similar to GABA, but the exact mechanism of this drug remains to be determined. That is, gabapentin does not appear to bind to the same receptors as GABA, and this drug does not appear to directly increase the release or effects of endogenous GABA. Nonetheless, gabapentin may decrease spasticity by raising the overall level of inhibition in the spinal cord, thereby decreasing excitation of the alpha motor neuron with subsequent skeletal muscle relaxation. The exact way that this drug exerts its antispasticity effects, however, remains to be determined.

Uses

Gabapentin is effective in decreasing the spasticity associated with spinal cord injury 102 and multiple sclerosis. Additional research should clarify how this drug can be used alone or with other agents to provide optimal benefits in spasticity resulting from various spinal, and possibly cerebral, injuries.

Adverse effects

The primary side effects of this drug are sedation, fatigue, dizziness, and ataxia.

Tizanidine

Tizanidine (Zanaflex) is classified as an alpha-2 adrenergic agonist, meaning that this drug binds selectively to the alpha-2 receptors in the CNS and stimulates them. Alpha-2 receptors are found at various locations in the brain and spinal cord, including the presynaptic and postsynaptic membranes of spinal interneurons that control alpha motor neuron excitability. Stimulation of these alpha-2 receptors inhibits the firing of interneurons that relay information to the alpha motor neuron; that is, interneurons that comprise polysynaptic reflex arcs within the spinal cord. Tizanidine appears to bind to receptors on spinal interneurons, decrease the release of excitatory neurotransmitters from their presynaptic terminals (presynaptic inhibition), and decrease the excitability of the postsynaptic neuron (postsynaptic inhibition). Inhibition of spinal interneurons results in decreased excitatory input onto the alpha motor neuron, with a subsequent decrease in spasticity of the skeletal muscle supplied by that neuron.

Uses

Tizanidine has been used primarily to control spasticity resulting from spinal lesions (multiple sclerosis, spinal cord injury), and this drug may also be effective in treating spasticity in people with cerebral lesions (CVA, acquired brain injury). There is some concern, however, that tizanidine might slow neuronal recovery following brain injury, and some practitioners are therefore reluctant to use this drug during the acute phase of stroke or traumatic brain injury. Because it may inhibit pain pathways in the spinal cord, tizanidine has also been used to treat chronic headaches and other types of chronic pain (fibromyalgia, chronic regional pain syndromes, and so forth).

As an antispasticity drug, tizanidine appears to be as effective as orally administered baclofen or diazepam, but tizanidine generally has milder side effects and produces less generalized muscle weakness than these other agents. Tizanidine is also superior to other alpha-2 agonists such as clonidine (Catapres) because tizanidine does not cause as much hypotension and other cardiovascular side effects. Clonidine exerts antispasticity as well as antihypertensive effects because this drug stimulates alpha-2 receptors in the cord and brainstem, respectively. Use of clonidine in treating spasticity, however, is limited because of the cardiovascular side effects, and clonidine is used primarily for treating hypertension.

Adverse effects

The most common side effects associated with tizanidine include sedation, dizziness, and dry mouth. As indicated, however, tizanidine tends to have a more favorable side effect profile than other alpha-2 agonists, and this drug produces less generalized weakness than oral baclofen or diazepam. Tizanidine may therefore be a better alternative to these other agents in patients who need to reduce spasticity while maintaining adequate muscle strength for ambulation, transfers, and so forth.

Use of Botulinum Toxin as a Muscle Relaxant

Injection of botulinum toxin is a rather innovative way to control localized muscle hyperexcitability. Botulinum toxin is a purified version of the toxin that causes botulism. Systemic doses of this toxin can be extremely dangerous or fatal because botulinum toxin inhibits the release of acetylcholine from presynaptic terminals at the skeletal neuromuscular junction. Loss of presynaptic acetylcholine release results in paralysis of the muscle fiber supplied by that terminal. Systemic dissemination of botulinum toxin can therefore cause widespread paralysis, including loss of respiratory muscle function. Injection into specific muscles, however, can sequester the toxin within these muscles, thus producing localized effects that are beneficial in certain forms of muscle hyperexcitability.

Mechanism of Action

The cellular actions of botulinum toxin at the neuromuscular junction have recently been clarified. This toxin is attracted to glycoproteins located on the surface of the presynaptic terminal at the skeletal neuromuscular junction. Once attached to the membrane, the toxin enters the presynaptic terminal and inhibits proteins that are needed for acetylcholine release. Normally, certain proteins help fuse presynaptic vesicles with the inner surface of the presynaptic terminal, thereby allowing the vesicles to release acetylcholine via exocytosis. Botulinum toxin cleaves and destroys these fusion proteins, thus making it impossible for the neuron to release acetylcholine into the synaptic cleft. Local injection of botulinum toxin into specific muscles will therefore decrease muscle excitation by disrupting synaptic transmission at the neuromuscular junction. The affected muscle will invariably undergo some degree of paresis and subsequent relaxation because the toxin prevents the release of acetylcholine.

It has been suggested that botulinum toxin might have other effects on neuronal excitability. This toxin, for example, might also inhibit contraction of intrafusal muscle fibers that are located within skeletal muscle, and help control sensitivity of the stretch reflex. Inhibiting these intrafusal fibers would diminish activity in the afferent limb of the stretch reflex, thereby contributing to the antispasticity effects of this intervention. Through its direct action on muscle excitability, botulinum toxin may also have other neuro-physiological effects at the spinal cord level. That is, reducing spasticity might result in complex neurophysiologic changes at the spinal cord, ultimately resulting in more normal control of

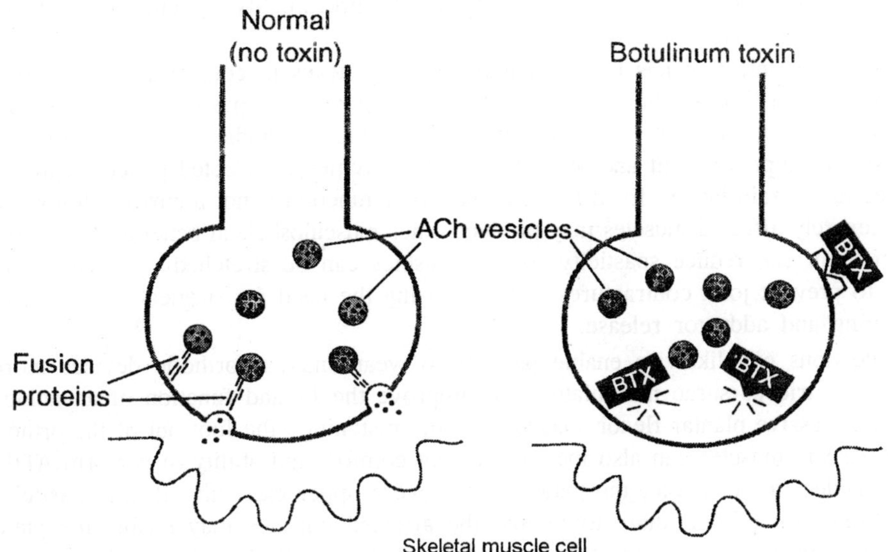

Fig. 18.2. Mechanism of action of botulinum toxin at the skeletal neuromuscular junction.

motor function in both the injected muscle and its antagonist. In other words, reduction of excessive afferent discharge from the spastic muscle might help reestablish a more reasonable level of excitation at the cord level, thus improving efferent discharge to the injected muscle and its antagonist. More research will be needed to help clarify how local administration of botulinum toxin can have direct effects on the injected muscle as well as reflex neurophysiological effects on the spinal cord.

Clinical Use of Botulinum Toxin

Seven strains (serotypes) of botulinum toxin have been identified, but only two types are currently available for clinical use: botulinum toxin types A and B. These types differ somewhat in their chemistry, duration of action, and so forth. The most commonly used therapeutic type is botulinum toxin type A; this agent is marketed commercially under trade names such as Botox and Dysport. Botulinum toxin type B (Myobloc) is also available, and can be useful in patients who develop immunity to the type A form of this toxin.

Botulinum toxin has been used for some time to control localized muscle dystonias, including conditions such as spasmodic torticollis, blepharospasm, laryngeal dystonia, strabismus, and several other types of focal dystonias. When used therapeutically, small amounts of this toxin are injected directly into the dystonic muscles, which begin to relax within a few days to 1 week. This technique appears to be fairly safe and effective in many patients, but relief may only be temporary. Symptoms often return within 3 months after each injection, necessitating additional treatments. Still, this technique represents a method for treating patients with severe, incapacitating conditions marked by focal dystonias and spasms.

More recently, there has been considerable interest in using botulinum toxin to reduce spasticity in specific muscles or muscle groups. This treatment has been used to treat spasticity resulting from various disorders including cerebral palsy, traumatic brain injury, CVA, and spinal cord injury. As with treatment of focal dystonias, the toxin is injected directly into selected muscles. If necessary, electromyography or ultrasonography can be used to identify specific muscles and guide the injection to the desired site within the muscle belly (e.g., the motor point of the muscle). There is also some evidence that electrical stimulation of the nerve supplying the muscle for the first few days following injection may help increase the efficacy of the toxin, presumably by enhancing its uptake by the presynaptic nerve terminals.

Botulinum toxin injection has been documented as a means to control severe spasticity in various clinical situations. This intervention, for example, can help remove spastic dominance in certain patients so that volitional motor function can be facilitated. For example, judicious administration of botulinum toxin can result in improved gait and other functional activities in selected patients with cerebral palsy, stroke, or traumatic brain injury. Even if voluntary motor function is not improved dramatically, reducing spasticity in severely affected muscles may produce other musculoskeletal benefits. For example, injection of botulinum toxin can reduce spasticity so that muscles can be stretched or casted more effectively, thus helping to prevent joint contractures and decreasing the need for surgical procedures such as heel-cord lengthening and adductor release.

These injections can likewise enable patients to wear and use orthotic devices more effectively. Injection into the triceps surae musculature can improve the fit and function of an ankle-foot orthosis by preventing excessive plantar flexor spasticity from "pistoning" the foot out of the orthosis. Injections into severely spastic muscles can also increase patient comfort and ability to perform ADL and hygiene activities. Consider, for example, the patient with severe upper extremity flexor spasticity following a CVA. Local injection of botulinum toxin into the affected muscles may enable the patient to extend his or her elbow, wrist, and fingers, thereby allowing better hand cleansing, ability to dress, decreased pain, and so forth.

Finally, local botulinum toxin administration has been advocated as a way to control muscle hyperexcitability in other clinical situations. There has, of course, been considerable interest in using this toxin for cosmetic reasons. Injection of botulinum toxin into specific facial muscles can paralyze these muscles, thereby reducing the appearance of wrinkles around the eyes, mouth, and so forth. Nonetheless, patients undergoing physical rehabilitation may also benefit from uses of this toxin. For example, patients with hyperactive (neurogenic) bladder following spinal cord injury can be treated by injecting botulinum toxin directly into the bladder detrussor muscle or external urethral sphincter. This intervention may help normalize bladder function and promote more effective voiding. Botulinum toxin has also been used to treat patients with chronic pain syndromes, including chronic headache, migraine, and various musculoskeletal disorders (back pain, whiplash injuries, and so forth). Clearly, this intervention has many potential benefits in many different clinical situations, and additional research will be needed to document how botulinum toxin can be used to reduce muscle hyperexcitability and improve function in various patient populations.

Limitations and Side Effects

Botulinum toxin does not cure spasticity and there are a number of limitations to its use. In particular, only a limited number of muscles can be injected during a given treatment because only a limited amount of botulinum toxin can be administered during each set of injections. For example, the total amount of botulinum toxin type A injected during each treatment session is typically between 200–300 units in adults, with proportionally smaller amounts used in children depending on his or her size and age. The typical dose of the type B form is 2500–5000 units. Exceeding these doses will cause an immune response whereby antibodies are synthesized against the toxin, making subsequent treatments ineffective because the patient's immune system will recognize and inactivate the toxin. The number of muscles that can be injected is therefore often limited to one or two muscle groups; for example, the elbow and wrist flexors in one upper extremity of an adult, or the bilateral triceps surae musculature of a child.

As indicated earlier, the relaxant effects of the toxin are likewise temporary, and these effects typically diminish within 2 to 3 months after injection. The effects apparently wear off because a new presynaptic terminal "sprouts" from the axon that contains the originally affected presynaptic terminal. This new terminal grows downward, reattaching to the skeletal muscle and creating a new motor end plate with a new source of acetylcholine. The effects of the previous injection are overcome when this new presynaptic terminal begins to function. Another injection will be needed to block the release from this new presynaptic terminal, thus allowing another 2 to 3 months of antispasticity effects. This fact raises the question of how many times the injection cycle can be repeated safely and effectively. At the present time, there is no clear limit to the number of times a muscle can be injected, providing, of course, that sufficient time has elapsed between each series of injections. Longitudinal studies will be needed to determine if there are any detrimental effects of long-term use of this intervention.

Consequently, botulinum toxin represents a strategy for dealing with spasticity that is especially problematic in specific muscles or groups of muscles. Despite the rather ominous prospect of injecting a potentially lethal toxin into skeletal muscles, this intervention has a remarkably small incidence of severe adverse effects when administered at therapeutic doses. Botulinum toxin can therefore be used as part of a comprehensive rehabilitation program to provide optimal benefits in certain patients with severe spasticity.

PHARMACOKINETICS

Most muscle relaxants are absorbed fairly easily from the gastrointestinal tract, and the oral route is the most frequent method of drug administration. In cases of severe spasms, certain drugs such as methocarbamol and orphenadrine can be injected intramuscularly or intravenously to permit a more rapid effect. Likewise, diazepam and dantrolene can be injected to treat spasticity if the situation warrants a faster onset. As discussed earlier, continuous intrathecal baclofen administration may be used in certain patients with severe spasticity, and local injection of botulinum toxin is a possible strategy for treating focal dystonias and spasticity. Metabolism of muscle relaxants is usually accomplished by hepatic microsomal enzymes; and the metabolite or intact drug is excreted through the kidneys.

Skeletal muscle relaxants are used to treat the muscle spasms that result from musculoskeletal injuries or spasticity that occurs following lesions in the CNS. Depending on the specific agent, these drugs reduce muscle excitability by acting on the spinal cord, at the neuromuscular junction, or directly within the skeletal muscle fiber. Diazepam and polysynaptic inhibitors are used in the treatment of muscle spasms, but their effectiveness as muscle relaxants may be because of their nonspecific sedative properties. Agents used to treat spasticity include baclofen, dantrolene, diazepam, gabapentin, and tizanidine. Each drug works by a somewhat different mechanism, and the selection of a specific antispasticity agent depends on the patient and the underlying CNS lesion (e.g., stroke, MS). Local injection of botulinum toxin can also be used to treat focal dystonias and spasticity, and this technique may help control spasms and spasticity in specific muscles or muscle groups. Physical therapists and other rehabilitation personnel will frequently work with patients taking these drugs for the treatment of either spasticity or spasms. Although there are some troublesome side effects, these drugs generally facilitate the rehabilitation program by directly providing benefits (muscle relaxation) that are congruent with the major rehabilitation goals.

19

METABOLIC ENGINEERING FOR CEPHALOSPORIN C

Improving product yield in an antibiotic fermentation relies on an understanding and exploitation of the basic biology of the producing microorganism. Traditionally, microbiologists and biochemical engineers optimize the productive phase of fermentations by manipulating the nutrition and environment of the producing microorganism. Genetic manipulation of the producing fungus or bacterium through natural selection or deliberate random mutation and screening for enhanced yield or favorable metabolite profile have been companions to fermentation optimization for decades. The success of these traditional techniques is typified by the two-orders-of-magnitude increase in the production of penicillin by *Penicillium chrysogenum* since the early 1950s.

Biochemical pathways leading from basic metabolic precursors to finished products are deduced through chemical structural analysis of the products and by-products coupled with biochemical and genetic investigation. Highly sensitive bioanalytical techniques allow biochemists to characterize many of the enzymes responsible for antibiotic production. Similar techniques also help to identify product precursor pools that can indicate rate-limiting steps in the production of an antibiotic. With the introduction of recombinant DNA techniques in the 1970s, the genes coding for the various enzymes responsible for the biochemical steps became targets for antibiotic yield improvement investigations.

The term *metabolic engineering* refers to the deliberate genetic manipulation of one or more steps in a biosynthetic pathway leading to a desired product. Such manipulations may include gene deletions to reduce or eliminate undesirable by-products, an increase in gene copy number to enhance conversion of rate- limiting precursor pools to end products, or the introduction of a non-natural gene resulting in a novel product. In this chapter we will discuss the metabolic engineering of the cephalosporin C (CPC) biosynthetic pathway for yield improvement and production of economically important intermediates for semisynthetic cephalosporin synthesis.

ENZYMES OF CEPHALOSPORIN C BIOSYNTHESIS

Cephalosporin C, characterized by β-lactam-dihydrothiazine fused ring, is produced via a multistep biosynthetic pathway by *Cephalosporium acremonium*. This pathway shares several steps with the pathway that diverges to penicillin produced commercially by *Penicillium chrysogenum* and again diverges and is extended by several steps to yield cephamycin C by *Streptomyces clavuligerus*. All of the enzymes in the CPC pathway have been purified and characterized, and the genes coding for each enzyme have been cloned using the so-called reverse genetics approach and by traditional genetic methodologies.

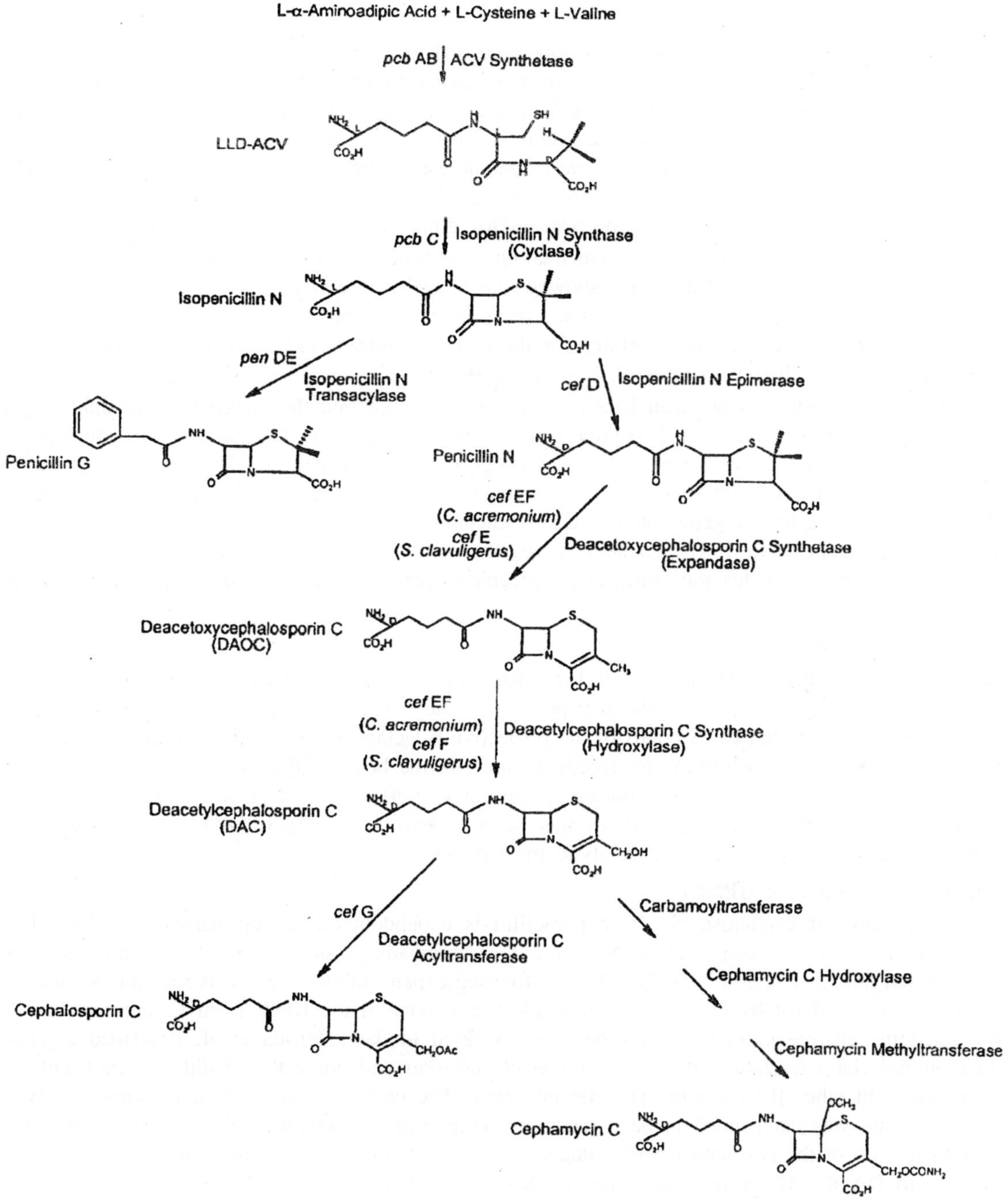

L-α-Aminoadipic Acid + L-Cysteine + L-Valine
pcb AB | ACV Synthetase
LLD-ACV
pcb C | Isopenicillin N Synthase (Cyclase)
Isopenicillin N
pen DE — Isopenicillin N Transacylase
Penicillin G
cef D — Isopenicillin N Epimerase
Penicillin N
cef EF (*C. acremonium*) *cef* E (*S. clavuligerus*) — Deacetoxycephalosporin C Synthetase (Expandase)
Deacetoxycephalosporin C (DAOC)
cef EF (*C. acremonium*) *cef* F (*S. clavuligerus*) — Deacetylcephalosporin C Synthase (Hydroxylase)
Deacetylcephalosporin C (DAC)
cef G — Deacetylcephalosporin C Acyltransferase
Carbamoyltransferase
Cephamycin C Hydroxylase
Cephamycin Methyltransferase
Cephalosporin C
Cephamycin C

Fig. 19.1. Biosynthetic pathway for cephalosporin C in C. acremonium, penicillin G in P. chrysogenum, and cephamycin C in S. clavuligerus.

Ingolia and Queener proposed the current nomenclature for the genes in this pathway. Genes common to both penicillin and cephalopsorin biosynthesis are named *pcb*, the genes unique to penicillin are designated *pen*, while those involved only in cephalosporin biosynthesis are named *cef*.

ACV Synthetase

In 1971 it was shown that incubating the dipeptide δ-(L-α-aminoadipyl)-L-cysteine (AC) with DL-[^{14}C]-valine and ATP in a particulate fraction from *C. acremonium* protoplast extracts yielded labeled δ-(L-α-aminoadipyl)-L-cysteinyl-D-valine (ACV), implying that AC was an intermediate in ACV biosynthesis. This notion was substantiated when Abraham identified AC from β-lactam-producing actinomycete. Later, soluble extracts of *C. acremonium* were shown to generate both AC and ACV from labeled amino acid precursors. These data led to the generally accepted conclusion that ACV synthesis was analogous to the two-enzyme process for glutathione biosynthesis.

Banko et al. speculated that the putative dual-enzyme process was instead catalyzed by a single, multifunctional enzyme. Their data clearly showed that in cell-free extracts of *C. acremonium* the rate of ACV synthesis was significantly greater when the precursor amino acids were provided than it was when AC and valine were used as substrates for the reaction. Jensen and her coworkers demonstrated a similar result using cell-free extracts of *S. clavuligerus*.

The issue was resolved when van Liempt et al. partially purified the enzyme responsible for the multifunctional synthesis of the ACV tripeptide from *Aspergillus nidulans*. The enzyme was later purified and characterized from *C. acremonium* and *S. clavuligerus* by Baldwin et al. The gene was cloned by reverse genetics from *A. nidulans* and by conventional methods from *P. chrysogenum* and *C. acremonium*. The name for the gene coding ACV synthetase, *pcb*AB, is reminiscent of the understanding of the biochemistry prior to 1987. To summarize, the enzyme activates the three component amino acids utilizing ATP, assembles the tripeptide, and epimerizes L-valine to D-valine prior to releasing the tripeptide.

Isopenicillin N Synthase (IPNS)

Isopenicillin N synthase (IPNS) or "*ACV cyclase*" catalyzes the oxidative cyclization of ACV by the removal of four hydrogens from the tripeptide with the consumption of one molecule of oxygen. The newly formed C—N and C—S bonds of the respective β-lactam and thiazolidine rings are putatively made in a stepwise manner while the intermediates are enzyme bound. IPNS from *C. acremonium* was purified and its N-terminal sequence reported in the early 1980s. Samson et al. utilized the sequence data to clone the IPNS gene *pcb*C. IPNS has been extensively characterized with respect to its enzymology, substrate specificity, and catalytic mechanism.

Isopenicillin N Epimerase (IPNE)

The generation of cephalosporin from penicillin is dependent on the epimerization of the L-α-aminoadipyl side chain of isopenicillin N to the D-α-aminoadipyl side chain of penicillin N, since penicillin N but not isopenicillin N is the substrate for ring expansion enzymes. This reaction is catalyzed by IPNE and is coded for by the *cef*D gene. While the activity of the IPNE from *C. acremonium* has been studied in cell-free extracts, it has not been purified to date. Jensen et al. described a partial purification and characterization of IPNE from *S. clavuligerus* and noted that it did not share cofactor requirements with other β-lactam biosynthetic enzymes. The enzyme was purified to homogeneity by Usui and Yu and was determined to be a racemase, converting isopenicillin N and/or penicillin N to an equimolar ratio of the two substrates/products, shifting to the direction of penicillin N by its further metabolism to DAOC. The gene was cloned by Kovacevic et al.

Ring Expansion/Hydroxylation Enzymes (DAOCS/ DACS)

The conversion of penicillin N to CPC is initiated by the oxidative ring expansion of penicillin N to deacetoxycephalosporin C (DAOC). Subsequent hydroxylation of the 3'-methyl carbon of DAOC generates deacetylcephalosporin C (DAC). Kohsaka and Demain described the enzymatic ring expansion activity from cell-free extracts of *C. acremonium*. Two reports of partial purification of the "*expandase*" enzyme by Kupka et al. and Scheidegger et al. and their respective co-workers suggested that ring expansion and hydroxylation activities were catalyzed by a single enzyme. They also described an inherent instability of the enzyme preventing sufficient purification to definitively determine the bifunctional nature of the enzyme. In contrast, ring expansion and hydroxylation activities from *S. clavuligerus* were clearly separable by anion-exchange chromatography. *S. clavuligerus* DAOC synthetase ("*expandase*") and DAC synthase ("*hydroxylase*") were subsequently purified to near homogeneity, biochemically characterized, and cloned and expressed in *E. coli*. Dotzlaf and Yeh devised a stabilizing cocktail that was modified as the purification progressed, allowing the purification of DAOC synthetase/DAC synthase from *C. acremonium*to near-homogeneity. The highly purified protein retained its bifunctional nature, an observation also reported by Baldwin et al. in a nearly simultaneous publication. The bifunctionality of the DAOC synthetase/DAC synthase from *C. acremonium* was conclusively demonstrated by cloning and expressing its structural gene in *E. coli*. The gene coding for the two activities in *C. acremonium* is named *cef*EF, while the separate genes coding for ring expansion and hydroxylation activities in *S. clavuligerus* are named *cef*E and *cef*F, respectively.

DAC Acyltransferase (DAC-AT)

The final step in the biosynthesis of CPC is catalyzed by acetyl CoA: deacetylcephalosporin C *O*-acetyltransferase (DAC-AT). Fujisawa et al. showed that cell-free extracts of a CPC-producing strain readily converted DAC and acetyl-l-[^{14}C]-CoA to labeled CPC. They utilized this novel assay system to characterize several mutants that accumulated DAC and correctly proposed that DAC was an intermediate in the CPC pathway and was converted to CPC by DAC-AT.

Scheideggar et al. purified DAC-AT approximately 15-fold and estimated the molecular mass of the enzyme to be ~70 kDa. By incorporating 7-aminocephalosporanic acid (7-ACA) in the purification buffers, Matsuyama and his co-workers were able to stabilize DAC-AT, allowing a 1300-fold purification to apparent homogeneity. They estimated the mass to be ~55 kDa based on gel filtration and determined that the enzyme was a heterodimer composed of 14-kDa and 27-kDa subunits based on SDS-PAGE. The difference in mass as measured by the two methods was not discussed by the authors. In a related article, the cloning of the *cef*G gene and expression of DAC-AT activity in *Saccharomyces cerevisiae* using the reverse genetics approach based on the amino acid sequence of the purified protein was reported. In a third paper the disruption of *cef*G gene expression by insertional mutagenesis causing an accumulation of DAC and a lack of CPC production in the mutant *C. acremonium* strain was described.

Gutierrez et al. and Mathison et al cloned the *cef*G gene using traditional genetics by first searching for potential open reading frames (ORF) flanking the *pcb*C (IPNS) and *cef*EF (expandase/hydroxylase) genes. A likely ORF was located upstream of the *cef*EF gene by DNA sequence analysis. Both groups demonstrated that the cloned gene complemented DAC-AT deficient mutants of *C. acremonium* by restoring CPC production. Gutierrez and his co-workers cloned and expressed DAC-AT activity in *P. chrysogenum*, while Mathison and her co-workers reported similar results in *Aspergillus niger*.

Based on DNA sequencing, the mass of the *cef*G gene product was deduced to be 49,269 Da, which correlated well with the value reported by Matsuyama et al. Subsequently, Velasco et al. demonstrated the mass of immunoaffinity purified DAC-AT to be 49–52 kDa based on SDS-PAGE and gel filtration. However, unlike Matsuyama et al., DAC-AT purified from three different *C. acremonium* strains by Velasco et al. was monomeric.

Metabolic Engineering for CPC Yield Improvement

Isolation and structural elucidation of the active components from antibiotic- producing microorganisms begins the study of the biosynthetic pathway leading to the desired end product. The abundance of the various intermediate products of an antibiotic biosynthetic pathway can be accurately determined throughout the fermentation cycle by techniques such as high-performance liquid chromatography (HPLC). This and other analytical techniques allow identification of potential rate-limiting steps in the pathway. Three rate-limiting steps in the CPC pathway that are catalyzed by ACV synthetase, DAOC synthetase/DAC synthase, and DAC acetyltransferase are discussed below.

ACV Synthetase

Mounting evidence established the formation of ACV to be a rate-limiting step in CPC biosynthesis. Because ACV synthetase catalyzes the transitional step between primary and secondary metabolism in the β-lactam-producing microorganisms, it is likely to be a major regulatory site for β-lactam biosynthesis. Martin and Liras documented that increased ACV synthetase activity paralleled higher levels of cephalosporin or penicillin production in sequential strains. Zhang and Demain showed that ACV synthetase from various cell-free extracts of *C. acremonium* and *S. clavuligerus* possessed from 1% to 10% of the specific activity of isopenicillin N synthase, isopenicillin N epimerase, and deacetoxy-cephalosporin C synthetase. Finally, analysis of a mathematical model of CPC biosynthesis based on *in vitro* enzyme kinetic data led Malmberg and Hu to conclude that ACV synthesis is the major rate-limiting step in the pathway. At this writing, there are no reports of improved CPC yields in industrial strains by increasing the copy number of *pcb*AB. However, MacCabe et al. described the restoration of penicillin production in *A. nidulans* transformed with the *pcb*AB gene or the *pcb*AB plus *pcb*C genes together. They also claimed that certain transformants expressed a higher level of antimicrobial activity than the corresponding wild-type strain and suggested that extra copies of *pcb*AB might improve yields in the wild-type *A. nidulans*. In related work, Kennedy and Turner overexpressed ACV synthetase when the promoter for *pcb*AB in *A. nidulans* was replaced with the ethanol dehydrogenase promoter and reported up to a 30-fold increase in penicillin yields.

Isopenicillin N Synthetase and Epimerase

Isopenicillin N synthase and epimerase have not been implicated as rate-limiting enzymes for CPC biosynthesis. Although ACV was found in the mycelia of *P. chrysogenum* and *C. acremonium*, an excessive accumulation of ACV in fermentation broths has not been reported. Furthermore, pools of excreted penicillin were determined to be mostly penicillin N, not isopenicillin N, favoring the synthesis of the next intermediate, DAOC. In addition, *in vitro* kinetic data exclude both IPNS and IPNE as potential rate-limiting enzymes.

DAOC Synthetase/DAC Synthase

Metabolite analysis of ultrafiltered broth from a high-yielding CPC fermentation showed, in addition to CPC, the accumulation of penicillin, DAOC, and DAC. Further analysis of the accumulated penicillin indicated that >80% was penicillin N, the substrate for the DAOCS. Skatrud et al. described the elegant first use of metabolic engineering of an industrially important antibiotic producing strain when they successfully cloned an additional copy of the *cef*EF gene into *C. acremonium* strain 394-4 (a derivative of *C. acremonium* ATCC 11550). Their cloning efforts resulted in a twofold increase in the DAOCS activity in 150-liter pilot-scale fermentations. Doubling the DAOCS activity translated into a 16-fold reduction in level of penicillin N, a 6-fold decrease of accumulated DAOC, and a 15% increase in CPC yields. There was no effect on the level of DAC. These data predated and confirmed the mathematical model of CPC biosynthesis of Malmberg and Hu.

DAC Acyltransferase

As stated above, Skatrud et al. clearly showed that, while penicillin N accumulation was significantly reduced and CPC yields were substantially enhanced, the level of DAC was unchanged. The authors suggested that limitation in the carbon flow at the DAC-AT step could be causing the accumulation of DAC; however, they cautioned that DAC present at the end of the fermentation could be the result of degradation of CPC. Cephalosporin C degradation to DAC can result from either or both enzymatic hydrolysis by an extracellular acetylhydrolase and chemical hydrolysis due to a rapid rise in pH at the end of the fermentation. Skatrud and his co-workers suggested that cloning and expression of the *cef*G gene in a strain similar to 394-4 would be a practical way to address this question, but DAC-AT had not been purified or cloned at that time. By 1993, the means to address this issue were available. The enzyme had been purified, characterized, and cloned in several laboratories by both traditional and reverse genetics. Mathison et al. and later Gutierrez et al. successfully cloned and expressed the *cef*G gene in *C. acremonium*. Both groups showed enhanced conversion of DAC to CPC compared to untransformed strains. Mathison and her co-workers speculated that, since the DNA fragment used by Skatrud et al. to clone the *cef*EF gene unknowingly contained the *cef*G gene, the reduced penicillin N pool and improved CPC yields reported could have been the result of enhanced DAC-AT rather than enhanced DAOCS activity. They suggested that increased DAC-AT activity might reduce DAC levels to a point below a theoretical repression level for *cef*EF expression. This interesting hypothesis would not account for the lack of reduction in the DAC pool in the Skatrud strain. Velasco et al. showed that the *cef*G gene is poorly transcribed during both early- and late-phase growth in three low-producing *C. acremonium* strains compared to the *cef*EF gene. Gutierrez and his co-authors reported that introduction of extra copies of the *cef*G gene with its native promoter region only marginally improved reduction of the DAC pool with a corresponding increase in the CPC product. However, when the promoter was replaced with four different promoters, including the promoter for the *P. chrysogenum pcb*C gene (IPNS), high steady-state levels of DAC-AT expression and activity for each construct were found. The report by Gutierrez et al. implies that Skatrud et al. correctly interpreted their data. However, to paraphrase Mathison et al., it will be interesting to see if incorporating an altered promoter region will increase *cef*G expression and improve titers in industrial production strains of *C. acremonium*.

Metabolic Engineering for Production of 7-ADCA

The manufacture of several semisynthetic oral cephalosporin antibiotics involves the chemical ring expansion of penicillin V to 7-aminodeacetoxycephalosporanic acid (7-ADCA). This is a costly and potentially environmentally damaging process. Cloning of the *C. acremonium cef*EF gene (DAOCS/DACS) and the *S. clavuligerus cef*D (IPNE) and *cef*E gene (DAOCS) opened the possibility for biosynthetic/enzymatic processes for production of 7-ADCA.

DAOC Generation

Early *in vitro* data indicated that ring expansion of adipyl-6-APA or penicillin G was either nonexistent or barely detectable. Therefore, an alternative route to 7-ADCA through the enzymatic deacylation of DAOC requiring the fermentative production of DAOC at economically feasible levels was pursued. Elimination of DACS activity would allow *C. acremonium* to produce DAOC as its end product. Before it was known that DAOCS and DACS activities in *C. acremonium* were catalyzed by a single bifunctional enzyme, Queener et al. conducted mutagenesis and screening for mutants blocked in DACS activity. They effectively eliminated CPC production in some mutants, but DAOC production was only slightly enhanced. Attempts to eliminate DACS activity of the bifunctional DAOCS/DACS by *in vitro* mutagenesis of the cloned *cef*EF gene always resulted in a concomitant loss of DAOCS activity as well. It was later revealed through the use of inhibition kinetics that the two activities probably share a common active site. A simple disruption or deletion of the *cef*F gene in *S. clavuligerus* would result in the desired effect, since DAOCS of that organism produces only minimal amounts of DAC; however, to date this result has not been reported. A second approach involved expressing the *S clavuligerus cef*D and *cef*E genes in *P. chrysogenum*. Cantwell et al. transformed *P. chrysogenum* with a hybrid *cef*E gene containing the promoter sequence from *P. chrysogenum pcb*C gene and reported DAOCS specific activities from 4.3% to 10.3% relative to *S. clavuligerus*. Cantwell et al. later cloned the *S. clavuligerus cef*D gene into the *P. chrysogenum* strain that contained the *S. clavuligerus cef*E gene and demonstrated IPNE activity. This pioneering work was the first demonstration of cephalosporin production by fermentation of *P. chrysogenum*. The DAOC production was at the expense of penicillin V production but much less than the normal end product. The authors concluded that DAOC production would be greatly enhanced if isopenicillin N-to-penicillin V conversion could be prevented.

DAOG Generation

A second potential biosynthetic/enzymatic route to 7-ADCA involves the enzymatic ring expansion of penicillin G or V *in vivo* followed by *in vitro* deacylation. Little or no *in vitro* ring expansion activity with these substrates was shown for either the bifunctional DAOCS/DACS or monofunctional DAOCS. It was proposed that, through site-directed mutagenesis, DAOCS could be "*enzyme engineered*" to convert penicillin G or V to DAOG or DAOV, which would then be enzymatically deacylated *in vitro* to yield 7-ADCA. Improved expression of native DAOCS in *P. chrysogenum* was the first goal in the proposed scheme. Queener et al. reconstructed the hybrid gene described by Cantwell et al. by inserting the *cef*E ORF between the *pcb*C promoter and terminator sequences. One *P. chrysogenum* isolate transformed with the new hybrid gene produced DAOCS specific activities 70-fold higher than the best transformant

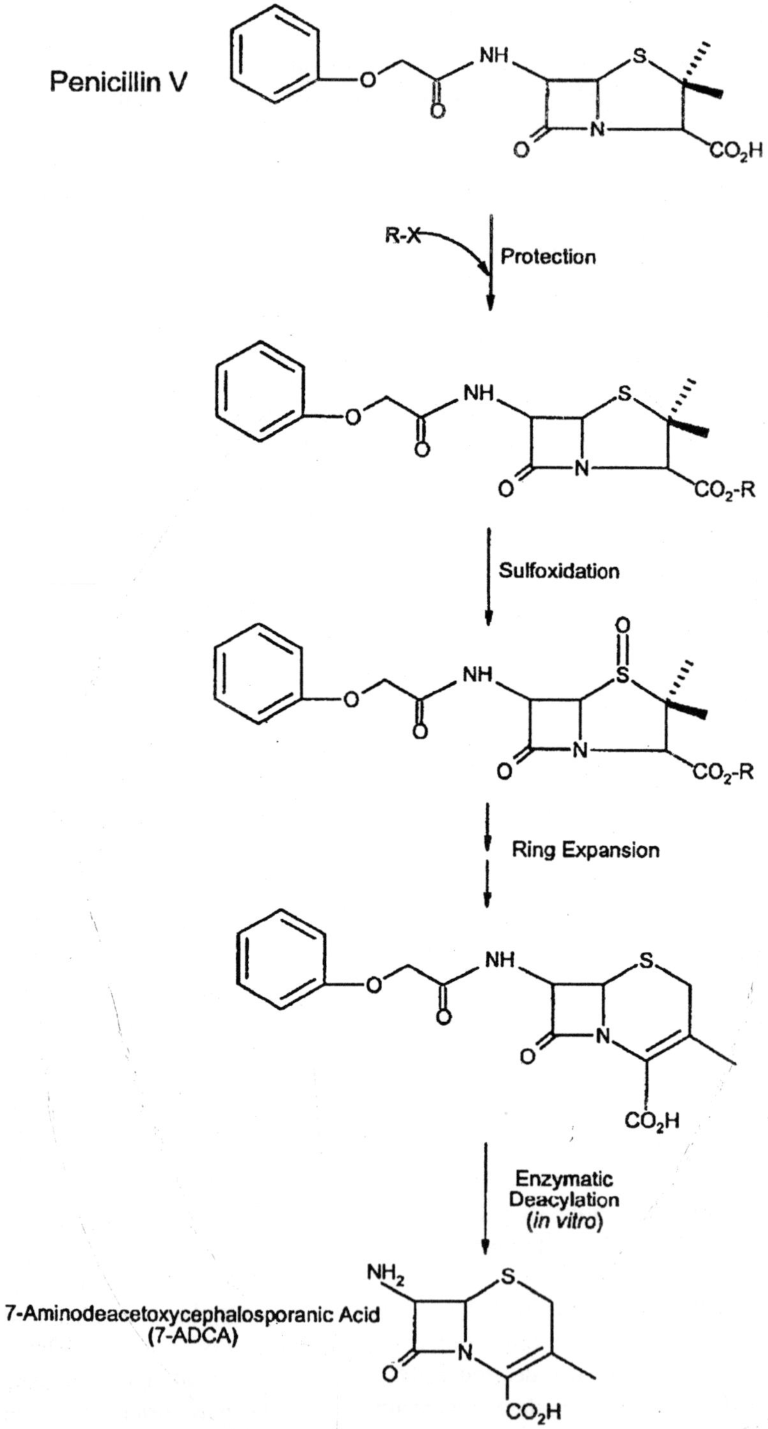

Fig. 19.2. The current chemical process for the production of 7-amino-deacetoxy-cephalosporanic acid.

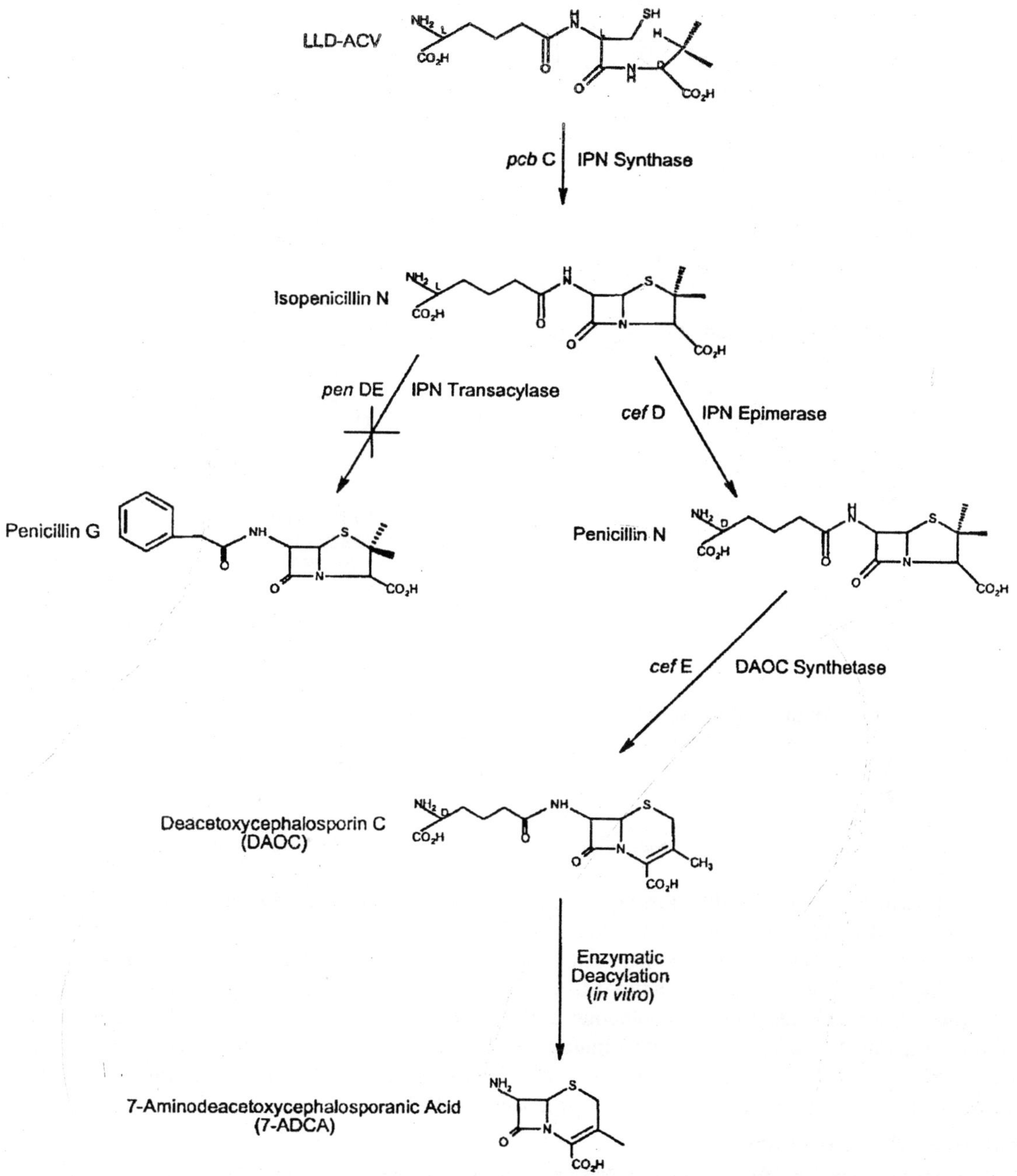

LLD-ACV

pcb C IPN Synthase

Isopenicillin N

pen DE IPN Transacylase

cef D IPN Epimerase

Penicillin G

Penicillin N

cef E DAOC Synthetase

Deacetoxycephalosporin C (DAOC)

Enzymatic Deacylation (*in vitro*)

7-Aminodeacetoxycephalosporanic Acid (7-ADCA)

Fig. 19.3. Metabolic engineering for deacetoxycephalosporin production in P. chrysogenum expressing the S. clavuligerus cefD and cefE genes.

previously reported, 4-fold higher than the parent *S. clavuligerus*, and about 75% of the activity of an industrial strain of *C. acremonium*. A similar tactic was used by Bovenberg et al to construct hybrid genes using the promoter and terminator regions of the *P. chrysogenum pen*DE gene and the *cef*E ORF from either *S. clavuligerus* or *Nocardia lactamdurans*. The *pen*DE promoter and terminator regions

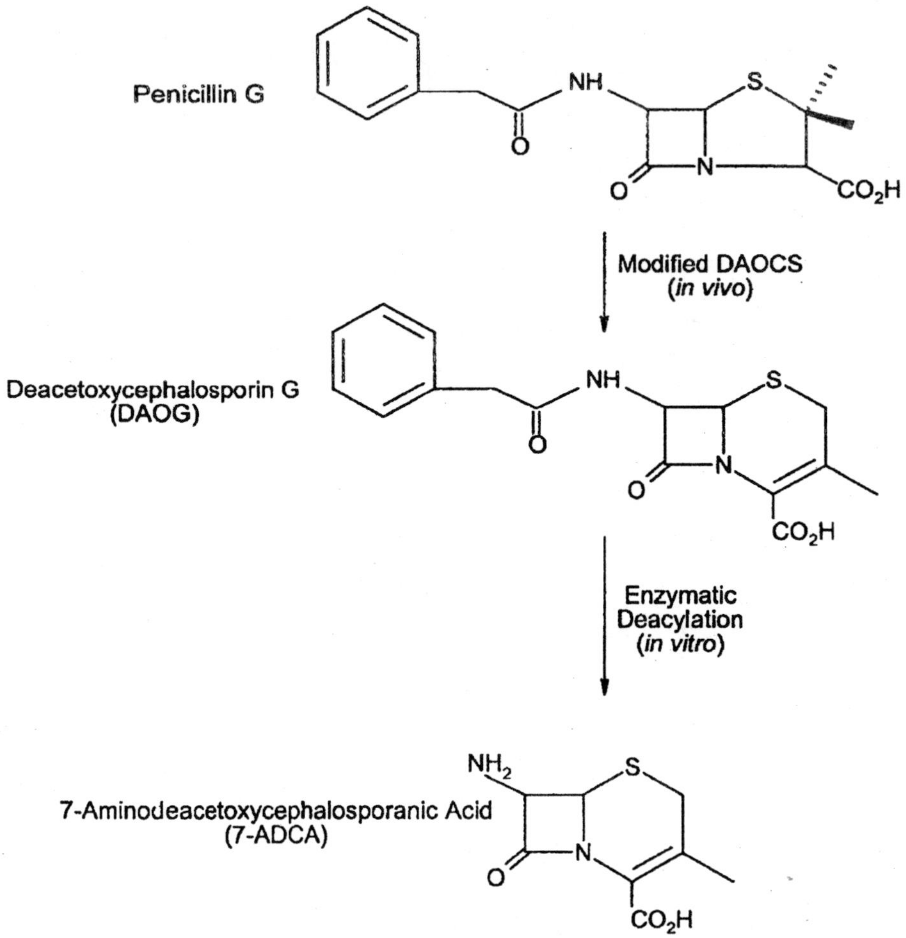

Penicillin G

Modified DAOCS
(*in vivo*)

Deacetoxycephalosporin G
(DAOG)

Enzymatic
Deacylation
(*in vitro*)

7-Aminodeacetoxycephalosporanic Acid
(7-ADCA)

Fig. 19.4. Metabolic engineering for ring expansion of penicillin G in P. chrysogenum expressing a modified S. clavuligerus DAOCS.

ensure expression of DAOCS after formation of isopenicillin N. Sutherland et al. reasoned that because IPNS and DAOCS were members of the same family of oxidase enzymes, they might share sequence similarity in the binding pockets for their respective substrates. In an elegant set of experiments, they analyzed the binding site of the L-α-aminoadipyl side chain of ACV from the structurally characterized *A. nidulans* IPNS and identified homologous amino acids in *S. clavuligerus* DAOCS responsible for binding penicillin N. Using site-directed mutagenesis, the *S. clavuligerus cef*E gene was modified to accept penicillin G as its primary substrate. *P. chrysogenum*, transformed with the modified gene hybridized as described above, successfully produced DAOG.

Production of Adipyl-7-ADCA

Yet another process for producing 7-ADCA utilizing expression of CPC pathway genes in *P. chrysogenum* was described by Conder et al. and Crawford et al. The process involved the generation of adipyl-6-amino penicillanic acid (adipyl-6-APA) by feeding disodium adipate in place of potassium phenoxyacetate to fermentations of *P. chrysogenum*, *in situ* ring expansion to adipyl-7-ADCA, followed by *in vitro* deacylation to the final product. The authors successfully gambled on the expandability of adipyl-6-APA *in vivo*, considering that *in vitro* expansion of the substrate was marginally detectable in one report using purified *C. acremonium* DAOCS/DACS and not detectable in other reports. Hybrid genes containing the promoter region from glyceraldehyde-3-phosphate dehydrogenase (GAP),*pcb*C (IPNS) or β-tubulin from *P. chrysogenum* fused to the *cef*E ORF of *S. clavuligerus* were constructed. Transformants were screened for the production of adipyl-7-ADCA and, although all isolates expressed mRNA for the hybrid gene and produced adipyl-6-APA, the level of product varied from undetectable to relatively high levels. The authors could not correlate product formation to gene copy number, and they concluded that expression was influenced more by site of gene integration than by the promoter sequence fused to the *cef*E ORF adipyl-7-ADCA. Finally, traditional strain improvement techniques with the highest-producing transformants significantly improved adipyl-7ADCA production, and the authors predicted a commercially viable process. In related work, Crawford et al. described the production of 7-aminocephalosporanic acid (7-ACA), another important intermediate in semisynthetic cephalosporin manufacture, in adipate fed *P. chrysogenum* transformed with a hybrid gene containing the *C. acremonium cef*EF gene.

The application of traditional microbiology, mathematical modeling, biochemical engineering, analytical chemistry, mutagenesis, and screening significantly improved the production of CPC by fermentation of *C. acremonium* from the early 1950s through the 1970s. With the advent of recombinant DNA technology combined with new, readily available analytical techniques and sophisticated enzyme biochemistry in the early 1970s, an unparalleled understanding of the biosynthetic process for CPC production was realized. Reducing or eliminating rate limitations in the biosynthesis of CPC through the application of gene cloning resulted in yield increases in production strains where the traditional methods were no longer proving to be successful. Cloning and expression of several CPC biosynthetic genes in *P. chrysogenum* has led to the novel, economical, and environmentally desirable biosynthetic routes to important precursors for the production of semi-synthetic cephalosporins. Interestingly, the traditional methods of fermentation optimization and strain improvement are successfully improving production of the semisynthetic cephalosporin intermediates by the newly created cephalosporin-producing *P. chrysogenum* strains. Metabolic engineering for improved biosynthetic production of intermediate and end products for economically important antibiotics has been firmly established as indicated by the pioneering work described in this chapter. Similar advances are discussed in other chapters of this book, and we believe that these gene/enzyme methodologies will be commonly applied to the production of other existing as well as newly discovered antibiotics in the future.

The authors had the privilege of working with Sir Edward P. Abraham and note with sadness the passing of this historically important scientist. EPA, as we affectionately knew him, helped elucidate the structure of penicillin during World War II. In 1940, with E. Chain, he discovered the β-lactamase enzyme. In the 1950s and early 1960s, with G.G.F. Newton and others, he discovered the cephalosporin antibiotics and described their isolation from the fungus provided to Oxford by Guiseppe Brotzu, culminating in the elucidation of the structure for CPC. EPA provided Lilly scientists with purified isopenicillin N synthetase, thereby enabling, via reverse genetics, the first cloning and characterization of the *pcb*C gene and the expression of recombinant IPNS in *E. coli*. Working with us, he helped demonstrate the transformation of *P. chrysogenum* with hybrid *cef*D and *cef*E genes from *S. clavuligerus* and the production of cephalosporins by the recombinant *P. chrysogenum*. Thus, his scientific career spanned the beta-lactam antibiotic story from first discovery to modern metabolic engineering. Throughout our interactions with him, he exhibited a mentoring, humble manner that inspired us and belied the greatness of this man from Oxford, England.

20

COSMETICS AND THEIR RELATION TO DRUG

Under the Food, Drug, and Cosmetics Act, the Food and Drug Administration (FDC) of the United States has the authority to regulate foods, prescription (Rx) drugs, over-the-counter (OTC) drugs, and cosmetics. The FDA also administers a second statute, the Fair Packaging and Labeling Act. In order to administer this complex task, the FDA depends on the legalistic and statutory definitions of drug and cosmetics in the FDCA. Nevertheless, the public's interpretation of what constitutes a drug or a cosmetic may differ somewhat from that of regulatory agencies. Philosophically and historically, a cosmetic is a product that nelps improve external appearance and has the ability to hide, or at least distract from, unwanted stigmata or skin defects.

A product that changes the color of hair is a cosmetic, as is a product intended to increase the skin's tendency to tan by exposure to sun. This traditional view remains ingrained in the consumer's mind but may not be judicially valid. A change in hair color, for example, can be effected by the following: (1) a wig, which might be viewed as an article of clothing; (2) a variety of dyeing processes, which are properly identified as cosmetic changes; and (3) possibly by a variety of ingested or topically applied substances that gradually alter the hair follicle's ability to synthesize melanin, which should be classified as a drug effect. The common goal of these three approaches is to effect a change in appearance, the key objective of all cosmetics. The method by which this goal is achieved differentiates the three hair "coloring" processes and makes a product a drug or a cosmetic. This can create some confusion, as is demonstrated by a consideration of sunscreen products. Sunburn prevention by topical products was for years considered within the scope of cosmetics, even though ultraviolet-B (UV-B) light absorbers were incorporated into these "*cosmetics.*"

The cosmetic industry responded rather calmly when the FDA's review of OTC drugs included suntan preparations and sunburn preventives. What for years had been a cosmetic suddenly became a drug by legislative or administrative fiat. The FDA's rationale is justifiably based on the concept that sunburn prevention is prevention of disease. Adding an ingredient that enhances the ability of melanocytes to produce melanin in the skin would be viewed as a cosmetic by the user. The FDA is likely to accept cosmetic (color change, appearance) claims for such a product, but a definition of a drug would become mandatory if the melanin is claimed to protect against sunburn. The implication that a parasol intended to prevent exposure to sun is a medical device has not been judicially examined. One must recognize that the differentiation between cosmetics and drugs is complex and is blurred by the interplay of consumer perception, commercial interest, and statutory interpretation by regulatory agencies, with the ultimate decision in the hands of the judiciary. For these reasons, differences between drugs and cosmetics are discussed in the next section on the basis of existing U.S. laws, the product's composition, and safety and efficacy. Laws and rules covering the distinction between cosmetics and drugs differ from country to country. For this reason, marked divergence from U.S. practices will be noted in this survey.

Comparison on the Basis of Law

Definitions

The sharpest distinction between a drug and a cosmetic is based on the statutory definitions in the Federal Food Drug and Cosmetic Act. Cosmetics are clearly defined as: (1) articles intended to be rubbed, poured, sprinkled, or sprayed on, introduced into, or otherwise applied to the human body or any part thereof for cleansing, beautifying, promoting attractiveness, or altering the appearance and (2) articles intended for use as a component of any such articles; except that such term shall not include soap.

On the other hand, drugs are defined as follows: The term drug means: (A) articles recognized in the official United States Pharmacopoeia, official Homeopathic Pharmacopoeia of the United States or official National Formulary or any supplement to any of them; (B) articles intended for the use in the diagnosis, cure, mitigation, treatment, or prevention of disease in man or other animal; (C) articles (other than food) intended to affect the structure or any function of the body of man or other animals; and (D) articles intended for use as a component of any articles specified in clause (A), (B), or (C); but does not include devices or their components, parts, or accessories.

Table 20.1. List of products (recognized as cosmetics)

Baby preparations	Creams, lotions, oil, powders, shampoos
Bath preparations	Bubble baths, capsules, oils, salts, soaps and detergents, tablets
Cleansing preparations	Creams, douches, liquids and pads, lotions, personal cleansing products
Dentifrices	Aerosols, breath fresheners, liquids, mouthwashes, pastes, powders
Fragrance products	Colognes and toilet waters, deodorants, fragrances, perfumes
Hair products	Depilatories, dressings, dyes and colors, grooming aids, lighteners, miscellaneous rinses, permanent waveproducts, shampoos, sprays, straighteners, tints, tonics, wave sets
Makeup preparations	Blushers, eyebrow pencils, eyeliners, eye makeup preparations, eye makeup removers, eye shadows, face powders, facial makeups, fixatives, foundation makeups, leg and body paints, lip glosses, lipsticks, mascaras, rouges
Miscellaneous products	Paste masks, powders (men's, women's, talcums)
Shaving preparations	Aftershaves, beard softeners, shaving creams (aerosol, brushless lather), preshaves
Skin care preparations	Body and hand preparations (moisturizers), eye creams, face and neck preparations, fresheners and astringents, suntan gels

These definitions may differ from the interpretation of the consumer or from generally accepted usage, but courts will adjudicate exclusively on the basis of these statutory definitions. It is clearly the intent of the product, not necessarily its performance, that is used judicially to classify a product as a drug or as a cosmetic. A skin-care product intended to beautify by the removal of wrinkles is both a cosmetic (alters the appearance) and a drug (affects a body structure). Historically and intuitively, the requirements for a drug are more stringent than those for a cosmetic, and the regulatory agency and the courts tend to apply the more stringent requirement to a product that may be perceived to be both a drug and a cosmetic. Some of the products are considered drugs or quasi-drugs in other countries.

Food and Drug Administration's Tasks

The FDA is authorized to enforce the FDCA and the FPLA. The FDA's tools include inspection and seizure, which may be applied equally to drugs or cosmetics. The FDCA prohibits the use (or presence) of poisonous or deleterious substances. Their presence makes a cosmetic "*adulterated*" or "*misbranded.*" In this regard, no significant distinction is made between drugs and cosmetics. Similarly, good manufacturing practices (GMPs) are applicable to drugs and with minor changes to cosmetics. Products that are manufactured under conditions that are in violation of the GMPs may become subject to seizure. In recent years, the FDA has not initiated formal cases against violators of cosmetic regulations; instead, the FDA has relied on so-called Warning Letters to obtain compliance without recourse to complicated legal action.

In contrast to Rx drugs, OTC drugs and cosmetics are not subject to pre-clearance. Preclearance is specifically designed to prevent the introduction of dangerous or undesirable drug entities into the market. The restrictions on ingredients are most severe in the case of OTC drugs and preclude introduction of untested drugs or combinations. In fact, a "new chemical entity," which might be entirely suitable for introduction as an OTC drug, requires workup via the new drug application (NDA) process. The approval of Rx and OTC drugs by the FDA is, in principle, based on the performance of the drug entity. Efficacy against the disease, bioavailability, and lack of adverse side effects are of primary importance. Thus, judicious choice of drug excipients is required for all drug approvals. Nevertheless, in the absence of an FDA- approved list of cosmetic ingredients, the cosmetic manufacturer has the responsibility to provide products that are not injurious to the user under the expected conditions of use. Some ingredients are specifically restricted, and a regulation requiring safety substantiation exists. These will be discussed in the section entitled "Restrictions on the Use of Ingredients."

Color Additives

Color additives are of particular importance to the formulation of cosmetics. Dyes and pigments not only make products more attractive but also are vital to any product that is intended to alter the color of any part of the body. Color additives are regulated meticulously by the FDA, and only some general information on the current regulatory status of colorants in the United States can be provided.

Certified color additives are synthetic organic dyes that are described in an approved color additive petition. Each manufactured lot of a certified dye must be analyzed and certified by the FDA prior to usage.

Color lakes are pigments that generally consist of an insoluble metallic salt of a certified color additive deposited on an inert substrate. These lakes are subject to the color additive regulations of the FDA and must be certified by the agency prior to use.

Color additives that are not classified as certified color or color lakes are identified as *non-certified color additives*. Each of these substances is the subject of an approved color additive petition, but individual batches do not require certification by the FDA prior to use.

The fourth major class of color additives is *hair colorants*. These compounds or their mixtures may be used only to color scalp hair and may not be used in the eye area. Use of these colorants is "exempt," that is, the so-called coal-tar hair dyes may be sold with cautionary labeling, directions for preliminary (patch) testing, and restrictions against use in or near the eye.

Soap Exclusion

Soap is specifically excluded from cosmetics in the FDCA, and no cosmetic or drug regulations are applicable to soap. The FDCA fails to define the term *soap*, but the FDA has ruled that a product is a soap if the bulk of the non-volatile matter is the alkali salt of a fatty acid and if its detersive properties are due exclusively to the fatty acid salt. In addition, the product must be labeled as a soap. A product is identified as a shampoo when it consists, e.g., only of aqueous potassium oleate. It then must conform to cosmetic regulations.

The term *soap* thus has two meanings. The first is the FDA's definition, which is used for legal purposes. The second is the generic sense, whereby soaps may refer to cleansing products that may not meet the specifics of FDA's definition. Such products must, therefore, be labeled as cosmetics. The Federal Trade Commission (FTC) and the Consumer Products Safety Commission (CPSC) handle the regulatory control for soaps.

Comparison on the Basis of Composition

Drug Ingredients Versus Cosmetic Ingredients

On the basis of the Drug Efficacy Study Implementation (DESI) review, which began in 1962, the FDA ultimately concluded that of about 16,000 claims made for 3400 Rx drugs, only about 2300 drugs were effective for at least one indication. Today, Rx drugs must undergo the NDA process, which, for all practical purposes, is a critical preclearance procedure. As the work on the DESI review neared completion, the FDA initiated the so-called OTC review in 1972. The FDA classified some 250,000 drugs into about 55 therapeutic groups. The panels that reviewed each group had the responsibility to establish the safety and efficacy of each OTC drug and to restrict claims for these drugs to those the panel considered appropriate for a given drug or combination of drugs. It is apparent that the marketability of a drug—Rx or OTC—requires the presence and bioavailability of an identifiable drug entity that can be expected to exert some therapeutic benefit. No such legal requirement for the use of raw materials exists in cosmetics. As a rule, the presence of and claim for any component in a cosmetic that may have a therapeutic effect converts such a cosmetic into a drug.

The FDA has classified the following topically applied products as OTC drugs on the basis of safety and efficacy review of the drug(s) constituents:

1. Acne products
2. Antidandruff products
3. Antimicrobial products
4. Antiperspirant products
5. Astringent products
6. Oral care products
7. Skin-protectant products
8. Sunscreen products
9. External analgesic products

In other countries, some of these products are considered cosmetics.

Some of the actives used in the past in such products have been classified as Category I, i.e., safe and effective. Usage of these agents and the claims made for the finished product make these products OTC drugs, not cosmetics.

The activities of the OTC panels are not yet completed, although most of the tentative final reports have been published. However, no definitive rulings have been made or subjected to judicial review. It appears at this time that the ingredients reviewed by the OTC panels can be used in cosmetics as excipients and the like. To repeat, their use, together with drug or therapeutic claims, transforms the cosmetic into a drug, in which case the labeling and claim structure must conform to those established for OTC drugs. The designation "*cosmetic*" places almost no restriction on the use of components.

However, claims for therapeutic efficacy convert any cosmetic into a drug, as interpreted by the FDA. The regulations do not restrict the use of a drug substance for purposes unrelated to its drug status.

Cosmetics and their Relation to Drugs

Restrictions on the Use of Ingredients in Cosmetics

The review of active drugs by the OTC panels was limited to relatively few drug entities, but the cosmetic industry employs thousands of ingredients, including many of plant and animal origin. Many typical cosmetic ingredients are identical to the components used in Rx and OTC drugs, but only very few cosmetic ingredients are subject to restrictions by the FDA. These include mercury compounds, except those used as preservatives in products intended for use in or near the eye. Others are bithionol, vinyl chloride, halogenated salicylanilides, zirconium compounds in aerosol products, chloroform, chlorofluorcarbon propellants, and hexachlorophene. With regard to cosmetic ingredients, the FDA has placed the responsibility for substantiating their safety squarely on the producer. Such safety substantiation also includes finished products. Each ingredient used in a cosmetic product and each finished cosmetic product shall be adequately substantiated for safety prior to marketing. Any such ingredient or product whose safety is not adequately substantiated prior to marketing is misbranded unless it contains the following conspicuous statement on the principal display panel: Warning—The safety of this product has not been substantiated.

These regulatory activities and the need to demonstrate to the public that the cosmetic industry as a whole is prepared to accept responsibility prompted the Cosmetics, Toiletries and Fragrance Association (CTFA) in 1976 to establish the Cosmetic Ingredient Review (CIR) for the purpose of evaluation and review of the safety of the ingredients used in cosmetics. The CIR process established a system for prioritizing ingredients based on frequency of use, concentration used, area of use, frequency of application, use by sensitive subgroups, likelihood of biologic activity, and consumer complaints. This is a scientific review of worldwide data, and non-voting members from industry and consumer groups participate in the deliberations. In order to speed up the review process and to avoid duplication, the CIR expert panel may defer study of substances that are already under review by other safety programs. The most important of these are those by the Research Institute for Fragrance Materials (RIFM) and the Flavor and Extract Manufacturers Association (FEMA). The former establishes the safety of fragrance components; its funding and concept permit expenditures for safety testing of substances. The latter addresses issues related to the safety of individual flavor materials. The reviews by the CIR panel are available from the CTFA and have appeared over a period of years in the Journal of the American College of Toxicology.

Although the CIR process is sponsored by the CTFA, the latter will conduct safety studies for substances considered crucial to the survival of the cosmetic industry. The CTFA will also establish and pay for research required to confirm the stability, chemical purity, and safety of various cosmetic ingredients. These activities are part of the cosmetic industry's technically oriented self-regulation program. Similar programs exist in the pharmaceutical industry. RIFM has recommended discontinuance of the use of acetylethyl tetramethyltetralin, 6-methylcoumarin, musk ambrette, and musk ketone. Another self- imposed ingredient restriction concerns the use of potential nitrosating agents in products containing various (secondary) alkanol amines, in light of the hazard of nitrosamine formation. In the European Union, the use of tri- and di-ethanolamine is restricted.

One of the key self-regulatory procedures in the cosmetic industry is the voluntary reporting process of adverse reactions. The program is intended to provide data on the type and frequency of adverse reactions reported by consumers or by their medical advisors to the industry. It is an important means of detecting problems that are not treated in hospital emergency rooms (i.e., documented in the National Electronic Injury Surveillance System, NEISS) or do not reach poison control centers.

Practical Aspects

For practicing formulators, the border between cosmetics and drugs is not clear. Drug entities for which claims are made on the label differentiate drugs from cosmetics. However, the same or chemically similar excipients and formulation aids are widely used in cosmetics and drugs. Finally, one must recognize that cosmetics may include groups of substances not normally found in drugs. Substances considered drugs by U.S. law have been excluded from the table. This listing is not comprehensive and is presented for illustrative purposes only. The overlap on the basis of ingredient usage is apparent from an examination of column 3.

Labeling of Cosmetics

An important ingredient-related topic is cosmetic ingredient labeling. Advocates of consumers' rights have suggested that the public would benefit from full disclosure of the composition of cosmetic products. Pursuant to the regulations by the FDA and the FPLA, all cosmetics are now required to carry the following information on labels: (1) a statement of the identity of the product; (2) a statement of the net quantity of contents; (3) a statement of the name and place of business of the manufacturer, packer, or distributor; (4) a list of the ingredients included in the product in order of predominance; and (5) cautionary or warning language.

Except the aforementioned labeling for item 4, similar requirements exist for Rx and OTC products at the time of this writing. Labeling of all constituents in OTC drug products is still under consideration. The listing of ingredients in cosmetics must be in descending order of predominance, with some exceptions for components present as minor constituent and color additives. In order to achieve uniformity for identification, the CTFA has continuously created shorthand nomenclature for all cosmetic ingredients. The "naming'' process is similar to that employed by USAN. Many names and chemical descriptions of cosmetic ingredients have been reviewed and accepted by the FDA (for the purpose of using these names on labels). As a result, cosmetics in the U.S. are now labeled in accordance with the nomenclature and the rules of the International Nomenclature of Cosmetic Ingredient Dictionary. This approach has been accepted in the E.U., where the same names (with minor modifications) are used. "Harmonization'' of names is a continuing process to make these names linguistically acceptable throughout the world.

Comparison on the Basis of Safety and Performance

Safety

Users know that, as a rule, Rx drugs are more likely to cause adverse side effects than OTC drugs. This is an obvious result of the nature and of the distribution system for these products. Prescription drugs are administered under the supervision of a physician, who has the responsibility and moral obligation to monitor the patient's progress. However, OTC drugs may be used ad lib by the uninformed, who may not always be competent to diagnose the underlying disease or to recognize adverse side effects. In this respect, cosmetics resemble OTC drugs except that cosmetics are used repeatedly and over extended periods of time. Thus, the requirements for the safety of cosmetics should be, in fact, much more stringent then those for many drugs. The level of side effects or adverse effects that can be tolerated by manufacturers of cosmetics is virtually nil. Of particular concern is the sensitizing potential of components during prolonged and repeated use. Photosensitization is another phenomenon that has led to the removal of some cosmetic ingredients from the list of routinely employed substances.

Elegance

Elegance is not a primary concern in the case of Rx drugs but impacts marketing of OTC drugs and helps to ensure patient compliance. By contrast, any feature that detracts from the elegance (appearance, odor, texture, etc.) of a cosmetic interferes with its marketability and acceptance. As a matter of fact, cosmetic elegance is the essential attribute of a successful cosmetic product.

Performance

Performance is the one issue in which cosmetics and drugs are different. Drug efficacy is assessed on the basis of cure or prevention of disease. The FDA has established that cosmetic products that exert therapeutic effects are drugs. As a result, some traditional cosmetics were converted into drugs via the OTC panel process. Any performance claims for these OTC products are limited to the wording approved during the OTC review process.

Claims for (non-drug) cosmetics may be, for example, fashion-oriented (color), beauty-oriented (hiding of blemishes), or texture-oriented (emollient or lubricant). These, and related claims, are easily perceived and can be readily documented. More complex issues arise when cosmetic claims are made for age-related or reparative skin-care preparations. In the past, various regulatory agencies have been permissive with regard to cosmetic puffery claims. More recently, claims made for some cosmetics suggest to consumers that the product may exhibit a drug-like effect, as defined by statute. A Commissioner of Food and Drugs has labeled these claims "daring." Advertising copy that implies that a product nourishes the skin, is active, causes tingling, tightens the skin, discourages wrinkle formation, is prepared by a pharmaceutical company, or performs like a face-lift may be false and misleading if the product does not perform. On the other hand, the product is considered a drug if it performs as claimed. Aside from drug results, claims for skin or hair benefits require documentation for commercial purposes (advertising and promotion). Thus, claims for performance are likely to run afoul of FTC rules. In the E.U., however, claims for efficacy require substantiation by regulation. Guidelines for documenting cosmetic performance exist in Europe but not in the United States. On the other hand, the FDA has a powerful tool for stopping unsubstantiated claims. A claim for wrinkle "removal," even on a temporary basis, may make a cosmetic product into a drug. Thus, the cosmetic industry is as tightly controlled as the Rx industry. Whenever a new indication for an existing drug constituent is claimed or whenever a drug-like claim is made for any ingredient, a new drug application is required.

Shelf Life

Cosmetic preparations need not be labeled for out-dating. This does not imply that cosmetic products must (or do) exhibit indefinite stability. The physical and chemical stability of cosmetics is routinely studied by the same procedures as those used for Rx or OTC drugs. Since cosmetic products do not contain active drug entities, the chemical stability of any component may be critical to the performance of the product: The components of a fragrance product require monitoring; the performance of a hair-waving preparation may depend on alkalinity and the chemical integrity of the reducing agent.

Physical stability affects cosmetic elegance, for example, by the breaking of an emulsion. Moreover, physical stability may also affect efficacy, as is the case during settling of a pigment in a nail lacquer that might then no longer be readily redispersible. A similar type of instability may occur as a result of the settling of an antiperspirant compound in a suspension aerosol. In these cases, neither the cosmetic (nail lacquer) or the OTC drug (antiperspirant) performs as claimed and may be considered misbranded or mislabeled. As a rule, therefore, the demands of chemical and physical stability are similar for drugs and cosmetics. Under certain circumstances, the demands on physical stability may be especially critical as, for example, in hand and body lotions that have to perform under tropical conditions after having been exposed to the heat of the sun on the beach or after storage under arctic conditions in a ski hut.

The criteria for microbiologic cleanliness of cosmetic products are especially complex. Like a drug, a cosmetic is deemed adulterated if: (1) it bears or contains any poisonous or deleterious substance which may render it injurious to users on the conditions of use as are customary or usual; (2) it contains in whole or in part of any filthy, putrid, or decomposed substance; and (3) if it has been prepared, packed, or held under unsanitary conditions where it may have become contaminated with filth, or whereby it may have been rendered injurious to health.

Cosmetic companies adhere to FDA-mandated GMPs or to GMPs promulgated by the CTFA with regard to housekeeping, cleaning, and sanitizing of equipment, and purity of raw materials and process water. Water is a particularly important component of finished cosmetics. Its purity is closely monitored to avoid the inadvertent introduction of contaminating biota into products. The GMPs established by the FDA are available in 21 CFR, Part 211, and the CTFA has published similar recommendations in the form of Quality Assurance Guidelines for Cosmetic Manufacture.

The final check on purity is on the finished product. The high water content and the inclusion of nutrients for unwanted microbiota make cosmetics subject to microbiological contamination. Thus, topical OTC products and cosmetics require preservation and a final check before distribution. Preservative systems and GMPs usually ensure delivery of essentially uncontaminated cosmetics. The microbiologic requirements recommended by the CTFA include the following: (1) baby products: less than 500 microorganisms/g; (2) eye products: less than 500 microorganisms/g; (3) oral products: less than 1000 microorganisms/g; (4) all other products: less than 1000 microorganisms/g; and (5) pathogens should be absent.

The use of preservatives to achieve the desired low levels of contaminating microorganisms is required. Some liquid cosmetic products do not support the growth of microorganisms (e.g., alcohol-based after-shave), while others are excellent growth substrates (e.g., a protein-containing hair conditioner). Because consumers frequently introduce microorganisms during normal product use, some cosmetic manufacturers may require that their products be self-sterilizing. This is a difficult task and not always achievable. A final check for levels of microorganisms is, nevertheless, desirable.

Relation to Health-Care Providers

Like the drug industry, the cosmetic industry requires animal toxicology and human testing to establish the safety of its products. As a rule, most cosmetic products are quite innocuous upon ingestion, even though they may cause laxation or act as emetics. The industry makes a deliberative effort not to market products that might elicit toxic syndromes when ingested or applied topically. The former type of problem is usually handled by poison control centers and routinely (in 90% of all cases) involves ingestion by children. The number of fatalities was reported as nil between 1971 and 1978.

Dermatologists see many patients who have used cosmetic products properly but still report adverse reactions. The cosmetic industry is conscious of the need to provide products that do not elicit irritation or allergic responses during use. For this reason, the cosmetic industry depends on all types of patch and related testing by dermatologic laboratories to establish the safety of a given product in a predictive fashion. A whole battery of test protocols is available, and hundreds of subjects are tested routinely by dermatologists before product marketing.

Topical drugs and cosmetics have the potential of penetrating the skin. In the case of a topical drug (e.g., an antiinflammatory steroid), localized permeation may be a desirable feature. Penetration of cosmetics into and through the skin may elicit undesirable effects, especially since consumers may apply two or more products to the same site. Thus, in contrast to topically used Rx drugs, cosmetics should be retained on the skin with minimal penetration. Dermatologists also recommend cosmetics to patients as, for example, in cases of dry or chapped skin. Clearly, the cosmetic industry–physician–user relationship is not very different from that existing in the drug industry.

Cosmetic or Drug?

Formulators and marketers require an answer to the question of whether a given product is a cosmetic or a drug. Some of the answers are almost obvious. In the United States, a product is a drug if a drug claim is made for the preparation. The inclusion of a new chemical entity on which a therapeutic claim is based requires filing of a NDA; a product containing such a substance is automatically viewed as a drug. A typical example is a suntan product that adds an UV light- absorbing substance that was not reviewed by the OTC panel but was previously used as a sunscreen. Although the product in question was labeled as a drug, the FDA ruled that this clearly constituted use of an unapproved new drug substance. The addition of an OTC-reviewed sunscreen into a cosmetic makeup preparation— without claims for sun-protective action but with the indication that the product contains a sunscreen for the purpose of reducing UV light-induced skin aging— could be considered a drug use in the United States.

A soap to which an OTC Category I antimicrobial agent has been added is converted into a drug. This raises an interesting secondary issue. Soaps may be tinted with non-certified color additives. This inclusion of the antimicrobial requires not only drug labeling but also reformulation with approved colorants. As a rule, the status of the product is determined by the claims made for it and its intended purpose. The use of aluminum chloride, a Category I OTC antiperspirant, as an astringent probably does not confer drug status on the product. It was already noted that certain OTC Category I skin protectants, such as petrolatum, can be used freely in cosmetics as long as no drug claims are made for the product. Numerous other issues might arise, and each one might require specific adjudication. An example is the use of an approved sunscreen in a cosmetic product to preserve it against UV light deterioration. Since the intent of the sunscreen's use is clearly not drug related, the product will probably be considered a cosmetic. Cosmetics and drugs are distinctly different on the basis of U.S. law. In principle, cosmetics may not contain ingredients that treat or prevent disease or alter the structure or function of the human body. The objective of cosmetics is limited to the enhancement of appearance. The ingredients used in cosmetics to a large extent are the same as those employed in drugs, with the exception of components that are intended to cure, alleviate, or prevent disease. The demands on product stability and manufacturing practices are essentially the same for cosmetics and drugs. Finally, important differences are seen in judging the performance of cosmetics and of drugs. Consumers assess cosmetics based on the products' performance vis-à-vis the demand for better appearance. On the other hand, drugs are assessed on their ability to prevent or improve a disease state.

21

Clinical Supplies Manufacture

The Federal Food, Drug, and Cosmetic Act (the Act), Title 21, U.S. Code, section 301 et. seq., establishes that a drug shall be deemed to be adulterated if "...the methods used in, or the facilities or controls used for, its manufacture, processing, packing, or holding do not conform to or are not operated or administered in conformity with current good manufacturing practice to assure that such drug meets the requirements of this article as to safety and has the identity and strength, and meets the quality and purity characteristics, which it purports or is represented to possess." This requirement is generally referred to as "CGMP" (current good manufacturing practice), or simply "GMP."

The requirement as written in the law is obviously very broad. It does not define the specific steps manufacturers must take to comply, or the controls that must be in place to ensure compliance. A later section of the Act gives the Secretary of Health and Human Services authority to promulgate regulations for the efficient enforcement of the Act. The FDA, acting in accordance with this authority, has promulgated regulations found in Title 21 of the Code of Federal Regulations (CFR) that sets forth the definitions to be used in specifying GMP requirements for all drugs (21 CFR Part 210) and the procedures and controls necessary for manufacturing of finished pharmaceuticals (human and veterinary), found in 21 CFR Part 211. Part 211 of the regulations is what is generally meant by the term "CGMP" or "GMP" (the acronym GMP will be used in this text). While FDA gives consideration to prevailing practice in regulated industry before specific requirements are written into the regulations as being "current, good practices," FDA's final basis used to establish GMP requirements is whether the practice is "feasible and valuable" in assuring drug safety, quality, and purity. We also point out that the final GMP regulations are the product of notice and comment rule-making through publication, first as a proposal in the Federal Register. The affected public, including the industry, has an opportunity to comment on the proposed rule before it is finalized.

Because the regulations apply to all "*finished pharmaceuticals*," and because of the statutory requirement to comply with GMP, there is no question that the regulations apply in a binding manner to the manufacture of clinical supplies. Nevertheless, a debate has existed for many years, and even continues today, regarding exactly how and in what respects a company may differ in its approach to the application of GMP regulations to clinical supplies vs. full-scale commercial production.

Background Information

Clinical supplies, also known as clinical trial materials, are those investigational new drug products intended for administration in human or veterinary (animal) patients during clinical trials. In many respects, there is no difference between the equipment and technology employed to manufacture clinical supplies and that used for commercial production. In other respects, for example, production scale, robustness of the manufacturing process, labeling for clinical trial materials, expiration period (and hence the need for supporting stability data), final container, and even formulation and dosage form, there are important differences that should be taken into account when designing appropriate GMP controls for clinical supplies.

Placebos used in medical treatment to bring about a therapeutic effect without a pharmacologically active ingredient, or placebos used as study controls in clinical trials for new drugs are also subject to the requirements in the current good manufacturing practice regulations (GMP). Because they lack any active ingredient, placebos clearly cannot be tested for potency, but their inactive composition can be confirmed. This and other considerations unique to placebos also call for some degree of interpretation of GMP.

Clinical supply manufacturing operations are those areas involved in the manufacture of Phase I–IV clinical trial materials, and may include laboratory (or table-top) scale activities, operations performed in a pilot plant (with batch sizes generally larger than lab scale, but smaller than commercial scale), clinical supplies produced in facilities manufacturing commercially approved products, as well as clinical supplies produced at contract manufacturing sites.

The GMP regulations apply to investigational new drug products produced for clinical trials in humans or animals, whereas those activities earlier in the product development life cycle such as "*basic research* " discovery or preclinical experimentation are not subject to GMP requirements.

FDA Inspections of Clinical Supply Manufacturers

Under the Federal Food, Drug, and Cosmetic Act, the FDA has the authority to "...enter, at reasonable times, any. . . establishment in which food, drugs, devices or cosmetics are manufactured, processed, packed, or held...". This authority clearly includes sites that manufacture or conduct analysis of clinical supplies (for lot release, stability, or in connection with failure investigations). The term "*reasonable time*" has been interpreted by the courts to mean any time-regulated operations are taking place, regardless of date, day of the week, or time of day or night. Inspections are typically not preannounced, but may be in certain cases.

In practice, FDA only occasionally inspects clinical supply manufacturing sites. However, that should not result in a false sense that an FDA inspection will never take place. Manufacturing sites should always be prepared to undergo FDA inspections. Factors that may cause FDA to inspect clinical supply manufacturers include: Review in connection with a pre-approval inspection of the commercial manufacturing site; routine inspections of contract manufacturers who manufacture only clinical supplies; inspections resulting from observed product defects, especially when such defects are linked to adverse reactions in patients (such as contaminated parenterals); in reaction to recalls of clinical supplies; or other factors. The FDA inspections of manufacturing operations for clinical supplies used in Phase III trials are more likely than for operations producing Phase I or Phase II clinical trial material.

Each site should have ready access to a person or persons highly knowledgeable in FDA inspection procedure who can prepare personnel for the inspection and manage it from the company's perspective when it occurs. It is not the purpose of this article to explain in detail how to manage an FDA inspection, but the authors highly recommend that key personnel at each site receive relevant training in preparation for an FDA inspection, and prepare detailed policies and procedures concerning the handling of FDA inspections.

Understanding and Using FDA Documents

To properly interpret and apply GMP requirements to a specific context require some research and a good deal of judgment. This process can be greatly aided by reference to a variety of FDA documents in the public domain. Examples of useful documents include: Guidelines; the so-called Points to Consider documents issued by the Center for Biologics Evaluation and Research (CBER); Compliance Policy Guides; Inspection Technical Guides; Compliance Program Guidance Manuals; and others.

A key document for interpretation of GMP in a clinical supply setting is FDA's 1991 Guideline on the Preparation of Investigational New Drug Products (Human and Animal). This Guideline illustrates when drug development activities are subject to GMP requirements, the degree of compliance expected at certain stages of drug development, and FDA guidance for several important sections of the GMP regulations.

FDA's position on the applicability of GMP to clinical supplies was clearly articulated in the Preamble to the September 29, 1978 revision of the Drug GMPs that stated: "GMP regulations apply to the preparation of any drug product for administration to humans or animals, including those still in investigational stages. It is appropriate that the process by which a drug product is manufactured in the development phase be well documented and controlled in order to assure the reproducibility of the product for further testing and for ultimate commercial production."

Compliance Policy Guides are FDA internal documents that provide precedent for GMP (and other) enforcement decisions by FDA's field offices. They are found on the "Field Operations" or "ORA" (Office of Regulatory Affairs) pages on FDA's website under the heading "Compliance References."

Points to Consider documents are topical policy statements by CBER on subjects such as viral inactivation, transgenic animals, and other specialized technology subjects. Compliance Programs provide FDA investigators with procedural guidance for performing inspections in a wide variety of industries.

Industry publications and seminars can also provide useful information, but users should be wary of placing too much weight on "*podium policy*" statements by FDA officials or reading inspection citations issued to other companies. These sources may be misleading when the reader may not know all the facts surrounding any statements.

Selected GMP Systems as Applied to Clinical Supplies

Quality Organization

21 CFR 211.22 is the regulation that sets forth the responsibilities of the "Quality Control Unit" (QCU). There is no difference in the required roles and responsibilities of the QCU in the manufacture of clinical supplies vs. commercial products. The FDA considers the presence of an adequately staffed and trained QCU, empowered with authority to carry out its responsibility effectively, as a critical factor in GMP compliance.

Companies should be aware that "*Quality Control Unit*" is a generic term, and the company-specific terminology may differ from the term QCU. For example, in most companies, this unit is referred to as Quality Assurance (QA). Other common terms include Regulatory Compliance, QA/QC, or in some cases, the Regulatory Affairs group fulfills many, if not all, of the listed QCU functions. In very small companies or "virtual" firms, the QCU may be as small as one person, while in large companies the number of QCU employees may be quite large, and the quality organization may have several subdivisions. Thus, the name given to the QCU and its members is not as important as the authority to implement the required roles and responsibilities.

The regulation requires that the QCU be responsible for the following, at a minimum:

1. Dispositioning (approval or rejection) of components, containers, closures, in-process materials, packaging, labeling, and finished products.
2. Review of production records to assure that no errors have occurred.
3. If errors have occurred, they have been fully investigated.
4. Approval or rejection of standard operating procedures (SOPs) and specifications.

5. Approval or rejection of changes.
6. Oversight of contracted manufacturing operations (including testing).
7. Approval or rejection of all activities having a potential impact on the safety, purity, potency, quality, and efficacy of the products being manufactured.

The FDA expects (and many other regulatory authorities require) that the QCU will have full independence from other units. This is to provide the maximum degree of assurance that the QCU's decisions will be free of conflicts of interest and other impediments. Normally, the expectation is that the head of the QCU will report to a very senior level person of the company, and that there will not be a situation where the head of the QCU reports to manufacturing, marketing, or other similar functions.

The GMP requires that the QCU should have a qualified laboratory. This may be an in-house laboratory that is part of the QCU itself, or it may be an outside contractor or another company site laboratory. Here again, there is an expectation of independence of the laboratory from manufacturing or other units, in order to assure the maximum degree of objectivity in the data that are generated.

Master (and Batch) Production and Control Records

The specific requirements for master production and control records, and batch production and control records outlined in sections 21 CFR 211.186 and 21 CFR 211.188, respectively, also apply to clinical supplies. Despite these requirements, the level and amount of available documentation for early developmental batches will generally be much less when compared to commercial products, until the manufacturing process becomes more fully defined. Batch production and control records for clinical batches produced will have an increased amount of notes, changes, and other information handwritten on them during execution of clinical batches. The amount of this extraneous information usually coincides with the stage of development for the drug product (e.g., early phase production = more notes and changes), and may include the following:

1. Notes of any situations arising during production.
2. Problems that occurred.
3. Modifications made to the formulation, processing step sequence, processing parameters, or equipment set points.

This information that is annotated on executed master production and control records should be evaluated, reviewed and, if necessary, approved, and incorporated utilizing an established change control system. In many cases, master production and control records used in the production of clinical supplies start out as "*batch cards*," which are sometimes printed on a heavier stock paper that may be colored (e.g., blue or green), in order to differentiate them as related to R&D production operations, and not commercially manufactured products.

Buildings and Facilities

While buildings and facilities are required to be of suitable size and construction, as well as maintained in a good condition for both approved products and clinical supplies, the level of protection these areas are required to provide is dependent upon the activities taking place inside a respective area. For example, sterile fill operations necessitate, among other things, high-efficiency particulate air (HEPA)-filtered air, temperature and humidity controls, and Class 100 (Class A) environmental conditions. It would be inappropriate to perform aseptic filling operations for even Phase I clinical supplies in a non-environmentally controlled laboratory suite under a hood certified to meet Class 100 conditions. As it will be noted later in this article, there is little to no difference in matters of sterility assurance when comparing clinical trial materials to approved products. Similar discretion should also be exercised for operations such as dispensing, mixing, and packaging because FDA expect buildings and facilities used to manufacture clinical supplies are the same as those for commercial products.

Equipment

As with buildings and facilities, equipment must also be of suitable size and construction, as well as suitably located to facilitate its operation, maintenance, and cleaning (21 CFR 211.63). While there is clearly no difference in regulatory requirements for equipment used to manufacture clinical supplies, when compared to commercial manufacturing (e.g., equipment must be maintained and cleaned at appropriate intervals, measurement devices calibrated, qualified, and operating according to written and approved procedures), cleaning is especially important, in as much as many compounds encountered during drug development are of unknown toxicities that pose additional risks. Generally, fully established and validated cleaning procedures will not be in place during Phase I and II clinical supply manufacture. However, the actual cleaning regimen should be robust enough to minimize the potential for contamination or product carry-over. This may be accomplished via visual inspection, or possibly by verification through actual sampling and analytical testing. Finally, 21 CFR Part 211.105 requirements regarding identification of equipment used in the manufacture of clinical trial material can be satisfied with a single sign, or placard, denoting the material in question, the phase of production, and batch number.

Control of Incoming Materials

General requirements related to incoming materials, which include components, drug product containers, and closures, include establishing and following written procedures for the receipt, identification, storage, handling, sampling, testing, and approval (or rejection) of said items (21 CFR 211.80). Research and development organizations will typically have receiving functions and areas that are separate from those used to receive incoming materials for commercial manufacturing operations. The quantities of components, drug product containers and closures, and the containers holding them are generally smaller when compared to the volumes and sizes of incoming materials received by commercial operations.

It is important to note that FDA expects incoming materials used in the manufacture of clinical supplies to be released by the Quality Unit (21 CFR 211.22). Attempts to circumvent the established receiving operation in order to expedite use of these materials should be avoided. Equally important is the requirement to ensure proper storage and segregation of incoming materials, such that quarantined, released, and rejected items are easily identified, and there is some level of separation among them. Different lots or item numbers of similar materials should not be comingled during storage, in order to avoid inadvertent mix-ups with their use in manufacturing (21 CFR 211.80). Finally, incoming components (e.g., raw materials) used to manufacture clinical supplies must be tested for identity using a specific identity test (if available). Specifications should be established and confirmed for each lot of components, drug product containers, and closures received (21 CFR 211.84 and 21 CFR 211.94), and all other provisions of 21 CFR Part 211, Subpart E, Control of Components and Drug Product Containers and Closures not noted in this section also apply to clinical supply manufacturing operations.

Qualification and Validation Activities

Qualification activities are normally associated with buildings, facilities, utility systems (e.g., water, air handling, Clean-in-place/Steam-in-place (CIP/SIP), and compressed gases) major equipment (including laboratory instrumentation), whereas validation likely is in reference to those confirmatory tasks related to processes and analytical methods. In simplistic terms, validation (and qualification) can be defined as documented evidence that a process, activity, or piece of equipment can consistently meet its predetermined acceptance criteria and quality attributes. This section will be dedicated towards outlining the requirements for validation of manufacturing processes, as the requirements for buildings, facilities and equipment, and the validation of cleaning processes have been discussed in previous sections.

The FDA has indicated that during development, processes are expected be validated, and this should be completed to the "*extent possible.*" Challenges with earlier stages of development include fewer batches from which to establish physicochemical characteristics (including toxicity and potency), processing parameters, and commensurate equipment set points. There is also a greater reliance on in-process monitoring and testing, and final product testing for Phase I, II, and possibly early Phase III clinical supply manufacture. This more intensive monitoring and testing is needed to supplant full process validation, where multiple batches have not been produced under replicated conditions. Once, as FDA puts it, "a growing body of scientific data and documentation" reaches a point, complete validation of the manufacturing process will be required.

While blending times and tablet press parameters may not be fully established for early phase clinical supply manufacturing of solid oral dosages, those variables have a much lower potential to directly affect product safety than sterility, endotoxin contamination, or objectionable types and levels of particulates do for sterile, parenteral clinical supplies. Because clinical supplies can be incompletely characterized, and are usually given to patients already in weakened conditions, those processes and their related validation data necessary to guarantee patient and product safety (e.g., sterilization and aseptic fill) are expected to be in place as early as Phase I clinical supply manufacture.

Production and Process Controls

Written procedures are required to be established and followed for production and process controls as specified in 21 CFR Part 211.100. Because the specific requirements regarding handling of changes, deviations, and equipment identification are addressed in other sections of this article, and all other provisions of Subpart F are required in order to meet CGMP requirements for clinical supplies, this section will focus on the other aspects of Subpart F that provide unique challenges during clinical supply manufacture. Yield calculations are not only required according to 21 CFR Part 211.103, but they also provide some measure of process, phase, or step consistency when compared on a batch-by-batch basis. This information may prove useful when continuing process development, process optimization, or in the investigation of any process problems encountered during clinical supply production. Actual yields and percentages of theoretical yield also one of many important measures used to evaluate the validation of a manufacturing process.

Time limitations on production may not be fully known or established during early clinical supply development. However, those operations that are time-sensitive such as mixing or blending times, and drying times should be supported by data that are obtained through developmental studies. Arbitrarily assigning time limits without the benefit of any data, or the working knowledge of the operation in question, should be avoided, and can result in costly developmental errors and product delays.

Reprocessing can be defined as the repeating of a defined step or sequence of steps outlined in a master production and control record, in order to achieve a predetermined endpoint. Written procedures should be established and followed for any reprocessing steps or operations that are incorporated into a developed manufacturing process. The effectiveness of any reprocessing activity should be demonstrated through validation studies and should be fully supported by data.

Sterility Assurance

During inspections, FDA places a great deal of emphasis on the following systems they feel most directly will impact the safety and efficacy of sterile products manufactured, namely:

1. Sterilization processes for the drug itself, any components, container/closures, product-contact equipment, and surfaces
2. Depyrogenation processes
3. Water systems

4. Air handling systems
5. Environmental monitoring programs
6. Handling of incoming components
7. Packaging and labeling operations
8. Laboratory controls
9. Lyophilization (if applicable).

In general, the above-mentioned, including procedures, systems and, if applicable, validation should be in place for clinical supply manufacturing operations. This would include validation of processes such as sterilization, depyrogenation, and lyophilization; qualification of water and air handling systems; establishing and following procedures for: environmental monitoring programs, handling of incoming components, packaging, and labeling operations; and CGMP compliance for laboratories performing analyses of raw materials, in-process and final product samples, environmental monitoring activities, and testing in support of clinical supply manufacturing. Additionally, those processes or activities that are product-specific (e.g., sterilization, depyrogenation, the manufacturing process for the finished drug product itself, and analytical testing related to raw materials, in-process and final product testing) should be validated to what has been previously noted as the "*extent possible*." For example, in the case of sterilization processes such as terminal sterilization using moist heat, all of the following validation and process control requirements would be necessary in order to avoid exposing a patient to a risk of non-sterility:

1. Equipment that is qualified, maintained, and calibrated.
2. Empty chamber heat distribution studies.
3. Heat penetration studies that are product and load pattern-specific.
4. Challenges with biological indicators.
5. Process controls and monitoring typical for steam sterilization (e.g., time, temperature, and pressure).

Similar logic can be applied to sterilization by filtration or depyrogenation by means of dry heat. In these and other cases, there will be little to no difference in the level of compliance necessary when comparing clinical supply manufacturing to that for the manufacturing for commercially approved products.

Change Control

Change control is one of the GMP systems that is applied somewhat differently in clinical supply manufacture than it is in the manufacture of commercial products. Change control does not have a separate and distinct section in the GMP regulations; however, the management of change is referenced or mentioned in several GMP sections.

In commercial manufacturing, the purpose of change control is two-fold:

1. Keep validated systems functioning in a validated state.
2. Maintain the accuracy of approved submissions to regulatory agencies.

In the manufacture of clinical supplies, normally, manufacturing processes are not robust (and therefore not completely validated) until Phase III, sometimes not until the later stages of Phase III. Therefore, the goals of change control in clinical supply manufacture are somewhat different. Those goals should include:

1. Assurance that equipment (including computer systems and software), which has been qualified (installation, operational, and performance qualification), is maintained in a qualified state.
2. Support systems (such as water for injection, air handling systems, compressed gases, vacuum, clean-in-place systems, and others) are likewise maintained in a qualified state.

3. Any significant modification of the Chemistry, Manufacturing, and Controls section of the IND is noted, and, where applicable, the approved submission is supplemented to provide for the change.
4. Key changes in the development of formulation, dosage form, manufacturing process, cleaning procedures, and other key operations are identified for the purpose of documenting them as part of the development history.
5. When significant numbers of batches are manufactured using replicate processes (usually in late Phase III trials), changes are evaluated in order to determine if process development is complete, and validation should commence.

Laboratory Controls

The majority of 21 CFR 211.160 (laboratory controls) and subsections can be applied in the same manner for clinical supplies as for commercial products. An exception, in many cases, is the time by which analytical methods validation is required. For new chemical entities or significant formulation changes, new analytical methods may need to be developed. As with manufacturing processes, until such methods are robust it is difficult (or impossible) to validate them to the full extent that is expected for commercial products. The factors normally considered in analytical methods validation include:

1. Specificity
2. Sensitivity
3. Linearity
4. Repeatability
5. Robustness
6. Ruggedness
7. Limit of detection
8. Limit of quantitation.

Analytical method validation should track closely to the stages of development of the method itself. However, it is not realistic to expect complete and thorough validation of the method until its development cycle is complete. An exception to this would be a situation where an accepted compendial method is applied to clinical material (such as a dissolution test or release testing of a compendial component). In these cases, companies must be prepared to demonstrate that consistent acceptable results can be obtained when using the compendial method in the company's laboratory (also known as methods verification). The obvious difference is that a compendial method is not a proprietary method, having been developed fully in a collaborative process. Therefore, transfer of a compendial method to a clinical supply context does not differ from a similar transfer to a commercial product.

Methods for the investigation of out-of-specification (OOS) results should be similar to what is required for commercial manufacturing. However, it is recognized that in many cases, specifications may be less exact and methods may still be under development; therefore, it may be considerably more difficult to determine assignable causes for OOS findings related to clinical supplies.

When considering OOS investigation procedures for clinical supplies, manufacturers must keep certain basic principles in mind. Those basic principles include:

1. OOS results must not be arbitrarily dismissed simply because they are unexpected and present obstacles to release of materials.
2. Consideration must be given as to whether analyst error, equipment malfunction, inappropriate reagents, or some other detectable and assignable cause was the reason for an OOS result.
3. Consideration must be given as to whether a detectable process error or non-process related (employee) error was the reason for the OOS result.

4. There must be a documented rationale for resampling or retesting, including documentation of the reasonableness of the number of retests that are needed to overcome an OOS finding.
5. Averaging of results should be avoided when the purpose of the test is to reveal variability in a batch (such as blend uniformity or content uniformity testing) because averaging tends to hide variability.
6. If averaging is employed, OOS results must be included along with within-specification findings, unless they may be discarded by an approved statistical outlier test (either approved in the compendia or in the IND).

Training records for analysts should demonstrate that they have the necessary combination of education, training, and experience to perform the specific methods they are assigned to perform. Stability testing will be guided mainly by the conditions approved in the IND. However, the manner in which the stability program is managed should be similar to that required for commercial products. For example (not an all inclusive list):

1. Procedures to ensure that stability samples are correctly collected and are representative of the batch.
2. Procedures to ensure that chambers are qualified (temperature mapped) and monitored for environmental parameters.
3. Procedures to ensure that test intervals are consistently met.
4. Procedures for the development of stability-indicating analytical methods.
5. Complete, clear, and accessible records of all testing, including the preservation of raw data.

Deviations and Failure Investigations

As with commercial manufacturing, product or process deviations, or the failure of any clinical batch or any of its components to meet any of its specifications must be handled by approved procedures and thoroughly investigated (21 CFR 211.192). The investigation report should include, among other things:

1. Nature of the deviation or failure
2. Date
3. Affected batch or batches
4. Root cause determination
5. Impact analysis
6. Recommended corrective actions
7. Approval by the Quality Unit.

Apart from being product or process-related, deviations can also be procedural in nature, meaning that certain requirements of a specific SOP were not adhered to. Sometimes the terms "unplanned" and "planned" deviations are also used. Unplanned deviations include those events, activities, or actions that are non-intentional. An example of an unplanned deviation could include shutdown of processing equipment during the manufacture of a batch due to safety concerns. Planned deviation, on the other hand, is a term that is not favorably looked upon by FDA. A conscious decision not to follow written procedures, manufacturing instructions, or other records required under the predicate rule is, at the very least, a CGMP issue. The FDA expects that deviations will be fully and thoroughly documented, including any decisions made and by whom.

In the clinical supply setting, systems and procedures should be established and followed for handling deviations and performing investigations. For deviations, this would also include trending (either according to defined categories such as equipment, process, etc. by product line or other predefined criteria), timely resolution of the issues, and re-evaluation of process or equipment parameters and specifications, procedural requirements, or other items bearing on the quality or purity of the finished drug product. This re-evaluation is especially important during new product development, where less information may be known about the drug product being studied, the method of manufacture, process capabilities, or sensitivities of test methods. In these and other cases, improperly or incorrectly defined product or process attributes could contribute to an artificially high deviation rate, and more importantly, could suggest that additional product development work is needed.

Complaints and Adverse Reactions

Section 211.198 of the GMP regulations sets forth the requirements for reporting and investigating complaints. This section is intended to assure that when a manufacturer is notified of a product defect, a thorough investigation will be performed to determine the cause of the defect, and whether a recall of the product from the marketplace should be initiated. Of course, these activities are all aimed at protection of patients from harm caused by defective products.

When the product in question is intended only for use in clinical trials, the fundamental purpose of the regulation, protection of patients from defective products, must still be of primary concern. However, the quantity of product at risk, and its limited distribution will impact the process of complaint investigation. For example, the generally smaller amount of product involved may make it difficult to identify low-level occurrences of manufacturing defects. The limited and more tightly controlled system of distribution of clinical trial supplies, however, will likely facilitate and limit the recall process should that be deemed necessary.

Complaints of adverse reactions to clinical supplies are typically seen as reportable events that impact the safety or efficacy of the test article. Companies should give consideration to the possibility that an increase in the frequency or severity of adverse reactions may be linked to a manufacturing defect. For example, a product that has been formulated such that it is super- potent in its final form can be expected to produce adverse reactions of greater severity or frequency than if it was properly formulated. Labeling mix-ups can have devastating impact on patients, or, at minimum, may seriously affect the validity of a clinical trial. Therefore, the following elements should be included in the complaint assessment system:

1. Complaints of observable (physical) defects should be promptly and thoroughly investigated to determine the root cause of the defect and the probable scope of its occurrence.
2. Complaints of unusual or severe adverse reactions, or significant and unexpected increases in the number of adverse reactions (including marked lack of efficacy) should be evaluated to determine whether manufacturing errors may have caused or contributed to the observed effects.
3. When a product defect is identified, the evaluation should include a health hazard assessment by a qualified person, usually a physician. The FDA's recall policy regulations contain a suggested rubric for performing a health hazard assessment.
4. Product defect complaints and adverse reaction data and trends should be periodically compared to determine if there is any correlation between unexpected numbers, types or severity of adverse reactions, and the number and type of reported product defects.
5. As with commercial products, careful records of reported complaints, their investigation and resolution are critical to GMP compliance.

Technology Transfer Plans and Reports

Technology transfer plans and reports are used by a research and development organization in order to document their official "transfer" of a newly developed or recently upgraded product/process from the developmental area and facilities to an operations unit and site, usually located in separate buildings, or at an entirely separate and different manufacturing sites. While the format and content has not been formally prescribed by FDA, companies generally include the following information in these documents:

1. Definition of responsibilities for key departments; documentation review, approval, and storage requirements.
2. Summary of developmental activities completed.
3. Summary of scale-up activities; summary of formulation, synthesis, process, and analytical method changes; establishment of impurity specifications; establishment of critical process parameters; identification of validation plans and activities.
4. Definition of component, container/closure, and product attributes.
5. Analytical methods development and validation summary.
6. Descriptions, specifications, design parameters and requirements of facilities, and major equipment and utility systems.
7. Definition of the manufacturing process.
8. Stability and expiry dating information.
9. Change control.
10. Reprocessing.
11. Cleaning processes, including methods development and validation of the processes and methods.
12. Summary of Regulatory Affairs activities, including regulatory commitments, key data and information to be summarized in regulatory filings.

Data Integrity Considerations

The integrity of GMP data should be a vital part of any company's compliance scheme. The term "data integrity" generally means that the raw (source) data and associated data summaries and reports are truthful, accurate, legible, indelible, complete, and readily accessible. This applies whether the data are in hard copy (paper) form or electronic form. The GMP rules allow for the preservation of data through photocopying or other optical reproduction process (microfilming, optically scanning, etc.); however, original documents should be preserved whenever possible.

The fundamentals of good data recording practices should be observed in clinical supply manufacturing in exactly the same manner as required for commercial materials. Those fundamentals include the following:

1. Data, and the identification of those responsible for it, should be recorded contemporaneously, or as close to the time of execution of a step or an observation as is practical. Transfer of data from one form to another should be minimized, and should include one hundred percent verification for accuracy by a second person. This serves to enhance the accuracy of the data.
2. Hard copy documents should be recorded in indelible ink. Errors are inevitable, and when they occur, the original entry should be struck out with a single line, initialed and dated, the correct information entered, and a brief explanation of the error should be appended as directed by the document and associated procedures.
3. Data should always be recorded on forms designed for the specific purpose. Extraneous notations on loose slips of paper should be strictly prohibited in a GMP environment.
4. Log books, laboratory notebooks (when used), batch production and control records, qualification and validation protocols and reports, investigations of deviations and failures, and other GMP documentation must be carefully identified, controlled, and archived in a manner that will facilitate its prompt retrieval.

5. Electronic records (and electronic signatures, if used) must comply with the provisions of 21 CFR Part 11. It is beyond the scope of this article to explain "Part 11" compliance in total, however, the general principle is to construct and maintain electronic records with the same degree of accuracy and linkage to the originator as is achieved with hard copy documents. Each company choosing to use electronic data capture techniques and electronic signatures must thoroughly understand Part 11 and ensure compliance with this regulation.
6. Each company should have a policy that strictly prohibits the deliberate falsification, mutilation, obliteration, or destruction of raw data and associated GMP documentation. Companies must insist on strict adherence to such policies and should take aggressive disciplinary action when lapses are detected. Failure to do so may subject the company and its corporate officers to severe regulatory sanctions, including criminal prosecution under the Federal Food, Drug, and Cosmetic Act, or the general criminal laws of the United States. Even inadvertent (non-deliberate) acts that result in loss of data or records should be prevented, and, if they occur, they should be promptly and thoroughly investigated.
7. Establishing and following policies and procedures for good documentation practices, numerical rounding, significant figures, and directed audits to ensure the integrity of data contained in records or other documents prior to submission of applications to FDA).

22

DENTAL PRODUCTS

A considerable number of products are now recommended for use in the oral cavity. Products for caries control are widely used and include fluorides in dentifrices and mouthwashes. Plaque control is achieved through the use of chemical agents such as chlorhexidine and quaternary ammonium compounds. Mechanical products for plaque control include dental floss, toothpastes, and mouthwashes. Products also exist to combat halitosis, act as topical anesthetics, desensitize sensitive teeth, act as tooth-bleaching agents, and assist in reducing xerostomia. More recently, products designed for the local delivery of antimicrobial agents to the oral cavity have also been made available. These, and other products, are reviewed in this article.

CARIES CONTROL USING FLUORIDES

Over 300 million people worldwide now consume optimally fluoridated water. The U.S. Public Health Service has established recommended levels for fluoride concentrations in water supplies in accordance with mean annual temperatures. The daily intake of fluoride not only comes from drinking water but also from food consumed or prepared with fluoridated water. Also, crops are frequently fertilized with phosphate fertilizers of high soluble-fluoride content, and food products including bone in animal feeds contain fluoride. Naturally fluoridated foods and water have been ingested for decades with no serious side effects. In addition, public fluoridation has been widespread in this country for over 30 years without serious adverse effects. The incidence of mottled enamel, one of the earliest and most sensitive signs of fluoride toxicity, has not increased significantly in the past 15 years of water fluoridation. The safety and efficacy of fluoride has definitely been established, with no scientific evidence against fluoridation.

Mechanism of Action

The mechanism by which fluoride prevents caries is not clearly understood. It is known that the fluoride ion (F^-) can replace the hydroxyl ion (OH^-) in hydroxyapatite, the major crystalline structure of enamel. The substituted crystal, called fluorapatite, is more resistant to acids, such as those produced by plaque bacteria, than the original hydroxyapatite. As the tooth develops and enamel is formed, ingested fluoride is incorporated into the enamel. Therefore, because enamel develops its outer layer first, more fluoride can be expected to be deposited on the outer layers as compared to the inner layers. It is this surface enamel layer containing fluoride that imports, in part, caries resistance to a tooth. Topical fluorides also become incorporated into enamel and provide protection against acid. A number of studies have now shown that topical fluorides may be most beneficial in early enamel caries and that there is an increased uptake of fluoride in early lesions, with some tooth remineralization occurring. This finding has caused some investigators to label fluoride as a remineralizing agent as well as a caries inhibitor. The incorporation of fluoride into enamel can be represented as a chemical reaction:

$$Ca_{10}(PO_4)_6(OH)_2 + F \rightarrow Ca_{10}(PO_4)_6F_2 + 2(OH)^-$$

Dental plaque also tends to concentrate fluoride. This could increase possible antienzymatic activity. Some caries protection from this may be expected. Additionally, studies have suggested that topical application of fluoride may also reduce smooth surface plaque, with a resulting beneficial effect on the periodontal tissues. In areas where there is no fluoridation of the community water supply, fluoride may be added to school water. This is not a substitute for community water fluoridation because fluoride intake from birth is important. In some areas where fluoride is absent from drinking water, the school water supply has been fluoridated as much as 4.5 times the level usually recommended for community water levels. These studies, conducted for 12 years in fluoride-deficient areas, revealed a 40% reduction in DMF surfaces. Essentially, no undesirable fluorosis resulted from this procedure. However, it should be noted that ingestion occurred only during part of each day and only on school days. This level (4.5 ppm) from birth (during major formation of permanent teeth) would cause undesirable fluorosis with continued intake.

Therapeutic Effects

Fluoridated water

The administration of fluoride in drinking water at concentrations of approximately 1 ppm significantly reduces dental caries. The anticaries benefits are similar to those due to natural fluoride in drinking water. Fluoridated drinking water produces the following: a 60% lower dental caries rate, a 75% decrease in the loss of 6-year molars, and a 90% reduction in the incidence of proximal caries of the four upper anterior teeth. Evidence suggests that greater inhibition of caries occurs when teeth receive fluoride throughout the calcification period. Therefore, maximum benefit may be expected from the continued use of fluoridated drinking water.

Dietary supplements/tablets

Maximum benefits to both deciduous and permanent teeth may result from daily fluoride supplements from infancy until approximately 13 years of age, at which time all permanent teeth except the third molars should have erupted. Because cariostatic benefits may tend to diminish gradually after fluorides are discontinued, periodic applications of topical fluorides may then be necessary. The use of dietary fluoride or topical applications of fluoride depends partly on the age of the child. Dietary supplements of fluoride are best for very young children, whereas topical fluoride applications are preferred for older children with permanent teeth. Younger children who are highly susceptible to caries may benefit from both measures. The natural level of fluoride in drinking water where the child lives should be known before dietary fluoride is prescribed. At present, it is suggested that fluoride supplements be limited to where drinking water contains 60% or less of the optimal level of fluorides recommended for community water in the geographic area.

As a precaution, no large quantities of sodium fluoride should be stored in the home. It is recommended that no more than 264 mg of sodium fluoride be dispensed at any one time, which is enough for at least a 4-month period. Each package dispensed should also bear the statement: Caution—store out of the reach of children. Although the optimal level of fluoride in drinking water is well documented, there is no established allowance for fluoride administered once a day. The standard allowance is 1 mg/day for a child over 3 years of age and one-half this amount for a child between the ages of 2 and 3. A more accurate method to use in calculating the daily fluoride needs of a child is to administer a dose based on the child's weight, for example, .025 mg/lb of body weight. However, for all children over 6 months of age, the dose should not exceed 1 mg/day of fluoride ion regardless of weight. In order to avoid the possibility of unesthetic dental fluorosis, the prescribed dietary allowance should be reduced in proportion to the fluoride levels in the drinking water. These allowances are for children over 6 years of age. The allowances should be reduced for children 6 years of age and under.

Table 22.1. Adjustment of prescribed fluoride relative to natural content of drinking water for children over 6 years of age

Water fluoride (ppm)	*Adjusted allowance sodium fluoride (mg/day)*	*Provides fluoride ion (mg/day)*
0.0	2.2	1.0
0.2	1.8	0.8
0.4	1.3	0.5
0.6	0.0	0.0

For children under 6 months of age, experts question the value of prescribing fluoride supplements. Dental caries have been prevented when fluoride tablets were administered in a school-based program. After two or more years of fluoride ingestion, protection against dental caries ranged from 20–40%. In an extended trial of fluoride tablets reported in the literature, there was a 36% reduction in dental caries after 8 years.

Table 22.2. Adjustment of prescribed fluoride ion relative to natural content of drinking water for children under 6 yr of age

	Content of water fluoride		
Patient's age	*0–0.3 ppm*	*0.3–0.6 ppm*	*>0.6 ppm*
0–6 mon	0.0	0.0	0.0
6 mon–3yr	0.25	0.0	0.0
3–6 yr	0.50	0.25	0.0

The use of fluoride tablets can provide both a preeruptive (endogenous) effect and a posteruptive (topical) effect. Therefore, tablets should be chewed or dissolved in the mouth and the teeth rinsed with the resultant solution before swallowing. One advantage of fluoride tablets compared to water fluoridation is that a specific dosage of fluoride is delivered. One disadvantage is that dietary supplements of fluoride taken once a day are rapidly cleared from the body.

Breast-feeding

Fluoride levels in human breast milk have been found to be less than 0.05 ppm. This concentration remains constant, regardless of drinking water and maternal plasma levels. Thus, breast-fed infants who receive no formula bottle feedings ingest considerably less fluoride than infants receiving formula mixed in 1 ppm fluoridated water. Fluoride supplementation for breast-fed infants should be considered. The administration of fluoride supplements to expectant mothers in an effort to benefit the teeth of the offspring has been evaluated in several studies. The evidence, however, is not sufficiently conclusive to warrant recommendation.

Vitamins

Vitamin preparations containing sodium fluoride are also available as drops, tablets, and chewable tablets. These forms of supplementation are useful in areas where the water supply contains less than 0.6 ppm, and they offer a way to provide fluoride to the child, if the parents are conscientious in dispensing the required amount daily and if the child does not object to taking oral medications. In recommending vitamins with fluoride, it is mandatory that one know the fluoride content of the child's water supply, as well as the fluoride content of the vitamin being recommended.

Topicals

Fluoride can be applied topically in various forms, offering the practitioner a number of options to choose for his or her patients. Topical agents are of lesser value in a caries reduction program when they are used in fluoridated communities. However, when used in non-fluoridated areas, they are more effective. In such areas, they often are the only form of fluoride therapy available. The dosage forms of topical fluoride currently available include varnishes, dentifrices, solutions, gels, mouthwashes, and prophylaxis pastes.

Table 22.3. Various topical fluoride preparations

Preparation	*Form*	*Formulation*
Acidulated phosphate fluoride	Topical solution	1.23% in 1% phosphoric acid
	Topical gel, foam	1.23% in 1% phosphoric acid
	Mouthrinse	0.02–0.04%
	Prophylaxis paste	1.2%
Amine fluoride	Dentifrice	1.6%
	Mouthrinse	2.5%
Sodium fluoride	Topical solution	2%
	Mouthrinse	2.5%
	Foam	0.2%
	Varnish	5% (every 3–6 months)
Sodium monofluorophosphate	Dentifrice	0.76–0.8%
Stannous fluoride	Topical solution	8%
	Mouthrinse	0.1%
	Prophylaxis paste	8%
	Dentifrice	0.4%
	Gel	0.4%

Dentifrices

The earliest fluoride dentifrices contained sodium fluoride. However, the fluoride was biologically unavailable because the calcium in the dentifrice abrasive bound the fluoride and thus inactivated it.

Although a number of dentifrices containing fluoride are on the market, not all provide available fluoride because the abrasive systems that some dentifrices contain inactivate the fluoride. Therefore, the product may contain as much fluoride as any other dentifrice but it is not available. Also, if the product has a short shelf life, it will be ineffective if poor marketing gets it to the consumer too late.

For these reasons, only dentifrices approved by the Council on Scientific Affairs of the American Dental Association (ADA) should be recommended. These products are listed in that association's publications and carry the ADA seal on their packaging.

Currently accepted dentifrices contain sodium monofluorophosphate, sodium fluoride, or, less frequently, stannous fluoride, all of which reduce caries by approximately 25% when used daily. In some clinical studies, stannous fluoride dentifrices stained teeth, particularly in pits and fissures. This stain is related to the tin in this compound, which adheres to plaque. The significance of this staining and its esthetic problems have resulted in a decreased usage in dentifrices. Stannous fluoride dentifrices are marketed in a plastic container because a reaction of stannous ions at an acid pH occurs when conventional soft metal tubes are used. The composition of some popular toothpastes is important for a proper understanding of this topic. With the exception of extra strength products, the various dentifrices are formulated to provide 1000 ppm of fluoride. Since children ingest most of the fluoride toothpaste when they brush their teeth, only a pea-sized amount should be placed on the brush.

Stannous fluoride

Dentifrices containing stannous fluoride as an active ingredient are no longer widely marketed; however, these formulations were the first to be evaluated for caries-reducing properties. Effectiveness in caries reduction varied from 23 to 34%. One stannous fluoride dentifrice containing a patented stabilized form of stannous fluoride is marketed with a claim of both caries and gingivitis reduction. However, this product is not ADA accepted. Currently, there are no ADA-approved, over- the-counter dentifrices containing stannous fluoride. However, there are a number of ADA accepted stannous fluoride prescription products approved for application by the dentist or by the patient.

Amine fluoride

Clinical data from several long-term studies in Europe have demonstrated the effectiveness of the use of a dentifrice containing organic amine fluorides. The amine fluorides also have strong plaque-reducing properties. However, although the amine fluorides may be more effective for caries reduction than other forms of fluoride, the FDA has not allowed these products to be extensively tested in this country.

Sodium fluoride

Sodium fluoride as an ingredient in dentifrices has been the subject of a number of clinical investigations. Recent studies of sodium fluoride dentifrices formulated to ensure ready availability of fluoride ions have shown anticaries benefits similar to those obtained in clinical caries trials with dentifrices containing stannous fluoride and sodium monofluorophosphate. Clinical caries trials conducted under well- controlled, daily supervised brushing conditions have reported reductions in dental caries of approximately 25–48%.

Sodium monofluorophosphate

A number of clinical studies have been conducted with dentifrices containing 0.76% monofluorophosphate (MFP). The data from these controlled clinical studies of sodium MFP dentifrices have indicated reductions in dental caries ranging from approximately 17–42%. Two studies indicating effectiveness were conducted in fluoridated communities. In clinical studies comparing this form of fluoride with sodium fluoride, the findings for caries reduction have been similar. Unlike dentifrices containing sodium fluoride, dentifrices containing MFP are compatible with a number of abrasive systems; this is one of the reasons why there are more ADA-accepted products in this category.

Solutions and Gels

In children, a reduction of 30–40% in dental caries is seen with the following: 2% sodium fluoride, 8% stannous fluoride, and acidulated phosphate-fluoride products. No one agent appears to be superior to any other when used as directed. Solutions of 8% stannous fluoride have been used to reduce caries. As with the other agents, the teeth are polished, dried, and isolated, and a 4-min application follows. The disadvantages of this solution are that it must be freshly prepared, some tooth discoloration (as discussed under dentifrices) has occurred, and it has an unpleasant taste that is difficult to mask.

Topical concentrated fluoride solutions are useful in children with high caries activity because they may have both a caries-arresting property and one of caries prevention. The frequency of application varies with the caries activity of the child. For children with an average incidence of caries, it can be applied annually between the ages of 3 and 13.

When gels are used, they are placed into a tray that is placed against the teeth so that the gel flows around all surfaces. Best results have been reported with custom-fitted trays. It has been estimated that about one-third of the total fluoride placed in a tray is actually available for uptake by teeth. The remainder is simply a filler for the tray, some of which is swallowed. The value of topical fluorides on adults has not been established. However, some studies have suggested that the acidulated phosphate fluoride types may offer some caries protection. Recent reports have suggested that polishing of teeth is not necessary prior to the topical application of fluorides. These studies have stated that deplaquing of teeth with a toothbrush is adequate and offers the advantage of not removing surface fluoride from tooth structure. This concept may be valid, and future investigations in this area should be encouraged.

Fluoride mouthwashes

Substantial research has been performed on the caries- inhibiting effect of fluoride mouthrinse products. The effectiveness of these topically applied fluorides varies with patient compliance. The daily use of fluoride rinses by young children should be carefully monitored, and it should be noted that the ADA does not recommend the use of fluoride mouthrinse for children under 6 years of age. Moreover, because these products, when brought into the home, present a potential danger, the ADA Council on Scientific Affairs has recommended that these rinses should not exceed 300 mg of sodium fluoride. Fluoride mouthrinse solutions for use in school or community programs, however, are available in larger volumes, based on the assumption that storing and dispensing of the products in public settings will be closely monitored. The potential dangers involved with unsupervised ingestion of these products should be made known to both parents and children.

Studies evaluating the effectiveness of mouthrinses containing sodium fluoride have shown the usefulness of these agents for children living in non-fluoridated areas. Most studies have been conducted using a mouthrinse containing approximately 0.05% sodium fluoride used daily or a 0.2% sodium fluoride used weekly. The Council on Scientific Affairs has accepted a number of fluoride mouthrinses. All products discussed below have ADA Council on Scientific Affairs acceptance. Some mouthrinses are marketed as a concentrate for dilution to recommended levels. If concentrates are used, special care should be exercised to keep them out of the reach of children. The products are not packaged in glass containers, because the pH becomes more alkaline in glass. Plastic is the container of choice. Examples of prescription and non-prescription products follow.

ACT

This product is an aqueous solution of 0.05% sodium fluoride. It also contains 8% glycerin, 7% alcohol, a detergent, a preservative, saccharin, coloring, and flavoring agents. It is intended to be used on a daily basis and is available without prescription.

Fluorigard

This product is available as a rinse containing an aqueous solution of a 0.05% sodium fluoride, 15% glycerin, 5% alcohol, a detergent, a preservative, saccharin, coloring, and flavoring agents. It is intended to be used on a daily basis and is available without a prescription.

Fluorinse

This product contains 0.2% sodium fluoride as the active ingredient. It also contains a detergent, a preservative, flavoring, and color agents. It is intended to be used on a daily basis and is available without a prescription.

Phos-Flur oral rinse supplement

This product is an aqueous solution containing 0.044% sodium fluoride, 0.055%, phosphoric acid, 1.35% sodium biphosphate, and flavoring and coloring agents. It is intended to be used once daily and is available by prescription.

Desensitizing Agents

A number of studies have reported that topical fluoride application may reduce dental hypersensitivity. These results have been found when concentrated dosage forms have been applied ranging from 8% stannous fluoride gels to 33.3% sodium fluoride paste. It has been shown that commercial dentifrices containing stannous fluoride may also decrease dental hypersensitivity. Also, a combination of stannous fluoride and potassium nitrate is marketed by one manufacturer to reduce sensitivity. Varnishes containing sodium fluoride have also been shown to reduce dental hypersensitivity.

Chemical Agents for Plaque Control

A number of chemical agents have been evaluated over the years in terms of their antimicrobial effects in the oral cavity and the importance of these effects on oral health. In 1986, the establishment by the ADA of guidelines for acceptance of these products has served to stimulate properly designed clinical studies for evaluating potential therapeutic agents.

Products that have earned the ADA's seal of acceptance are Peridex, Listerine, some generic copies of Listerine, and Colgate Total. In this section, data on various available agents are presented according to chemical agent category. When the term *substantivity* is used, it refers to the ability of an agent to be retained in the area cavity and to be released over an extended time period with a continued antimicrobial effect.

Chlorhexidine

Of the products included in this report, chlorhexidine appears to be the most effective agent. Long-term studies in over 700 subjects showed reductions in plaque averaging 55% and in gingivitis 45%.

The mechanism of action of chlorhexidine is related to a reduction in pellicle formation, alteration of bacterial absorption and/or attachment to teeth, and an alteration of the bacterial cell wall so that lysis occurs. Chemically, it is classified as chlorhexidine digluconate and the U.S. Adopted Name (USAN) designation is chlorhexidine gluconate. It has high substantivity. Adverse effects reported included staining of teeth, reversible desquamation in young children, alteration of taste, and an increase in supragingival calcified deposits. Long-term and microbiologic studies do not demonstrate the development of resistant strains. It is sold in the United States in a 0.12% concentration as a prescription mouthrinse (Peridex, PerioGard, and generically), which contain 11.6% alcohol with a pH of 5.5 and is approved by the ADA for control of plaque and gingivitis. Recommended usage is twice daily.

Fluorides

Fluorides are purported to have some antiplaque properties. The most widely used topical fluorides are stannous fluoride, acidulated phosphate fluoride, and sodium fluoride. Of the fluorides, short-term studies of stannous fluoride have been promising. However, long-term published studies showed lower plaque scores, but the differences were not significant. No effect on gingival health was noted with the exception of one study. With stannous fluoride, the mechanism of action appears to be related to an alteration of bacterial aggregation and metabolism.

In summarizing the properties of this agent, it can be stated that it has moderate substantivity, that the antibacterial activity may be related to the tin ion, and that a 0.4% concentration may be the most effective. Stannous fluoride is the most toxic of the products considered and has the shortest shelf life. Adverse effects have been taste and black stain lines on teeth. Usage of once or twice daily favors compliance. Stannous fluoride is most often available as an aqueous gel.

Stannous fluoride products are accepted by the ADA for their ability to deliver fluoride but have not been approved for their plaque-reducing properties. Examples of accepted products are Activux Basic Control, Gel-Kam, Gel-Tin, Perfect Choice, Pro-Dentx, Schein Home Care, and Super-Dent.

Oxygenating Agents

In evaluating the efficacy of oxygenating agents, one must evaluate the endpoints selected for efficacy and their measurement. Oxygenating agents have anti- inflammatory properties. Therefore, less bleeding on probing, a major sign of inflammation, would be expected following their use, but the bacteria producing the disease process would not necessarily have been reduced. Peroxides are found in dentifrices in combinations with sodium bicarbonate in concentrations of 1.5% or less. Also, they are found in bleaching agents discussed later in this chapter. As long-term studies of the effect of oxygenating agents are unavailable and short-term studies offer contradictory findings, questions of safety have been raised with regard to chronic use.

Phenolic Compounds

Listerine

Short-term studies of phenolic compounds have shown plaque and gingivitis reductions averaging 35%, and long-term studies have shown plaque reduction averaging 35% and gingivitis reduction averaging 30%. The only product in this category that has been adequately studied is Listerine. Listerine is a mixture of essential oils—thymol, menthol, a eucalyptol, and methylsalicylate. The mechanism of action appears to be related to alteration of the bacterial cell wall. This product is uncharged and has a low substantivity. Adverse effects reported have been a burning sensation and bitter taste. It is available in a 21.6–26.9% alcohol vehicle with a pH of 4.2. Recommended usage is twice daily, and the ADA accepts the product and some of its generic copies for the control of plaque and gingivitis.

Plax

Only short-term, clinical studies with small numbers of patients have been published. These pilot studies suggested some reduction in plaque when this product was used as a prebrushing rinse. Effects on gingivitis have not been reported. Additional long-term studies have questioned the efficacy of this product to reduce plaque and gingivitis. The active ingredient is stated to be sodium benzoate. However, the product also has about 30% of some of the ingredients (oils) found in Listerine. It contains 7.5% alcohol. Usage is as a prebrushing rinse. It is not ADA accepted.

Quaternary Ammonium Compounds

Quaternary ammonium compounds have been evaluated in a number of short-term studies relative to their effect on plaque and gingivitis. In these studies, an average plaque reduction of 35% has been reported, with mixed effects on gingival health. A 6-month study has been reported showing a 14% reduction in plaque and a 24% reduction in gingivitis. Cepacol, Scope, and Advanced Care Viadent are well-known representatives of this group, each with concentrations of approximately 0.05% cetylpyridium chloride. In addition, Scope contains 0.005% domiphen bromide. The mechanism of action is related to increased bacterial cell wall permeability, which favors lysis, decreased cell metabolism, and a decreased ability for bacteria to attach to tooth surfaces. These agents are categorized as being cationic, which favors their attraction to anionic surfaces of teeth and plaque. They are surface-active agents that alter surface tension and have some substantivity. Adverse effects have been some tooth staining and a burning sensation in the oral cavity. These agents are available in a 14–18% alcoholic vehicle with a pH range of 5.5–6.5. Recommended usage is twice daily, and they are not ADA accepted.

Sanguinarine

Short-term studies of sanguinarine have shown some plaque and gingivitis reduction. In the long-term studies of the product in a dentifrice form, no significant reduction in plaque or gingivitis occurred, with the exception of one study in which the product was used as a dentifrice and as a mouthrinse.

The proposed mechanism of action is by alteration of bacterial cell surfaces so that aggregation and attachment is reduced.

Sanguinarine (benzophenathradine) is derived from the bloodroot plant (*Sanguinaria canadensis*). The extract concentration in the product is 0.03%, which equals 0.10% sanguinarine. It also contains 0.2% zinc chloride. The product may be cationic, and the degree of substantivity is unclear. Adverse effects have been a burning sensation and a question of epithelial cell dysplasia. It is available as Viadent toothpaste and Viadent mouthrinse. The mouthrinse pH is 4.5, the dentifrice pH is 4.8, and the alcohol content of the rinse is 11.5%. It is not ADA accepted.

Triclosan

Triclosan (2,4,4'-Trichloro-2'-hydroxdiphenyl ether) is a new antiplaque/antigingivitis agent available in dentifrices. The addition of a copolymer, vinylmethyl-ether maleic acid (Gantrez), has been shown to improve the effectiveness of triclosan by enhancing its retention (substantivity) by hard and soft surfaces. This formula (Colgate Total) has been approved by the FDA for sale in the United States, and is ADA accepted. Claims allowed are for the reduction of plaque, gingivitis, calculus, and caries. Studies as early as 1973 showed that this chemical agent had a broad spectrum, antimicrobial effect against a wide range of gram-positive and gram-negative bacteria found in the mouth. The minimal concentration of triclosan for oral pathogens is 0.3 mg/ml. Triclosan' s antibacterial activity is not affected by anionic agents, such as lauryl sulfate, which are essential to dentifrice and mouthwash formulations—a fact that broadens its range of use. In doses lower than 0.5%, taste perception is minimally affected; however, at concentrations of greater than 0.5%, undesirable effects on taste occur.

Zinc citrate

This agent is found in some tartar control dentifrices and also has some plaque- and gingivitis-reducing properties as found in Mentadent and Advanced Care Viadent. ADA does not accept dentifrices with this ingredient for reducing plaque and gingivitis.

Mechanical Products for Plaque Control

Good control of plaque is accomplished by mechanical procedures, which include brushing, flossing, and professional prophylaxis. A professional cleaning is recommended at least twice a year to remove plaque and tartar (calculus), both supragingivally and subgingivally.

Brushing

A recent survey of brushing habits in the United States showed that only 60% of the public follow a strict brushing regimen. Clearly, motivation and education are needed in this area. For the average adult, a soft brush with rounded bristles is most efficient in removing plaque from supragingival tooth surfaces (with the exception of the surfaces between the teeth). Most bristles are made of nylon, and the bristle ends are rounded. Subgingival plaque can be removed only to a depth of a few millimeters. For patients with a highly developed gagging reflex, a child's toothbrush is recommended. In addition, these patients sometimes find that placing a small amount of salt on the tongue is helpful in checking the desire to gag.

Studies of toothbrushing methods indicate that thoroughness is more important than technique. In the United States, the most widely used technique is one in which the bristles are directed into the gingival crevice at a 45° angle, and a gentle, jab-jiggle action is used. The motion is elliptical, rather than a back-and-forth scrubbing. Power toothbrushes are of special value for people who have motor coordination problems or difficulty in properly removing plaque by manual brushing. For children, the novelty effect of the powered brush is sometimes of motivational value. Also, a number of studies have shown advantages of 10–15% better plaque removal than manual brushing.

Flossing

Surveys find that only 25% of the population questioned use dental floss regularly. Flossing is essential for removal of plaque from the surfaces between teeth and under the gumline, where the toothbrush does not reach. Because plaque has a propensity to build up in these areas, some dentists feel that flossing is actually more important than brushing. Patients who do not have the manual dexterity to use dental floss can use the various types of dental floss holders or powered interdental cleaners. Dental floss is available in waxed, lightly waxed, and unwaxed varieties. Most dentists feel that lightly waxed and unwaxed types are the most efficient in plaque removal. If the floss shreds or splits during use, this may be a sign of decay between the teeth or a defective filling margin. However, new flosses have been introduced that do not shred and are easier to use. The first of these new flosses was Glide Floss, followed by similar products from Colgate and Oral B.

Disclosing Agents

Disclosing agents are dyes similar to those in food colorings that, when introduced into the oral cavity, color the supragingival plaque and make it easily visible. Various dyes are available in both liquid and tablet form. They are used in the dental office and at home both to increase the patient's awareness of plaque and to demonstrate where self-care has been ineffective in removing plaque.

Toothpastes

The majority of toothpastes advertised as specially formulated to control plaque contain (in addition to fluoride) a foaming agent and a mild abrasive, both of which facilitate plaque removal. However, the only toothpaste accepted by the ADA as possessing an active ingredient with proven ability to prevent or control plaque formation and reduce gingivitis is Colgate Total, with Triclosan as the active ingredient. Toothpastes claiming to be effective against plaque are simply more effective than brushing without any toothpaste because the use of toothpaste motivates people to brush longer and more thoroughly. In fact, it is mainly the mechanical action of brushing that removes plaque.

Toothpastes are effective as vehicles to deliver fluoride and Triclosan to the tooth surface, and although fluoride may have some effect against plaque bacteria and their enzymes, its major effect is to make the tooth surface more resistant to destruction by plaque bacteria. With the exception of Colgate Total, other tooth-pastes are accepted by the ADA for their fluoride content and effectiveness against tooth decay but not for their plaque-and gingivitis-reducing properties.

Other Oral Hygiene Aids

A number of devices aid in the removal of plaque from surfaces between teeth, around bridgework, and in other areas that are difficult to reach. The limitation of many of these devices is that they are effective for control of supragingival plaque but, at best, can remove subgingival plaque only to a depth of few millimeters. Therefore, they are of minimal value against subgingival plaque located deeper within the gingival crevice, as is the case in periodontal disease.

Various oral irrigators on the market remove some loosely attached plaque and particles of debris present around teeth and dental appliances, including braces. Because they are not effective in removing all attached plaque, they are not substitutes for brushing and flossing; rather, they should be used as adjuncts to these procedures. In addition, oral irrigators are limited in their ability to reach subgingival plaque. However, the introduction of subgingival applicator tips allows solutions to be delivered 6–7 mm apically.

Some studies have suggested that irrigators may alter plaque composition by eluting bacterial endotoxins. Patients with severely inflamed gum tissues should be cautioned to use irrigators at low pressures to guard against tissue laceration (if the tissue is severly inflammed), which may aggravate the existing problem.

Tartar (Calculus)-Reducing Products

A number of products, both dentifrices and mouth- rinses, are available for reduction of supragingival calculus (tartar) in dental patients. Calculus reduction has been shown with dentifrices containing pyrophosphates, zinc salts, triclosan, and papain. The incidence of calculus formation ranges from 45 to 66%, with some variation between males and females and different age groups. Although supragingival calculus is not a major etiologic agent for gingivitis or periodontitis, its surface porosity provides an environment for plaque formation. In addition, it serves as a plaque-delivery system by holding plaque against gingival tissues. Although plaque formation has been well correlated with gingivitis and periodontitis, a similar correlation for calculus has not been reported. For this reason, the ADA does not offer an acceptance program for products that reduce calculus formation because this is considered to be a cosmetic issue, rather than an issue of disease. The mechanism of action of the calculus-reducing chemicals is related to the latter's ability to inhibit crystal growth and interrupt the transformation of calcium phosphate (found in foods and saliva) into dental calculus. This effect may occur as follows:

1. The agents complex on the tooth surface to block receptor sites for calcium phosphate that precipitates from saliva and chemically absorbs to initiate calculus formation.
2. This same receptor site blockage also occurs in the calculus matrix as it begins to form.
3. The pyrophosphate complexes combine with free calcium in saliva to inhibit the attachment at the tooth surface (probably a secondary mechanism).

Because these products offset mineralization, there has been concern over demineralization of teeth. All manufacturers have addressed this issue and have reported that this has not been a problem, probably because of the positive effect of fluoride on remineralization of dentin and enamel. Some patients cannot use tartar control toothpastes containing pyrophosphates because they develop tooth sensitivity and sloughing of tissue. These adverse effects have not been reported with nonpyrophosphate-containing tartar control products such as those made by Den-Mat Corporation.

Crest tartar control dentifrice

This dentifrice contains 3.4% tetrasodium pyrophosphate and 1.37% disodium dihydrogen pyrophosphate to reduce calculus. Also, 0.243% sodium fluoride is included for caries reduction and prevention. It was the first calculus-reducing dentifrice introduced into the United States. On the basis of various clinical studies, a reduction of 30–40% can be expected. It has also been shown to significantly reduce the tooth staining seen in some patients who use chlorhexidine.

Crest tartar control mouthrinse

This mouthrinse provides 1.6% ionic pyrophosphate from di sodium and tetrasodium pyrophosphate to act against calculus formation and 0.05% sodium fluoride as a caries-reducing agent. Data on the extent of calculus and caries reduction were not available when this article was written because the product was in test market.

Colgate tartar control dentifrice

This product contains 5% tetrasodium pyrophosphate and a polymeric fatty acid with the company-patented name of Gantrez as the calculus-reducing agents. Also, 0.243% sodium fluoride is included for caries reduction and prevention. On the basis of various clinical studies, a calculus reduction of 35–50% can be expected. It is equal to Crest in terms of calculus reduction, with some clinical studies even suggesting a superiority to Crest.

Colgate tartar control mouthrinse

This mouthrinse contains tetrasodium pyrophosphate and tetrapotassium pyrophosphate, which provide 1% ionic pyrophosphate. It also contains 0.02% fluoride. Calculus reduction has been reported to be 35–40% with twice-a-day rinsing, with no claim made for caries reduction.

Listerine tartar control mouthrinse

This mouthrinse contains 0.09% zinc chloride to reduce calculus and also contains the same ingredients as Listerine mouthrinse.

Rembrandt mouth-refreshing rinse

This product has been shown to reduce tartar due to a formulation of surface-active agents and citroxain, a form of papain.

Targon

This mouthrinse reduces staining due to a formulation of surface-active agents. With the introduction of these products, the practitioner is offered a variety of dosage forms and flavors. If one decides to recommend a calculus-reducing agent, the product selection should be based on the product the patient likes to use best and one that will not diminish his awareness of the importance of plaque control. For example, if he is not already using a mouthrinse, would its introduction de-emphasize the mechanical methods of brushing and flossing as a means of plaque and/or calculus reduction?

Halitosis

Local factors, systemic factors, or a combination of both can cause halitosis. It is estimated that 80% of all mouth odors are caused by local factors within the oral cavity, and these odors are most often associated with caries, gingivitis, and periodontitis. Oral malodors occur because of the action of various microorganisms on proteinaceous substances, such as, exfoliated oral epithelium, salivary proteins, food debris, and blood. Studies have shown that saliva from individuals who are free of dental disease produces malodor less rapidly than saliva from patients with dental disease. It has also been observed that after prolonged periods of decreased salivary flow and abstinence from food and liquid malodors tend to be most severe.

Various oral bacteria produce products that are degraded to a number of compounds, foremost of which are sulfides and mucoproteins. These compounds have been most often associated with oral malodor. Specifically, it appears that oral malodor usually results from the bacterial-mediated degradative processes of methyl mercaptan and hydrogen sulfide in oral air. Ammonia is also produced but does not appear to contribute significantly to halitosis. It has even been suggested that ammonia production may improve the odor of mouth air. Control of halitosis is directed at its etiology. If systemic factors are the problem, a medical consultation is indicated. If local factors are responsible, efforts should be directed toward their elimination. However, for many patients, systemic or local factors cannot be identified. Tongue scraping has been shown to reduce malodor in some patients. Mouthwashes and dentifrices can serve an esthetic function by reducing halitosis. They can accomplish this by masking malodors, acting as antimicrobial agents, or both. There are no ADA-accepted products to reduce halitosis at this time.

Topical Anesthetics

Topical anesthetic agents are selected for their ability to diffuse into the oral mucosa. Because many anesthetics used effectively for nerve block or infiltration do not adequately cross the mucosa, they cannot be used for topical anesthesia. The concentration of anesthetic used for surface application is 2–5%. The rate of onset of topical anesthesia ranges from 2 to 5 min, is of relatively short duration, and has minimal effects deep to the area of application. One exception is a mucosal patch containing 10.4 mg of Lidocaine that gives anesthesia deep into the gingiva after a 5-min application period. Systemic absorption of topical anesthetics applied to the oral mucosa is rapid, and blood levels may approach those seen following injection. Several drugs used as topical anesthetics are not readily soluble in water but are soluble in organic solvents. They are, thus, prepared in alcohol, propylene glycol, polyethylene glycol, volatile oils, and other vehicles suitable for surface application. Their slower absorption rates make them safer for topical use on abraded or lacerated tissue. They produce anesthesia for short periods.

Topical anesthetics are useful to temporarily relieve the pain of ulcers, wounds, and other injured areas. The topical use of anesthetic agents before injection may produce superficial anesthesia. They are also of value in taking impressions or intraoral radiographs in patients with an excessive gag reflex.

Patients who are allergic to parenterally administered local anesthetics will also be allergic to topical application of these agents. In addition, as the agents may be absorbed into the systemic circulation, careless application of excessive amounts can result in signs of systemic toxicity. Symptoms of toxicity should be treated, as they would be for injectable agents. One can minimize the absorption of these agents by limiting the concentration of the drug, the area of application, and the total amount applied. In general, for topical anesthesia, one should use no more than one-fourth to one-half the maximum recommended dosage for injection of the agent. Some topical anesthetic preparations are marketed in spray containers. These containers make it difficult to control the amount of material expelled and to confirm the agent was applied to the desired site. If these agents are applied to the posterior part of the mouth, a patient may inhale enough of the aerosol spray to provoke a toxic reaction. Use of topical anesthetics on the posterior pharynx may alter the swallowing reflex.

Benzodent

This ester-type anesthetic is poorly absorbed. Because it contains benzocaine, which has a low water solubility, it is prepared in a base containing petrolatum and sodium carboxymethylcellulose. Eugenol is included for its antiseptic and anodyne properties. Hydroxyquinoline sulfate is a preservative. This ointment can be directly applied to abraded or ulcerated lesions with minimal systemic effects. It is sometimes used to temporarily relieve denture sores and painful lesions.

Hurricaine

This ester-type anesthetic also contains benzocaine and is prepared in a polyethylene glycol base with flavoring agents added. It is available as a liquid, gel, or spray. The propellant for the spray is A 70.

Butyn

This ester-type anesthetic contains butacaine, with benzyl alcohol as a preservative. It is available as an ointment. The maximum dose is 5 ml of a 4% solution or 200 mg.

Cetacaine

This ester-type anesthetic is a combination of tetracaine HCl (2%), butyl aminobenzoate (2%), and benzocaine (14%). Benzalkonium chloride and cetyl dimethylammonium bromide are included as surface-active agents to facilitate the passage of benzocaine into the mucosal tissues. Tetracaine is rapidly absorbed through biologic membranes and requires no facilitating agents. Because of its high toxicity and absorption, agents containing tetracaine should be used with caution and should not be placed under dentures. Spraying this agent is dangerous because the patient may inhale the aerosol. The maximum amount to be applied is 20 mg or 1 ml of a 2% solution. Cetacaine is available as a liquid, ointment, spray, or gel.

Xylocaine

This amide-type anesthetic contains a lidocaine base in a monoaqueous vehicle. It is available as a 2% viscous product containing lidocaine 2%, sodium carboxymethylcellulose, sodium saccharin, methylparaben, propylparaben, flavors, and purified water. It is also available as a liquid containing 4% methylparaben, sodium hydroxide, and flavoring agents. Another dosage form is a 5% ointment containing lidocaine 5%, polyethylene glycol, propylene glycol, and flavoring. The maximum dose is 300 ml of a 5% liquid form or 15 ml of the 2% viscous preparation.

Dentifrices and Sensitive Teeth

Sometimes a patient will complain of teeth that are hypersensitive to heat and cold. These teeth usually have exposed root surfaces, sometimes with a loss of cementum. Most teeth, when in an ideal position in the mouth, have only the enamel surface exposed to the oral cavity. On occasion, such teeth may even respond with pain to extreme heat or cold. However, in true dentinal hypersensitivity, the response to thermal and tactile changes is more pronounced, sometimes eliciting severe pain. Root surface exposure that allows contact with stimuli may occur because of gingival recession or following periodontal therapy.

Several theories have been advanced to explain the mechanism of dentinal hypersensitivity: innervation of the dentinal tubules, permitting transmission of impulses to the pulp, or the presence of lymph fluid in the dentinal tubules. In the latter case, exposure of dentin results in increased colloidal pressure on the tubules (thereby increasing pressure on the odontoblastic cells). Also proposed is a hydrodynamic mechanism involving the movements of tubular fluid in either direction, which elicits pain in the nerves of the pulp. Although no one theory has been proved, occlusion of the dentinal tubules by various methods brings relief. Various dentifrices are recommended for the treatment of sensitivity, with some success.

The greatest success occurs with dentifrices containing 5% potassium nitrate, and some fluoride-containing dentifrices. Recently, a dentifrice containing potassium nitrate and stannous fluoride has been introduced to treat this problem (Colgate). The primary mechanisms postulated for these dentifrices are that they occlude dentinal tubules, preventing stimuli from the oral cavity from irritating the dental nerve via these tubules. Also, those containing potassium may depolarize nerve fibers resulting in decreased impulse conduction and an associated decrease in pain. For maximum effect, a patient must use only one of these dentifrices for at least a month. If no benefit occurs after a month, a different dentifrice should be recommended or other methods employed. Topical varnishes containing sodium fluoride have also been shown to reduce dentinal hypersensitivity (e.g., Duraphat and Fluor-Protect) as well as reduce root surface caries.

Bleaching Agents

Tooth-bleaching agents can be classified as to whether they are used for external or internal bleaching and whether the procedure is performed in the office by a dentist or at home by a patient. For tooth bleaching, hydrogen peroxide (H_2O_2) is used alone at levels of 30% or at 10–22% levels in a stable gel of carbamide peroxide (urea peroxide) that breaks down to form hydrogen peroxide (3.35% H_xO_2 from 10% carbamide peroxide), urea, ammonia, and carbon dioxide. The FDA has not approved peroxide solutions for use as a home bleach, however.

Internal Bleaching

Internal bleaching produces reliable results when used to eliminate intrinsic stains in dentin caused by blood breakdown products or endodontics or for stains in receded pulp chambers. Internal bleaching is always an in-office procedure.

External Bleaching

External bleaching is indicated for teeth that are disclosed from aging, fluorosis, or staining due to the effects of tetracycline. External bleaching can be applied by the dentist or staff or can be applied by the patient in home-use bleaching. When dentist-administered and home-use bleaching are both used, it is called "*dual bleaching*."

Dentist-applied external bleaching can be done with periodic repetitions of an office-bleaching agent using Superoxol or 30% H_2O_2. An etching gel containing phosphoric acid applied to selected dark areas increases the penetration of the bleach. Light is used to produce heat, which accelerates the bleaching process. External bleaching may need additional treatment every 1–2 years to touch up relapses. Severely stained teeth may require more frequent retreatment. Home bleaching, supervised by the dentist, is done by the patient at home using a custom-made carrier that holds the bleach against the patient's teeth. After the desired result is achieved, overnight use on a periodic basis (1–4x month) can maintain the lightening that has been achieved.

External bleaching is seldom permanent, lasting approximately 1–4 years, after which teeth gradually return to their original color. Usually the younger the patient, the longer the bleaching will last. The more difficult it is to bleach a tooth, the more likely it is to discolor again. Bluish–gray stains seem to reappear more quickly than yellow stains. Because reoccurrence of staining is unpredictable, promises about longevity should not be made. Internal bleaching usually lasts longer than external bleaching.

Whitening Formulas

Whitening of teeth can occur by two mechanisms. One method is mechanical, in which an abrasive is used to remove debris from the tooth. The other method involves either the use of peroxides, which react with water to form free oxygen radicals that help to whiten the teeth or a combination of mechanical and chemical actions. This latter mechanism is found with bleaching agents and is longer lasting than whitening procedures.

XEROSTOMIA

The widely held belief that saliva production significantly decreases with age is not well supported in the literature dealing with this subject. Aging does not appear to play a major role as a single contributing factor in causing xerostomia. However, senior citizens may receive medication that produces the side effect of xerostomia. The aged also develop medical problems that can diminish salivary production. For these reasons, most of the studies of xerostomia have focused on older patients. One study reported a direct correlation between the intake of anticholingergic drugs, sedatives, and hypnotics and xerostomia. Over 400 drugs have been identified as potential reducers of salivary flow by acting on the cholinergic (parasympathetic) system either directly or indirectly. Another study found that the use of drugs producing xerostomia increases with age and, as expected, is highest in institutionalized patients. There are over 30 classifications of prescription and non-prescription medications that can reduce salivary flow.

Other factors that can cause xerostomia are systemic disorders and radiation. These factors must be considered in the differential diagnosis of xerostomia.

Clinical Problems with Xerostomia

Clinical problems associated with reduced salivary flow include difficulty chewing foods, reduced denture retention, recurrent caries, root surface caries, and oral candidiasis (low grade). When any of these conditions are found in a patient, regardless of age, reduced salivary flow should be considered in a differential diagnosis of the problem.

Treatment

Treatment of patients with reduced salivary flow should include the following: (1) drug and dosage changes by the patient's physician in consultation with the patient's dentist; (2) use of artificial saliva in a spray form; (3) use of mouth moisturizers and lip balms; (4) use of sugarless hard candy; (5) frequent sipping of water; (6) use of decaffeinated products; (7) use of pilocarpine (Salagen) 3–5× daily; and (8) inclusion of citrus and pineapple flavors in the diet.

Local Delivery of Antimicrobial Agents

In the past decade, significant research and product innovations have focused the attention of dental practitioners on the concept of the local application of antimicrobials to treat periodontal diseases. Three local delivery agents are now available in the United States, and two additional products are available in other parts of the world. Though the rationale of antimicrobial approaches to treatment is evident, their limitations have also been evident. With systemic therapy, it may be difficult to achieve bacteriostatic or bactericidal antibiotic concentrations in pockets without using doses that evoke systemic side effects. The development of bacterial resistance is also an issue. The rise of antibiotic resistant, disease-producing bacterial strains is currently a major public health concern. Prolonged, repetitive courses of antibiotics for recurring dental infections is discouraged, because such practice can more readily lead to the development of resistance. Preferably, the cause of the infection should be eliminated rather than merely "managed" with antibiotics. Once antibiotic therapy is initiated, however, the importance of compliance with dosage and duration of treatment must be stressed with the patient. With poor patient compliance, under-dosing may occur, which, in turn, can favor the emergence of resistant bacteria.

Controlled Medication Delivery

The limitations of systemic therapy have prompted extensive research for the development of alternative delivery systems. Local, controlled delivery systems are available to release pilocarpine to the eye for a week after single placement for treatment of glaucoma. The oral cavity offers another relatively accessible disease site for localized therapy. In localized therapy for periodontal disease, the concern is the difficulty in reaching deep pockets and sustaining bacteriostatic or bactericidal levels long enough to be effective but not causing the development of resistance.

Tetracycline-containing fibers (Actisite)

The first local delivery product available in the United States, one which has been extensively studied, is an ethylenevinyl acetate copolymer fiber, diameter 0.5 mm, containing tetracycline, 12.7 mg/9 in. When packed into a periodontal pocket, it is well tolerated by oral tissues, and for 10 days, it sustains tetracycline concentrations exceeding 1300 μg/ml, well beyond the 32–64 μg/ml required to inhibit the growth of pathogens isolated from periodontal pockets. In contrast, crevicular fluid concentrations of only 4–8 μg/ml are reported following systemic tetracycline administration, 250 mg, 4× daily for 10 days (total oral dose, 10g). Thus, controlled site-specific tetracycline delivery can achieve a bactericidal effect at approximately 1/1000th of the dose administered systemically.

Studies demonstrate that the tetracycline fibers, applied with or without scaling and root planing, reduce probing depth, bleeding on probing, and periodontal pathogens and provide gains in clinical attachment level. Such effects are significantly better than those attained with scaling and root planing alone or with placebo fibers. The fibers used in conjunction with scaling and root planing have also provided a statistically significant improvement in probing depth reduction and clinical attachment level gains of over 60% and in bleeding on probing reductions over scaling and root planing alone at 6 months after therapy. Actisite was the first local delivery system cleared by the FDA for the adjunctive treatment of recurrent periodontal disease. Although 6-month studies have demonstrated their value, longer-term studies are needed.

Chlorhexidine delivery system (PerioChip)

A newer development in controlled local delivery, one that utilizes the antiseptic chlorhexidine as the antimicrobial agent, has been introduced in a number of countries and was recently cleared by the FDA for use in the United States. This delivery system, Perio-Chip, was developed in Israel and has been tested in the United States as well as in Europe.

The PerioChip is a small chip (4.0 × 5.0 × 0.35 mm) composed of a biodegradable hydrolyzed gelatin matrix into which has been incorporated 2.5 mg chlorhexidine gluconate per chip. It is rounded on one end and inserts easily and in less than a minute into periodontal pockets that are 5 mm or greater in depth. The PerioChip releases chlorhexidine and maintains drug concentrations in the gingival crevicular fluid greater than 100 μg/ml for at least 7 days, concentrations well above the tolerance of most oral bacteria. Because the PerioChip biodegrades in 7–10 days, a second appointment for removal is not needed. Studies with the PerioChip were as long as 9 months. At 9 months, significant decreases were observed in probing depth from baseline favoring the active chip plus scaling and root planing compared with controls (scaling and root planing only): chlorhexidin chip plus scaling and root planing, –0.95 ± 0.05 mm; placebo chip plus scaling and root planing, –0.69 ± 0.05 mm ($p = 0.00056$); scaling and root planing alone –0.65 ± 0.05 mm ($p = 0.00001$). The proportion of pocket sites with a probing depth reduction of 2 mm or more was increased in the chlorhexidine chip group compared with scaling and root planing alone, a difference which was statistically significant on a per patient basis ($p < 0.0001$). Improvements favoring the chlorhexidine chip compared with controls were also observed for clinical attachment levels at 9 months, improvements that were significant when the data were pooled ($p < 0.05$). Bleeding on probing was reduced in the active chip group compared with both controls, differences which were significant in one of the two studies ($p < 0.05$) and when the data were pooled ($p = 0.012$).

The results of these studies suggest that the Perio Chip may be a valuable adjunct to scaling and root planing in the treatment of periodontal disease. This product is easily placed, requires no appointment for removal, and provides reductions in probing depths similar to subgingivally placed antibiotics now available in various countries across the world. In addition, a major advantage of this system is that its active agent is an antiseptic instead of an antibiotic.

Subgingival Delivery of Doxycycline (Atridox)

Atridox is a recently developed gel system that incorporates the antibiotic doxycycline (10%) in a syringeable gel system. An animal study in beagle dogs initially suggested some benefit to locally delivered doxycycline, and it is used in the veterinary population.

A recent 9-month, multicenter study was designed to study the effects of subgingivally placed doxycycline compared to subgingival placement of the vehicle and an herbal agent (Sanguinaria). No scaling or root planing was performed in any of the groups, and there was no untreated group. The patients were instructed in oral hygiene and randomly assigned to one of three groups: vehicle control, 5% sanguinarine in the vehicle control, and 10% doxycycline in the vehicle control.

Treatment with doxycycline was more effective than the other treatments at all time periods, with the exception of the 3-month clinical attachment level value. Also, when the authors evaluated the effect based on initial probing depth, the differential effect in the doxycycline group in comparison with the other two groups was greater as pretreatment probing depth increased. For the doxycycline group, the reduction in clinical attachment level at 9 months showed a gain of 0.4 mm compared to vehicle control, the reduction in probing depth was 0.6 mm greater than vehicle control, and the reduction of bleeding on probing was 0.2 units greater than vehicle control. Although the differences were small, they were statistically significant. The patient's oral hygiene scores (plaque index) averaged between 0.7 and 1.1 in all three groups throughout the study. Although resistance was not evaluated in this study, the local application of doxycycline has previously been reported to show transient increases in resistance in oral microbes and no overgrowth of foreign pathogens.

Data have recently been presented from two multicenter clinical trials. All treatment groups showed clinical improvements from baseline over the 9-month period. The results for all parameters measured were significantly better in the doxycycline group compared with vehicle control and oral hygiene only. Compared with scaling and root planing, the effects of doxycycline on clinical attachment level gain and probing depth reduction were equivalent. Clinical study results suggest a potential periodontal benefit from the subgingival application of doxycycline. However, the value of this agent as an adjunct to scaling and root planing is untested. This product is cleared by the FDA for use in animals and humans.

Host Modulation

In 1998, the first non-antimicrobial drug to treat periodontal disease, Periostat, was approved by the FDA. Nonetheless, in the antibiotic family, the dose of the drug used is too low to kill bacteria. Periostat acts through its effects on inhibition of metalloproteinases, such as, collagenase and gelatinase. The therapeutic objective is to modulate the inflammatory host response. Periostat, available as a 20 mg capsule of doxycycline hyclate, is prescribed for use by patients twice daily. The mechanism of action is by suppression of the activity of collagenase, particularly that produced by polymorphonuclear leukocytes. Although this drug is in the antibiotic family, it does not produce any antimicrobial effects because the dose of 20 mg twice daily is too low to affect bacteria. As a result, resistance to this medication cannot develop. Four double-blind, clinical, multicenter studies in over 650 patients have demonstrated that Periostat improves the effectiveness of professional periodontal care and slows the progression of the disease process.

23

VIRTUAL SCREENING

Identification of viable chemical leads is one of the key tasks of the early stage of drug discovery. Historically, the lead discovery phase was mainly supported by in vivo experiments that usually resulted in compounds with acceptable efficacy and suitable pharmacokinetic profile at least in animal models. On the other hand, however, lead optimization was slow and rarely successful that gave significant role to serendipity. Because in vivo based, purely intuitive approaches yielded hardly predictable results; drug discovery faced a paradigm shift in the early 1980s. Limitations of animal models and the lack of the molecular mechanism were found to be critical factors when analyzing attrition rates that initiated research groups to introduce in vitro tests at the frontline of discovery programs. Application of rational approaches was also facilitated by in vitro screening supplying reliable data-sets for the first time for computer aided drug discovery (CADD) methods. In vitro assays serve the basis of structure- activity relationship that drives medicinal chemistry during active-to-hit and hit-to-lead processes. Dramatic developments in molecular biology, detection methods, computer technology, and robotics made high-through-put in vitro screening (HTS) to be a characteristic tool of lead discovery. In the 1990s, the brut-force HTS was the ultimate technology of lead discovery. Today, however, it became clear that productivity of lead discovery could not be increased by screening more compounds against more targets even in more and more sophisticated assays. In addition to limitations in target validation, assay development, compound and data quality and despite ultra high throughput, the number of available, or ever synthesized compounds is still negligible relative to the drug-like chemistry space. Random screening should, therefore, be replaced by methodologies that combine the capacity of HTS approaches and the rational basis of CADD techniques. Virtual screening (VS) methods exemplify this idea, as high-throughput CADD tools are capable to investigate huge compound collections in reasonable time and cost.

Application of the HTS technology requires the selection of the target, the development of the assay, and the definition of the screening library in a suitable format. In vitro HTS campaigns are then typically performed in a highly automated environment and generates huge amount of data that should be stored, treated, and analyzed. In these contexts, VS techniques can be considered as "*in silico*" analogues of in vitro HTS technologies. After defining the target, VS also requires the development and optimization of the prediction technique (i.e., the in silico analogue of the assay) applied for affinity predictions. Databases that serve as screening library should be preprocessed to use in VS. The screening process itself is performed in the computer memory and should, therefore, be fully automated while generating data similar to HTS data-sets both in quantity and quality. In addition to similarities between the procedures, HTS and VS have a common conceptual framework as well.

Both methods have limited accuracy that is compensated by the number of compounds investigated. VS and HTS, are rather classification techniques that separate actives from inactives, than a method of choice when quantifying biological affinity. These methods could identify candidates rather than validated hits. Some of the promising candidates could never be validated, these are false positives. Both high-throughput technologies surely miss some active compounds that are called "*false negatives.*" Although every reasonable effort should be done to minimize false positive and negative rates, the common philosophy behind these techniques suggest that if we identify even a single interesting compound, then false positives and negatives can be tolerated.

Finally, candidates identified by HTS or VS should be experimentally validated before starting active-to-hit and hit-to-lead processes. The most characteristic difference between HTS and VS is that the former identifies the candidates experimentally, while the latter derives them computationally. The computational strategy applied in VS suggests that: (i) it could be more effective in time, resource, and cost; (ii) it could explore a significantly larger part of the drug-like chemistry space; and (iii) it could yield higher hit rate than random screening. Although these potential advantages suggest VS being more favorable than HTS, comparative studies demonstrated that these approaches are rather complementary than competitive. In one hand, VS techniques could be useful when designing target specific screening libraries. On the other hand, distinct structural classes identified by VS and HTS are clearly the observations that most straightforwardly support complementarities between VS and HTS. While the underlying disciplines of HTS are bioinformatics and biochemistry, VS is based on cheminformatics and computational chemistry.

In fact, there are computational approaches–most of them are CADD methods–already applied in drug discovery that were transformed to VS tools. Similar to CADD techniques VS methods can be divided into ligand-based and structure-based approaches. Ligand-based techniques operate exclusively in the small molecule space using chemical and biological information encoded in known active compounds to identify new candidates with similar properties. Structure-based methods require the three-dimensional structure (3-D) of the target protein that is used for docking small molecules into the binding site. Evaluation of binding modes and protein-ligand interactions finally allows ranking of docked compounds by their binding affinity. This entry summarizes the background of both approaches, gives case studies for supporting practical applications, and collects success stories to demonstrate capabilities.

Data Base Filtering

Physicochemical Filters

One of the early physicochemical filters is the famous rule-of-five (ROF) introduced by Lipinski et al. ROF is based on the distributions of easily accessible and interpretable physicochemical properties obtained from known drugs. Compounds fulfilling ROF do not violate more than one rule out of the followings: molecular weight (MW) < 500, calculated log P (clogP) < 5, number of hydrogen bond acceptors (HBA) < 10, and number of hydrogen bond donors (HBD) < 5. These ranges of properties define a chemistry space containing molecules without serious absorption, distribution, metabolism, and elimination (ADME) problems that are expected to be orally bioavailable. This chemistry space is usually referred as drug-like space and its content is called drug-like molecules. Consequently, drug-likeness of compound libraries (both virtual and physical) can be easily investigated by assessing their members by ROF. In addition to properties included to ROF, Oprea proposed further limitations in features when searching for drug-like molecules. His analysis suggested that the number of rotatable bonds (RB) should be lower than eight while the number of rings ideally smaller than four. Kelder et al. introduced polar surface area (PSA) as a relevant descriptor for predicting oral bioavailability. PSA was defined as the sum of the van der Waals surface of polar atoms including oxygen, nitrogen, and sulfur with attached hydrogens. PSA showed significant impact on membrane penetration including intestinal (PSA < $140A^2$) and blood–brain barrier permeabilities (PSA < $80A^2$). As PSA can be approximated from the 2-D structure, these approaches are now considered as filtering methods for VS of large compound libraries. Although purely statistical approaches are still dominating on this field, Gillet, Willett, and Bradshaw used a genetic algorithm (GA)-based weighting scheme for property and shape descriptors when discriminating between drugs and non-drugs.

The concept of lead-likeness has been established by Hann and Oprea, analyzing lead molecules and corresponding drugs. Comparative studies on leads and drugs revealed that leads are typically less complex molecules than drugs. Consequently, their physicochemical properties should differ significantly from that of the drugs. In fact, effective leads have lower MW and clogP, have a smaller number of rings (RNG), and RB. The original ROF was therefore modified to rule-of-three (ROT: MW < 300, clog P < 3,H-bond donors (HDO) < 3, rotatable bond (RTB) < 3) by Astex reflecting to the reduced complexity of leads. Based on these findings, Leach et al. established a filtering scheme of MW < 350, RTB < 6, number of heavy atoms < 22, HDO < 3, high-activity moleucle (HAC) < 8, clogP < 2.2 when selecting compounds for reduced complexity screening. Surveying medicinal chemistry literature Oprea and coworkers have drawn less strict conclusion, when formulating the criteria of lead-likeness MW < 460, –4 < LogP < 4.2, RTB < 10, RNG <4, HDO < 5, HAC < 9.

As similar to HTS, the basic objective of VS is to identify interesting starting points for medicinal chemistry programs. We believe that lead-likeness would be a useful concept for filtering compound libraries before more sophisticated approaches. Nevertheless, it should be emphasized that limits applied for both drug-like and lead-like compounds are based on statistical analyses of known examples. Although these simple filters demonstrated significant classification accuracy when discriminating drugs and non-drugs, leads and drugs–their fully empirical nature warns against unconditional applications.

Functional Group Filters

Functional group filters are mainly utilized to remove unstable, reactive, toxic, or otherwise unsuitable compounds from compound libraries. The rapid elimination of swill (REOS) method. introduced by Vertex was the first realization of this concept. REOS effectively combines physicochemical filters with a set of functional group filters. Databases are first subjected to property filtering similar to ROF that is followed by checking a set of rules based on the presence of functional groups expected to be problematic. It is important to note that REOS allows the user to customize each functional group filter as well as the set of rules applied.

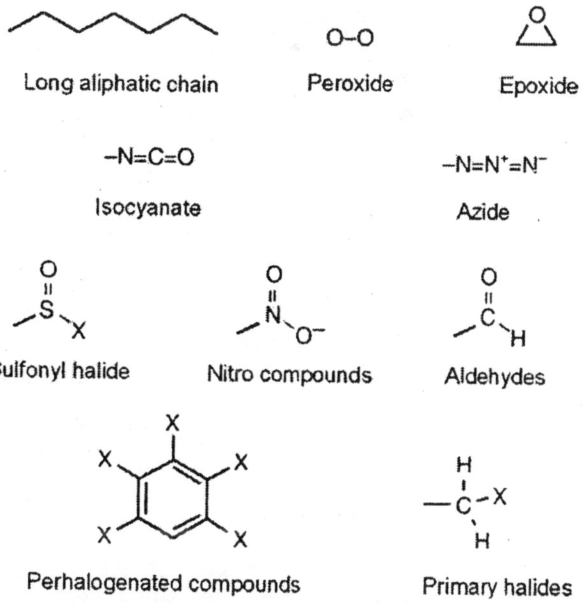

Fig. 23.1. Examples of functionalities filtered out by REOS.

Hann et al. used a similar, multilevel approach when pooling compounds for HTS. These authors applied three types of filters. Basic filters were used to remove molecules with non-drug-like features. Next functional group-based hard filters were utilized comprising filters for reactive functional groups, unsuitable leads (i.e., compounds which would not be initially followed up), and unsuitable natural products (i.e., derivatives of natural product compounds known to interfere with common assay procedures). Finally, soft filters represented by a GA trained to identify unsuitable compounds that the other filters would fail to find. This algorithm scores compounds for drug-likeness, relative to a training set classified by medicinal chemists. Andrews and coworkers used a set of 200 drug molecules to derive a set of "*intrinsic binding energies*" for the 10 functional groups. The inherent binding affinity of compounds was then estimated by summing the intrinsic binding energies and subtracting an entropic factor. Muegge, Heald, and Brittelli described a functional group filter to discriminate between drugs and non-drugs. The authors assigned a score to each molecule that is based on the presence of fragments typically found in drugs. Each non-overlapping drug-like fragment counts one point in this scheme. Molecules with a score between two and seven are classified as drugs, otherwise they are classified as non-drugs. As it was noted that CNS active compounds are relatively small and typically contain only a single pharmacophoric group, they defined a second filter. This filter ensured that compounds containing a single drug-like functional group could only be classified as drugs if they contain one of the distinguished groups.

Topological Filters

It is generally accepted that structural similarity to known drugs significantly increases the drug-like character of compounds. Therefore, molecular topology of known drugs in comparison to non-drugs served as suitable starting point for a number of approaches. One group of methods utilized neural networks for discriminating between drugs and non-drugs. Compounds in drug databases such as World Drug Index (WDI), Comprehensive Medicinal Chemistry (CMC), and MDL Drug Data Report (MDDR) and databases of chemical suppliers (typically Available Chemical Directory; ACD) were represented by structural descriptors. Sadowski and Kubinyi reported the application of Ghoose–Crippen atom types as input neurons, while the output neuron was set to one for drugs and zero for non-drugs when training the net by 5000 WDI and 5000 ACD compounds. The trained net was able to classify about 80% of test compounds.

Murcko and coworkers reported a similar approach based on drugs collected from CMC and non-drugs from ACD. Molecules were represented by 166 binary ISIS keys and the authors added further physicochemical descriptors, including MW, number of HBD and acceptors, number of RBs, aromatic density, clog P, and one additional descriptor reflecting the degree of branching. A Bayesian neural network (BNN) was trained using 3500 molecules from both the CMC and the ACD databases. The trained network was then tested on CMC and ACD compounds that were not included in the training set. A subset of the MDDR library was used for external validation. The classification accuracy of both CMC and ACD approached 90%, while external validation revealed 78% of the MDDR compounds being drug-like.

Frimurer et al. also reported a neural network based approach trained on a larger dataset. These authors partitioned the MDDR database into drug- like (compounds that have progressed to at least Phase I of clinical trials) and lead-like (compounds labeled as "*Biological Testing*") sets. Diversity selection from these sets resulted in 4400 MDDR drug-like compounds (3000 training and 1400 test compounds), and 90,000 ACD compounds (60,000 training and 30,000 test molecules) dissimilar to the drug-like set. The 60,000 lead-like MDDR compounds were used exclusively for external validation. All compounds were represented by 77 CONCORD atom types and three further descriptors including the number of atoms, number of heavy atoms, and total charge. Predictive power of the trained neural network was first assessed in the test set. Using a threshold of 0.15 as a criterion to discriminate between drugs and non-drugs, the neural network was able to classify 88% of the MDDR drug-like set and ACD databases correctly. External validation on lead-like compounds predicted 75% of these molecules as drug-like. Although neural network based methods are extremely fast and successfully identified the majority of known drugs, these models are hardly interpretable for medicinal chemists and, therefore could rather be used as high-throughput filters than driving chemistry to the drug-like space.

Wagener and Geerestein applied recursive partitioning to distinguish of drugs and non-drugs. Analyzing tolerated and non-tolerated functional groups in both WDI and ACD databases the authors were able to recognize almost 75% of drug-like molecules in MDDR and CMC databases.

Limited number of structural frameworks represented in known drugs can also be used for the identification of drug-like compounds. In their pioneering work, Bemis and Murcko analyzed shapes of existing drugs and identified drug-like molecular frameworks. A graph-theoretical approach was used to decompose molecules into fragments. Rings and linkers together form the framework, while acyclic side chains were removed. Based on this analysis, the authors concluded that almost the 50% of known drugs in the CMC could be described by only the most frequent 32 frameworks. The diversity of drug-like side chains was found to be similarly low, only 20 different side chains account for over 70% of all the side chains appeared in CMC.

It is interesting to note that this approach is also useful for designing target-based libraries when the topological framework analysis is applied to active compounds within a target family. One realization of this concept is the retrosynthetic combinatorial analysis procedure (RECAP) algorithm that was also utilized for the analysis of drug-like fragments. RECAP first identifies active or drug-like fragments using retrosynthetic analysis applying any of the 11-retrosynthetic reactions defined. In the next step, the resulting fragments are usually clustered and transformed into monomers that can be used for designing targeted libraries. As fragments were extracted from known actives, it is expected that compounds enumerated from the derived monomers will be also active and are synthetically accessible because of the retrosynthetic approach applied. A similar method, TOPology-Assigning System (TOPAS) has been reported by Schneider et al. These authors developed an evolutionary algorithm for fragment-based de novo design. This stochastic method utilizes a set of ~25,000 fragments that serves as building blocks obtained by a rule-based fragmentation procedure applied to 36,000 known drugs.

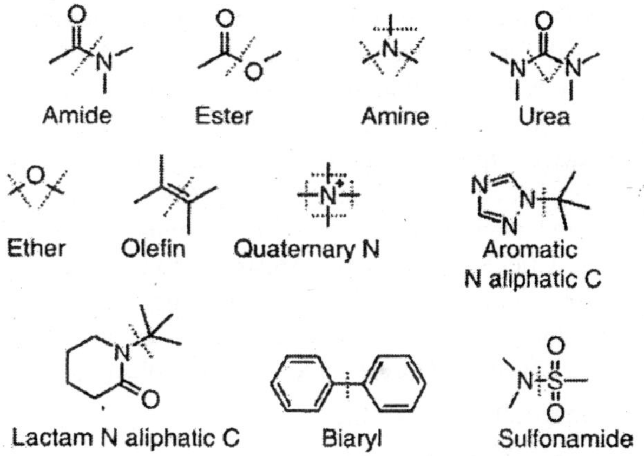

Amide Ester Amine Urea

Ether Olefin Quaternary N Aromatic N aliphatic C

Lactam N aliphatic C Biaryl Sulfonamide

Fig. 23.2. Retrosynthetic reactions defined in RECAP.

Ligand-based Screening

Similarity Searches

Similarity searching is one of the simplest methodologies of ligand-based VS, when screening databases against a query using chemical similarity principles. During a similarity search, the query molecule is compared to members of the database and a similarity measure is calculated quantifying the similarity between the query and each molecule in the screened database. For 2-D similarity searches, the query structure and members of the screened database are typically represented by molecular fingerprints that encode molecular structure and properties in binary format. Each bit of the fingerprint detects the presence or absence of molecular fragments or connectivity pattern, can encode descriptor value ranges or binary transformed descriptors. Fingerprints can be divided into two major groups: structural keys and hashed fingerprints. Structural keys associate a specific descriptor (structural fragment or property) with each bit, while hashed fingerprints assign overlapping bit segments to descriptors.

Generation of structural keys requires a predefined fragment library that collects the fragments searched in each molecule of the database. MACCS key (MDL Information Systems) is a typical example for a structural key. In contrast, there is no fragment library needed for hashed fingerprints. These fingerprints are derived algorithmically from all possible linear paths of the limited number of connected atoms. Paths define a pattern of atoms and bonds that are used to generate a set of bits during the hashing procedure that typically produces 4–5 bits per pattern. Although hashed fingerprints are not physically interpretable, they show highly characteristic bit patterns for molecules. Bit strings vary in length and complexity but Daylight and UNITY are the most popular hashed fingerprints used in similarity searches.

Analysis of molecular similarity is based on the quantitative determination of the overlap between fingerprints of the query structure and all database members. As descriptors of a given molecule can be considered as a vector of real or binary attributes, most of the similarity measures are derived as vectorial distances. Tanimoto and Cosine coefficients are the most popular measures of similarity In addition to binary descriptors, molecular holograms are also useful for similarity searches. Similar to fingerprint, hologram is a vector that contains numerical properties, e.g., number of occurrences for atoms or fragments.

3-D similarity searches utilize 3-D information including shape, steric, and electrostatic properties obtained for the query molecule and the database screened. High-throughput molecular alignment techniques of this kind superpose all database entries onto the query molecule. FlexS, one of the most popular approaches, keeps the query rigid and considers test molecules as flexible when offering several alternative superpositions–each scored and ranked by similarity. Genetic algorithm similarity program (GASP) is a superposition tool using GA that handles both the query and the test molecules as flexible. Wild and coworkers described an alignment tool utilizing GA-based fitting of molecular electrostatic potential fields. In MIMIC, Mestres, Rohrer, and Maggiora represented molecules as sets of Gaussian functions, modeling property fields. Alignment is optimized and scored assessing the overlap between corresponding fields. Rapid overlay of chemical structures (ROCS) performs a shape-based superposition using a Gaussian representation of the molecular volume and allows to combine 2-D and 3-D similarity.

Pharmacophore Searches

Pharmacophore mapping

Pharmacophore is an arrangement of steric and electrostatic features in the 3-D space that are crucial for the biological action. These kinds of feature- based pharmacophore models were found to be useful for ligand-based VS because they can effectively fish very different chemotypes from virtual libraries. Pharmacophore models usually consist of a number of pharmacophore points including a group of atoms, or features such as HBDs and HBAs, charged groups, hydrophobic centers, and corresponding geometric constraints. Pharmacophore features can be derived from both the structure of the target protein or from the collection of known ligands.

Structure-based pharmacophores are typically explored by analyzing binding site interactions formed between ligands and protein atoms within the active site of the target. In addition to direct structural information, site directed mutagenesis data are also useful when identifying most important residues responsible for ligand binding. LigandScout uses ligand-bound target structures to extract structure-based pharmacophore models. Hydrogen bonding features, as well as electrostatic and hydrophobic interactions, are utilized to derive the most important interactions within the active site. Starting from the protein structure, LUDI generates interaction sites that are preferable to occupy for ligand atoms. This methodology is the basis of the structure-based focusing (SBF) technique available in Cerius2. The identification of the interaction sites by LUDI is followed by the clustering of interaction vectors. The obtained clusters are the starting point for generating the pharmacophore hypothesis. POCKET realizes a similar approach to LUDI when identifying grids within the active site to characterize favorable ligand interactions. Considering the flexibility of the active site, Carlson et al. suggested a molecular dynamics approach when generating a diverse set of protein conformations to develop structure-based pharmacophore models. Reflecting to multiple potential binding modes, geometric constraints between pharmacophoric points are here defined as ranges rather than values. Pharmacophore constraints can include not only distance, angles, and dihedrals, but also excluded volumes; surface volumes and spatial restraints might also be used in the UNITY program. Molecular Operating Environment (MOE) also allows queries containing locations of features, chemical groups, or shape constraints.

In the absence of structural information on the target, pharmacophore could be developed using a set of actives that are expected to realize similar binding modes when interacting with the target. Ligand-based pharmacophore generation that is also called as pharmacophore mapping usually consists of three elementary steps. In the first step, the pharmacophore features, common in all of the actives, are identified. The second step involves the generation of putative bioactive conformations that might be explored by the actives. Finally, alignments of these conformations are prepared that ensure matches of pharmacophore features. Identification of possible bioactive conformations is clearly the greatest challenge in pharmacophore mapping. There are two basic strategies to achieve this goal. The first one generates only low energy conformations for all of the actives and then searches for common features. The other one, however, enumerates all possible conformations of each ligand and evaluates the orientation of pharmacophore features previously identified.

Although pharmacophore mapping can be completed manually in simple and straightforward cases, most of the applications require the automated generation of pharmacophore. There are several software suites available for this purpose. HipHop and HypoGen are both featured by the Catalyst package. In Catalyst, the random search algorithm used for the identification of low energy conformers is conducted with a pooling function that allows the in-depth coverage of the conformational space. Features are then identified by analyzing the surface accessibility of the actives followed by the definition of the pharmacophore using the absolute coordinates of all conformations. HipHop is useful to generate qualitative hypotheses, while HypoGen is the method of choice for more predictive quantitative models. The initial model is based on the features of the two most active molecules that serve as a starting point to generate all the possible pharmacophores. Models are then evaluated by analyzing the overlay between the pharmacophore hypotheses and the geometric arrangement of features in all conformations of the actives.

For quantitative models, Catalyst assigns weight descriptors to each feature that correspond to its importance in explaining the biological activity. Disco and Disco-Tech, both characterize actives by ligand and site points. Ligand points include HBDs and HBAs, and hydrophobic and charged features. Site points are generated on the basis of complementarity principles using the atomic coordinates of the corresponding ligand atom. Similarly to the Catalyst approach, a set of low energy conformers is first generated that are aligned as rigid objects. Alignment of the conformers represented by interfeature distances to a reference molecule having the fewest conformation is carried-out by a click detection algorithm. Disco produces a ranked list of hypotheses that contains all of the common features identified in actives. Alignment parameters calculated by Disco drive the users to select good quality pharmacophore maps. In GASP, the conformational analysis of actives takes place on the fly that is followed by the assignment of pharmacophore features including both the ligand points and site points. The molecule with the least number of features serves as reference.

The alignment procedure is carried out by a GA utilizing chromosomes that encode dihedrals of RBs in all actives and mapping of the reference's pharmacophore features to other actives. The fitness function generates conformations for each active that are then fitted to the reference using the mapping information. The best possible overlay is achieved by calculating the internal van der Waals energy of each molecule, the number, and similarity of the overlaid features in combination of the volume integral of the overlay.

Pharmacophore search

The pharmacophore model obtained by the mapping procedure allows 3-D database searching. Database searching can identify actives in different chemotypes relative to those utilized for pharmacophore generation. This procedure is often termed as scaffold hopping or lead hopping that is not limited to lead discovery programs but might contribute to back-up/follow-up strategies.

Pharmacophore searches are usually realized in two steps. Search algorithms first check the availability of pharmacophore features encoded in the query and next they evaluate the overlay of the spatial arrangement of features and the query. The fastest way of the second step is matching database entries as rigid objects. As flexible molecules can adopt a number of different low energy conformations, this set of conformers should be precomputed before screening. Another option for rigid searches is the on the fly generation of conformers that is followed by the subsequent structural alignment. Conformational flexibility is more explicitly considered in flexible 3-D searches that, however, require significantly higher resources. Pharmacophore queries that include constraint ranges could partially compensate conformational changes occurring upon ligand binding. There are a number of codes available for database searching. 3D-SEARCH divides the searches into two parts, a fast pre-screen using an inverted key system and a slower atom-by-atom geometric search using the Ullman algorithm. Features to handle angle/dihedral constraints and to take into account "excluded volume" are implemented as part of the geometric search. Catalyst utilizes both multiconformer databases and the on the fly conformer generation. ChemDBS-3D generates low energy conformers that are filtered by conformational rules. Root mean square (RMS) deviation from the pharmacophore constraint can be minimized by torsional minimization. The flexible 3-D search available in UNITY realizes this concept based on the Directed Tweak algorithm that could match the constraints of the query. A recent review by Langer and Wolber compares these technologies when used for pharmacophore searches.

Case Study: Ligand-Based VS against Kv1.5 Potassium Channel

Peukert et al. reported VS experiments using different ligand-based techniques against the voltage-dependent potassium channel Kv1.5. In their first attempt, the authors utilized similarity searching to identify new actives. A potent indane derivative first published by Eli Lilly was used as a query in a 2-D similarity search performed in UNITY. Compounds in the corporate collection were represented by 2-D UNITY fingerprint and the fingerprint of the query was compared to that of the library members. Compounds with Tanimoto coefficient larger than 0.8 were considered to be similar and was subjected to biological testing. This protocol led to the identification of a structurally novel hit with moderate potency (9.5 μM) and limited chemical stability. Suboptimal physicochemical properties and stability prompted the authors to replace the central naphthalene moiety that resulted in the discovery of a good

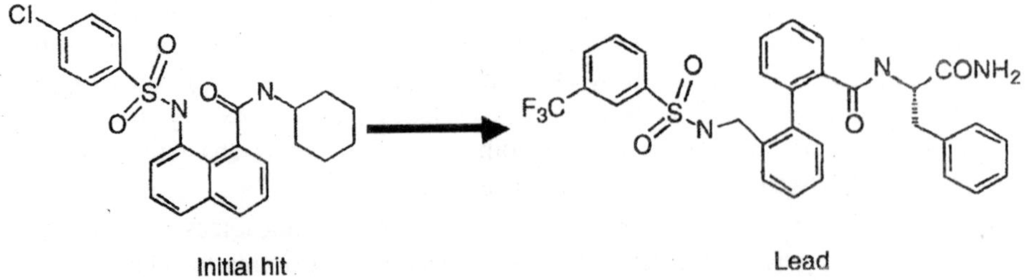

Initial hit

Lead

Fig. 23.3. The initial hit from similarity searching was converted a viable lead.

quality lead with improved potency (4.8 μM). Optimization of this lead was supported by solid phase parallel synthesis that enabled the authors to identify a set of highly potent and selective Kv1 .5 potassium channel blockers.

Structure-activity information gained for this compound series and also that obtained in a parallel lead optimization program allowed the development of a pharmacophore model for Kv1.5 potassium channel blockers. Seven potent molecules from each series were used to derive the model that consists of three hydrophobic centers in a triangular arrangement. The seven compounds were first subjected to an exhaustive conformational search utilizing the Monte Carlo (MC) Multiple Minimum algorithm as available in MacroModel. The resulting conformers were then clustered using distances between the potential pharmacophore features. A minimum energy conformation in each of the clusters was used as input to DISCO algorithm. DISCO models were visually inspected and one of them was used as a 3-D query in the subsequent UNITY 3-D flexible search.

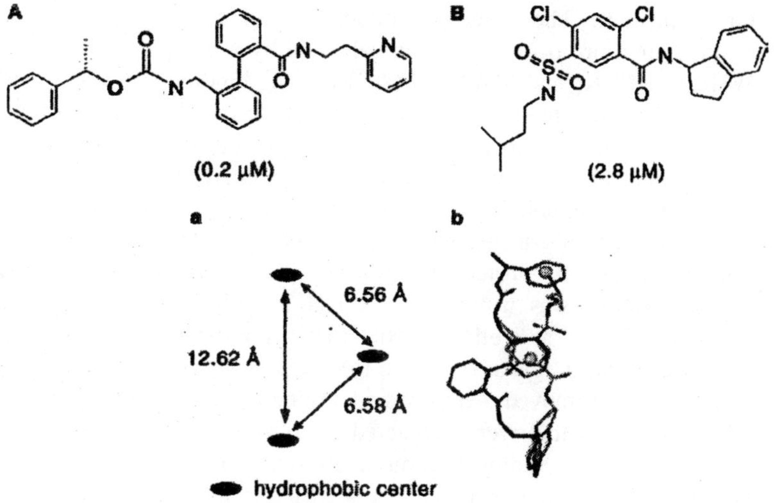

Fig. 23.4. Definition of the pharmacophore query for the Kv1.5 channel.

The performance of this ligand-based VS tool was first evaluated against an in-house set of known Kv1.5 potassium channel blockers. This test revealed that the methodology was able to retrieve 58% of known actives. VS was performed on the Aventis compound collection and identified 4234 virtual hits that were first subjected to filtering. Compounds with reactive or non-tolerated features regarding the Kv1.5 potassium channel inhibitory activity, with non-drug-like character, as well as known blockers were removed during this process. The final set of 1975 compounds was submitted to hierarchical clustering that resulted in 27 clusters in total. Representatives of the available 18 clusters were tested against Kv1.5 potassium channel that identified one structurally novel compound with an IC_{50} of 5.6 μM. This hit was considered as a starting point for optimization that led to the identification of a series of compounds with remarkable activity (best IC_{50} was found to be 0.5 μM) and acceptable pharmacokinetics.

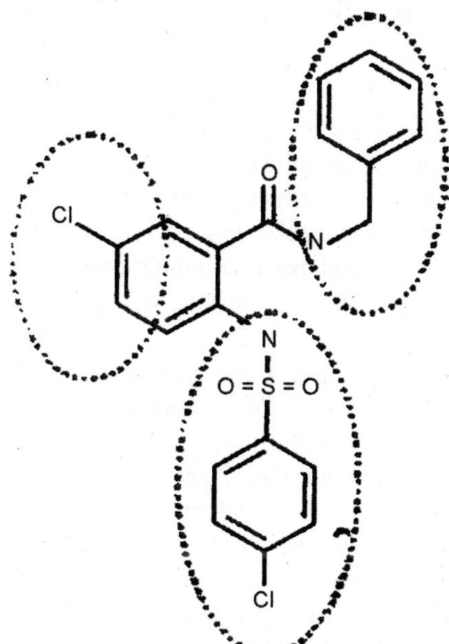

Fig. 23.5. The structurally novel lead identified by the pharmacophore search.

In the final round, the authors reported the development of a structure-based pharmacophore that was also used for VS. To achieve this goal, a homology model of the Kv1.5 potassium channel has been developed. The pore domain of the target protein was built using the crystal structure of the bacterial KcsA channel. A single subunit of the Kv1.5 channel was generated by the COMPOSER program as implemented to SYBYL software that was used to create the tetrameric structure arrangement of the target protein. The resulting model was then subjected to structural refinement using a two-step minimization protocol and it was validated by a number of protein analysis tools including PROCHECK, WHATCHECK, and MATCHMAKER. The binding site was identified by applying geometrical criteria on the validated model using the putative active site for spheres (PASS) algorithm. Visual inspection of PASS results led to the selection of a binding site that has been further characterized by the GRID force field. Pharmacophore features were derived by the calculation of molecular interaction fields using the hydrophobic, the amide nitrogen, and the carbonyl oxygen probes. Local minima of the fields were visually inspected and the selected minima of GRID energy maps in addition to the exclusion volume defined by protein atoms were used to define the pharmacophore query. This structure-based pharmacophore was utilized for a UNITY Flexsearch-based VS that resulted in 3102 hits in total. Drug-like filters, as well as partial match constraints (at least 3 out of the 12 features), were applied. Compounds with reactive or non-tolerated features regarding the Kv1 .5 potassium channel inhibitory activity were removed. After visual inspection of the hits by medicinal chemists, the authors identified 244 compounds that were subjected to in vitro screening. Biological evaluation of the hits revealed 19 actives in total including 5 compounds with an inhibition concentration (IC_{50}) under 10 μM, while the best compound having an IC_{50} of 9 μM. As all of the ligand-based efforts described in these papers were carried out on the same screening library (i.e. the Aventis compound repository), hit rates of different approaches could directly be compared.

Based on this comparison, one can conclude that pharmacophore search–both with ligand-and structure- based pharmacophores–outperformed 2-D similarity search. Although the two latter techniques gave similarly good result in hit rate, the authors found no overlap between their hit lists. Comparing the number of chemical series identified it is clear that screening by the structure-based pharmacophore hypothesis outperformed the ligand-based approaches. It should be noted, however, that the effectiveness of different VS protocols obviously depends on the target and the quantity and quality of structural and structure-activity relationship (SAR) information actually available. The multiple chemotypes identified by different strategies suggest the usefulness of parallel VS programs against the same target but with different approaches.

Structure-based VS

The functions of drug molecules and protein targets are regulated by the principles of molecular recognition. The rational drug development requires the understanding of molecular recognition in terms of structure and energetics. Structure-based VS tools study the binding between the ligand and protein structures with respect to structural and energetic considerations. In the earlier era of the structure-based drug discovery process, the low resolution of protein structures and poor computational power hindered the rapid improvement of the method. Today, these techniques have experienced a comeback because drastic changes occurred.

Genomics have resulted in a huge number of potential therapeutic targets that are available for investigation. However, learning the sequence of a genome is a long way from understanding its biological function. Predictions of protein function can be attempted from the knowledge of the structure alone or other additional information can be used to gain information about functional predictions. In many respects, it is still early days for seeing the fruits of this process in the products offered on the market by pharmaceutical companies. Therefore, there are still large investments in functional genomics, HTS methodologies, combinatorial chemistry, predictive ADME methods, and structural biology.

VS, and structure-based VS, has emerged as an inexpensive and straightforward method for identifying lead molecules. The investments in structural biology prompted the improvement of structure-based VS. Structure-based VS involves explicit molecular docking of each ligand into the active site of the target protein. Hereby, a predicted binding mode is produced, and then the quality of the fit of the molecule in the active site is scored. This scoring information is used to rank the compounds and only the top solutions can be investigated further. Without the need of completeness, we discuss the most state-of-the art structure-based VS that are generally used at pharmaceutical industries during the drug discovery process. Our attempt was also to give a picturesque overview on the structure-based VS process and show its effectiveness or its failures through a case study and some success stories during the CADD processes.

Preparation of Protein Structures

The first step in the structure-based VS process is to obtain the coordinates of a protein. Generally, structures solved by X-ray crystallography or nuclear magnetic resonance (NMR) are used, but protein structures, which have difficulties in the crystallization process e.g., membrane proteins such as G-protein coupled receptors (GPCR) can be modeled based on homology. Currently, 3-D structure information can be generated for up to ~56 % of all the known proteins. However, there is considerable controversy concerning the real value of homology models for structure-based VS. Recently published results on ligand-supported homology modeling might be able to provide reasonable quality homology models that are suitable for structure-based VS.

The definition of the active site is needed for docking into a target protein because scanning the entire surface of the protein would hardly be feasible with most of the currently used docking algorithms. On the other hand, ignoring biochemical information or structural data on the active site is unreasonable, although, in some cases information about binding sites is not available. These cases-binding sites can be identified by algorithms detecting geometric cavities, or algorithms based on physicochemical and geometrical characterization. The preparation of the active site depends on the docking tools being used. This step involves the addition of hydrogen atoms avoiding atomic clashes; assignment of appropriate protonation states of titratable residues and correct tautomers of histidine residues, and involvement of structural water molecules in the binding cavity. The conformational flexibility in the active site has to be evaluated. Commonly used docking methods, however, are able to consider the flexibility to a limited extent. Therefore, the selection of the target structure is a crucial point in the docking procedure, so target-binding sites should be as representative as possible, mimicking a real and general binding conformation.

Docking Algorithms

In spite of the fact that only a specified part of the target protein is considered during the docking procedures, the representation of atomic coordinates is not a practical choice. Thus geometric space descriptors alone or combined with physicochemical descriptors, sphere images and interaction points/surfaces are commonly used instead. Otherwise, a complete representation of ligands in atomic coordinates is definitely feasible. The central problem in ligand handling is the flexibility. Two generally used strategies can be applied: whole molecule and fragment-based methods. Earlier rigid docking, when the whole molecules are docked, was commonly used. An extension of rigid body docking is the incorporation of conformational flexibility. Historically, the DOCK algorithm addressed rigid body docking using a geometric matching algorithm to superimpose the ligand onto a negative image of the binding pocket. Important features that improved the algorithm's ability to find the lowest energy-binding mode, including force field-based scoring, on the fly optimization, an improved matching algorithm for rigid body docking, and an algorithm for flexible ligand docking, have been added over the years. This multiconformer docking can be an effective tool, however, for flexible molecules that have significantly higher number of conformers it may not be straightforward. Fragment-based methods provide an alternative solution for the docking problem; molecules are dissected into fragments that can be docked individually, either separately or incrementally. Now there is a driving force to treat protein flexible because ligands requiring larger conformational changes in the active site upon binding cannot be placed correctly by these methods. The degree of the applied flexibility varies in a wide range. Small adjustments of rigid structures, explicit side chain flexibility, or the use of protein ensembles are very popular methods, however, the full consideration of flexibility still remains as the domain of the molecular dynamical simulations.

Systematic methods

These kinds of algorithms make an attempt to explore all the degrees of freedom but face the problem of combinatorial explosion:

$$N_{\text{conformations}} = \prod_{i=1}^{N} \prod_{j=1}^{n_{increment}} \frac{360}{\theta_{i,j}}$$

$\theta_{i,j}$-the size of incremental rotational angle j for bond i

N-the number of rotatable bonds

Thus ligands are often incrementally built within the active site. The principle of the FlexX algorithm is that, physicochemical properties provide the most useful information for ligand placement. Once a set of favorable placement of the base fragment (the core part of the ligand from where the incremental construction starts) has been computed, the ligand building can be started. The incremental construction is formulated as a tree search problem. As the search tree grows exponentially, a complete search is definitely not feasible to calculate. Instead the binding energy values, approximated by the scores, which are represented by the interior nodes, can be used to guide the search. Conversely, DOCK 4.0 algorithm divides ligands into rigid (core fragment) and flexible parts (side chains); the core parts are docked prior to the flexible parts. The steric complementarity is the guideline during the ligand construction. Another method of systematic search is the use of databases of pregenerated conformations. Conformations are calculated once and the search problem is reduced to a rigid body docking procedure. This is the main concept of FLOG docking program.

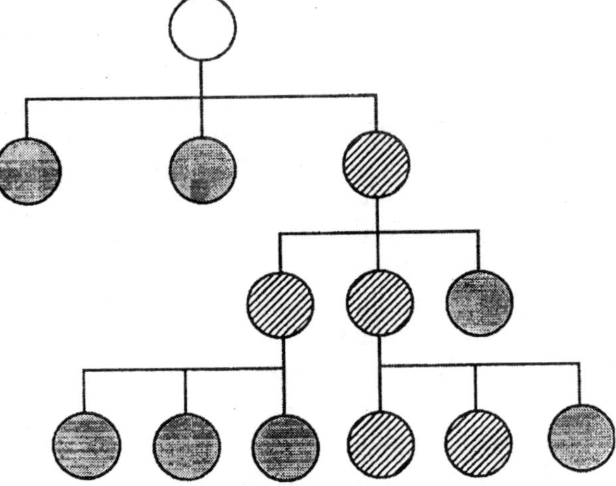

Fig. 23.6. The schematic representation of the search tree. Red nodes indicate energetically unfavorable conformations during the ligand building.

Random or stochastic methods (MC, GA, and tabu search)

The most widely used random approaches are the MC, genetic, and tabu search algorithms. MC algorithms generate initial random conformations of a ligand in the binding cavity then calculate scores for these initial configurations. The generation and scoring of configurations are repeated until the Metropolis criterion, which is used to determine whether the new configuration is retained. According to the Metropolis criterion, the new solution is accepted if the score of the new configuration (E_{new}) is better than the older one's (E_{old}). If the configuration is not a new minimum, it has to pass the Boltzmann-based probability function test, otherwise the solution is rejected.

$$P = \exp\left[\frac{-(E_{new} - E_{old})}{kT}\right]$$

P - probability for the acceptance of the new configuration

Internal coordinated mechanics (ICM) uses global MC minimization docking procedure, describes both the relative positions of two molecules and their conformations by a uniform set of internal variables and uses a pre-calculated grid of interaction energy values to speed up the computation. GAs form a class of computational problem solving methods adapting the main principles of biological competition and population dynamics. GAs are stochastic optimization methods; the problem is encoded generally in the language of genetics.

Initially, a random population is generated that composes a set of the potential solutions for a given problem. The members of the population are represented by chromosomes; the genes correspond to certain variables. When docking into protein structures, the variables for translation, rotation, and torsion angles are encoded in the chromosome. Then genetic operators (crossing over and mutation) are applied for the generation of new populations. The members of the new population are decoded and the estimation of the binding free energy is evaluated. The generation of new populations is terminated when a fixed number of population generation or a given score is reached. A prominent example for the GA using docking algorithms is the genetic optimization for ligand docking (GOLD) program. Its special characteristic is the direct encoding of H-bonding motifs. The latest version of AutoDock uses a Lamarckian GA, which is a combination of a traditional GA with local search method to perform energy minimization.

Besides MC and GA methods, further heuristic algorithms have been developed for the docking problem. Tabu search was found to perform well and provided a straightforward searching strategy of the PRO_LEADS program. This method operates on randomly generated positions and these positions are examined on the basis of the tabu list. This latter list contains pregenerated solutions and provides restriction on the search process. A random move of the ligand is "tabu" if it generates a solution that is not sufficiently different from the stored ones, unless its energy is more favorable, therefore, the revision of the search space is avoided.

Simulation methods (molecular dynamics and energy minimization)

Molecular dynamics simulation methods are currently the most popular approaches. This method is for the analysis of protein flexibility and dynamic properties of molecular systems. With respect to docking, these simulations could provide a realistic view of the docking process, however, these calculations are still out of reach. Therefore, dynamical simulations during the docking process are limited to the protein-ligand complexes. Molecular dynamical simulations are often unable to cross high-energy barriers as well, so an attempt is generally made to simulate different parts of a complex at different temperatures or molecular dynamical simulations can be started from different starting ligand positions. In contrast to molecular dynamical studies, energy minimization methods are rarely used as search techniques but often complement other methods such as MC methods. DOCK performs an energy minimization step after fragment addition, followed by a final minimization step before scoring.

Scoring Functions

The interaction between protein and ligand is a reversible equilibrium reaction. The quantity to characterize this reaction is the free energy of binding. Binding free energy values with reasonable accuracy can only be calculated requiring large computational resources. For scoring thousands of ligands, functions to estimate the binding free energy must be computed fast and without much computational power. Generally used scoring functions estimate the binding free energy for only one position/ conformation, and all of them share the assumption that the full energy term can be decomposed into a sum of terms.

However, the free energy of binding is a state function so, in a strict physical sense, additivity is not allowed. These scoring functions at low computational cost are suitable for the calculation of an estimation of the binding free energy. Three main classes can be separated: force field-based methods, empirical methods, and knowledge-based methods.

All fast scoring functions share several deficiencies. First of all most of them are fitted to or derived from some kind of experimental data. Consequently, the functions reflect the accuracy of these measurements. Molecular size can influence the scores as well, generally the larger the molecule the better the score is, however biological measurements do not support this observation. As scoring functions are derived from X-ray structures, only the favorable interactions are rewarded but unfavorable interactions are not penalized because information from the crystal structures cannot be obtained. Uncertainties in the protonation states and the involvement of water in ligand binding further complicate scoring. Some of the failures can be corrected using consensus-scoring schemes, when the disadvantages and advantages of the various scores might provide a combination, which is able to describe the main characteristics of the protein-ligand binding.

Force field-based scoring functions

The force field is a function expressing the energy of a system as a sum of e.g., diverse molecular mechanics terms. Non-bonded energy terms of molecular mechanics force fields were first used to score protein-ligand complexes. The binding energy between a ligand and a protein is most often estimated by the summation of the electrostatic and van der Waals energy terms. Standard force field scoring functions have major limitations because they were developed to model enthalpic gas phase contributions to structure and energetics, and do not involve solvation and entropic terms either. These scoring functions are restrained by the fact that in VS, significant steric clashes cannot be avoided because the energy terms have steep form at short interatomic distances, the Lennard- Jones potentials used for modeling van der Waals interactions can lead to very strong repulsion, therefore, these terms are often scaled down. Recently developed scoring functions contain entropy terms to increase the potential of specific molecular recognition, H-bonding are often designed in different ways. Below, two generally applied scoring functions are detailed in terms of use.

The GOLD score (G-score) is based on the work of Jones et al. and concentrates on H-bonding interactions. The H-bonding term contains desolvation of donors and acceptors. A pairwise dispersion term involves the contribution of hydrophobic interactions and a molecular mechanical equation is used to calculate the internal energy of the ligand. Therefore, this scoring function performs well when polar interactions are dominant and has difficulty with ligands that are primarily non-polar in nature.

Gold Score

Protein-ligand:

$$E_{vdW} + E_{\text{H-bond}} = \sum_{\text{protein}} \sum_{\text{ligand}} \left[\left(\frac{A_{ij}}{d_{ij}^{8}} - \frac{B_{ij}}{d_{ij}^{4}} \right) + \left(E_{da} + E_{ww} \right) - \left(E_{dw} + E_{aw} \right) \right]$$

Internal-ligand:

$$E_{vdW} + E_{\text{torsion}} = \sum_{\text{ligand}} \left(\frac{C_{ij}}{d_{ij}^{12}} - \frac{D_{ij}}{d_{ij}^{6}} \right) + \sum_{\text{ligand}} \frac{1}{2} V \left[1 + \frac{n}{|n|} \cos(|n|\omega) \right]$$

where A_{ij}, B_{ij}, C_{ij}, and D_{ij} are van der Waals parameters for atoms i and j, and d_{ij} is the interatomic distance. E_{da}, E_{ww}, E_{dw}, E_{aw} are the donor–acceptor individual energy values, V is the torsional barrier, $|n|$ is the periodicity, ω the torsion angle.

GOLD score is the original GOLD scoring function implemented in GOLD docking program package. An optional H-bonding energy term can be added.

Protein-ligand:

$$E_{vdW} + E_{\text{electrostatic}} = \sum_{\text{protein}}\sum_{\text{ligand}}\left[\left(\frac{A_{ij}}{d_{ij}^{a}} - \frac{B_{ij}}{d_{ij}^{b}}\right) + 332\frac{q_i q_j}{\varepsilon(d_{ij})d_{ij}}\right]$$

Internal-ligand:

$$E_{vdW} + E_{\text{electrostatic}} = \sum_{\text{ligand}}\left[\left(\frac{A_{ij}}{d_{ij}^{a}} - \frac{B_{ij}}{d_{ij}^{b}}\right)\right] + 332\frac{q_i q_j}{\varepsilon(d_{ij})d_{ij}} + E_{\text{H-bond(optional)}}$$

where q_i and q_j are atomic partial charges and $\varepsilon(d_{ij})$ is a dielectric function.

Dock score (D-score) considers both electrostatic and hydrophobic contributions to the binding energy but entropic terms. A distance dependent dielectric attenuates polar interactions.

Protein-ligand:

$$E_{vdW} + E_{\text{electrostatic}} = \sum_{\text{protein}}\sum_{\text{ligand}}\left[\left(\frac{A_{ij}}{d_{ij}^{12}} - \frac{B_{ij}}{d_{ij}^{6}}\right) + 332\frac{q_i q_j}{\varepsilon(d_{ij})d_{ij}}\right]$$

$\varepsilon(d_{ij})$ - a distance-dependent dielectric function

The scoring function implemented in DOCK Version 4.0:

Protein-ligand:

$$E_{vdW} + E_{\text{electrostatic}} = \sum_{\text{protein}}\sum_{\text{ligand}}\left[\left(\frac{A_{ij}}{d_{ij}^{a}} - \frac{B_{ij}}{d_{ij}^{b}}\right) + 332\frac{q_i q_j}{\varepsilon(d_{ij})d_{ij}}\right]$$

Empirical scoring functions

Empirical type functions form the second group of the scoring functions. The binding energy is approximated by a weighted sum of explicit hydrogen bonding and hydrophobic contact terms. Many additional terms and different functional forms are used for the scoring. Some functions describe H-bonds with, e.g., distance terms while others penalize angular deviation from the idealized values. The binding free energy can be estimated as: $\Delta G_{\text{bind}} \cong \sum \Delta G_i f_i$, where f_i corresponds to a weighting factor and ΔG_i represents an interaction term. The weighting factors are obtained from regression analysis using experimentally determined binding energies and 3-D structural information. The appeal of empirical scoring functions is that their terms can be simple to evaluate but they are based on approximations similar to force field functions.

The disadvantage of this class of scoring functions is the dependence on the dataset used for the regression analysis and fitting. Empirical scores contain a rotor term, which estimates entropy penalties on binding from a weighted sum of the number of RBs in ligands. Currently used terms involve an incomplete description of solvation/desolvation energy upon ligand binding. In the next paragraph, three of the most commonly used scoring functions are discussed in terms of their use.

LUDI separates the H-bonding term into neutral and ionic H-bonds and calculates the hydrophobic contributions based on the molecular surface area.

$$\Delta G_{\text{bind}} = \Delta G_{\text{H-bond}} \sum_{\text{H-bond}} f(\Delta R, \Delta\alpha)$$
$$+\Delta G_{\text{ionic}} \sum_{\text{ionic}} f(\Delta R, \Delta\alpha)$$

$$+\Delta G_{\text{hydrophobic}} \sum_{\text{hydrophobic}} \left|A_{\text{hydrophobic}}\right|$$
$$+\Delta G_{\text{rotor}} N_{\text{rotor}} + \Delta G_0$$

where $A_{\text{hydrophobic}}$ is the molecular surface area, ΔR is the deviation from the ideal H-bond length, $\Delta\alpha$ is the deviation from the ideal H-bond angle, ΔG_0 is a regression constant.

FlexX score is based on Bohm's work. This equation is basically the ΔG for an ideal H-bond, ionic, aromatic, etc., interaction, adjusted by a penalty function that depends on the deviation from the ideal geometric values of two interacting elements.

$$\Delta G_{\text{bind}} = \Delta G_{\text{H-bond}} \sum_{\text{H-bond}} f(\Delta R, \Delta\alpha)$$
$$+\Delta G_{\text{ionic}} \sum_{\text{ionic}} f(\Delta R, \Delta\alpha)$$
$$+\Delta G_{\text{aromatic}} \sum_{\text{aromatic}} f(\Delta R, \Delta\alpha)$$
$$+\Delta G_{\text{contact}} \sum_{\text{contact}} f(\Delta R)$$
$$+\Delta R_{\text{rotor}} N_{\text{rotor}} + \Delta G_0$$

ChemScore is based on a diverse training set of 82 receptor-ligand complexes. It uses four terms that estimate contributions to binding energy from lipophilic interactions, metal-ligand binding, hydrogen bonding, and loss of ligand flexibility. ChemScore is more accurate and robust than many other widely used functions.

$$\Delta G_{\text{bind}} = \Delta G_{\text{H-bond}} \sum_{\text{H-bond}} f(\Delta R, \Delta\alpha)$$
$$+\Delta G_{\text{metal}} \sum_{\text{metal}} f(\Delta R, \Delta\alpha)$$
$$+\Delta G_{\text{lipo}} \sum_{\text{lipo}} f(\Delta R)$$
$$+\Delta G_{\text{rotor}} \sum_{\text{rotor}} f(P_{nl}, P'_{nl}) + \Delta G_0$$

where P_{nl} and P'_{nl} are the fraction of non-lipophilic atoms on either side of the frozen bond.

Knowledge-based scoring functions

In knowledge-based functions, the "knowledge" that is implicitly encoded in the protein-ligand complexes is tried to be captured. These scores are based on the concept of the inverse formulation of the Boltzmann law:

$E_{ij} = -kT \ln(p_{ijk}) + kT \ln(Z)$

E_{ij} – potential of mean force

p_{ijk} – probability density

Z – partition function

This approach has been applied to assemble potentials from databases of protein structures to score protein models in the context of protein structure predictions. To establish a function for scoring, the i, j, and k variables are assigned to protein and ligand atom types and their interatomic distances. The occurrence frequency of their contacts is a measure of the energetic contribution to the binding.

DrugScore and potential of mean force (PMF) are popular implementation of this type of scoring functions:

DrugScore:

$$\Delta W = \gamma \sum_{\text{protein}} \sum_{\text{ligand}} \Delta W_{ij}(r) + (1-\gamma) \times \left[\sum_{\text{ligand}} \Delta W_i(\text{SAS}, \text{SAS}_0) + \sum_{\text{protein}} \Delta W_j(\text{SAS}, \text{SAS}_0) \right]$$

SAS — solvent accessible surface area

W_{ij} — distance-dependent pairwise potential

γ — adjustable weight factor

Parametrized pairwise potential PMF score:

$$\text{PMF} = \sum_{\text{protein}} \sum_{\text{ligand}} A_{ij}(d_{ij})$$

$$A_{ij}(d_{ij}) = -k_B T \ln \left[f^{j}_{\text{volume\_corr}}(r) \frac{\rho^{ij}_{\text{seg}}(r)}{\rho^{ij}_{\text{bulk}}} \right]$$

k_B - Boltzmann constant

$f^{j}_{\text{volume\_corr}}(r)$ - ligand volume correction factor

$\rho^{ij}_{\text{seg}}(r)$ - the number density of a ligand-protein atom pa of type ij at a certain atom pair distance r

ρ^{ij}_{bulk} - the number density of a ligand-protein atom pair of type ij in a reference sphere with a radius of 12Å

Post-processing

Filters such as the ones used for preparing the input screening databases can also be applied here. Although after docking, this step does not save time, e.g., compounds not suitable for further drug development can be filtered out. Currently used scoring functions are inadequate for the precise binding affinity predictions. Therefore, additional postprocessing strategies are often advised to apply for the minimization of the number of false positives in the ranked database and to propagate the true hits to the top of the list.

A popular strategy is the consensus scoring. In this approach, scoring functions first can be separately applied for selection of the best docked position and then for ranking the best positions. The top ranking molecules then can be rescored by other scoring functions, and can be ranked again. Scoring functions can be weighted, so a linear combination of the scores can also be applied. An appropriate scoring scheme for the particular protein target can be worked out. Several variety of consensus scoring approaches have been frequently applied to increase the performance of VS.

Besides the consensus scoring and 1-D filters (MW, log P etc.) can decrease the artificial enrichment, which occurs as larger molecules are usually scored better. Thereby normalized scores can be calculated with e.g., solvent accessible surface, MW etc., so as to compensate the large molecular surface.

From the visual inspection of the docking solutions to the involvement of solvation or entropic effects, scores are often corrected to improve the prediction of the binding free energy and as a direct consequence the enrichment of active compounds.

Case Study: VS for Checkpoint Kinase-1 Inhibitors using Knowledge-Based VS

Kinase inhibitors have recently become a major area of drug discovery and structure-based design. Novel inhibitors for kinase targets such as cyclin-dependent kinase, and epidermal growth factor receptor kinase have recently been discovered. As many 3-D structures are publicly available for kinases, they seem to be an ideal target for VS studies. Although only a few case studies have been published in the pharmaceutical industry, VS is often performed for kinase targets. As kinases share a conserved ATP binding site, the discovery of truly novel inhibitors can be limited. The existence of the conserved ATP binding sites does suggest that a general VS strategy can be employed in searching for kinase inhibitors.

Lyne et al. proved an evidence for the above assumption using knowledge-based strategy for checkpoint kinase-1 (ChK-1). Their strategy exploits the chemical and structural information available for kinase inhibitors. Compounds with a minimal kinase-binding motif were docked; only then the docked poses were rescored using a scheme customized for a kinase, the CDK-2. High scoring compound were further investigated visually and selected for biological testing. Thirty-six effective inhibitors out of the 103 best ranking compounds were found.

The screening library was first prepared for docking. The preprocession of this database involved a filtering step of molecules having MW greater than 600 Da, and having rotatable bonds more than 10. Large, non-drug-like, and flexible molecules were excluded. Flexible molecules are often docked improperly using the FlexX algorithm. Tautomeric and protonation states of the ligands were generated using Leather face. 3-D coordinates were computed using Corina. Compounds without an appropriate kinase-binding motif were filtered out by using Plurality (H-bond donors/acceptors).

The ChK-1 crystal structure was protonated at crystallization pH. Active site contained all the residues within 6.5Å of the bound inhibitor. Essential pharmacophore constraints for the Cys87 (backbone NH) and Glu85 (backbone CO) residues were given.

CDK-2 was chosen as a surrogate for ChK-1 because more activity data were available for the CDK-2 that time. An enrichment study using a screening database of 8000 inactive and 100 of active compounds was performed. Three hundred docked poses per molecule were saved. For rescoring, the Cscore module of SYBYL was used. Z-scores were calculated for all the possible scoring functions combinations:

$$Z = \sum_i \frac{x_i - \bar{x}}{\sigma}$$

where x is the raw score for a pose, $\bar{x}$ average raw score for all the poses, and σ is the standard deviation for all the raw scores. For CDK-2 PMF and FlexX, scoring functions were found to give the best enrichment factors (EF). Thus this scoring scheme was applied for ranking the docked solutions for ChK-1. Enrichment factor (EFs) assess the quality of the rankings:

$$\mathrm{EF}(\%) = \left(\frac{N_{\mathrm{active}(\%)} / N_{(\%)}}{N_{\mathrm{active}} / N_{(\mathrm{all})}} \right).$$

where EF(%) is given at the percentage of the ranked database, $N_{\mathrm{active}(\%)}$ is the number of active compounds in a selected subset of the ranked database, $N_{(\%)}$ is the number of compounds in the subset, and N_{active} and Nall are the number of active molecules and the number of compounds in the screening database. EF were not scaled, i.e. absolute values depend on the ratio of active and inactive molecules and should be compared to the maximum (ideal) achievable EFs.

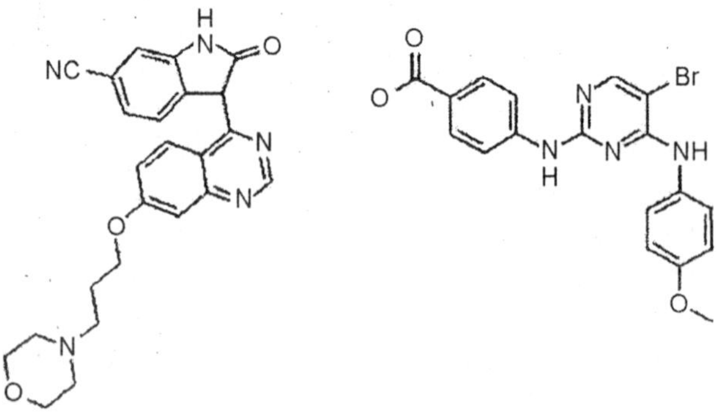

This study proves to be a successful case study in the field of protein kinase inhibition with ATP competitive compounds. The hit rate was

Fig. 23.7. Two examples of the hits found by virtual screening for ChK-1.

36%, and was achieved by screening 103 compounds. Hits corresponded to four chemical classes. These are the results for this particular study only and it is not premised that these could be observed in general with VS for protein kinases. However, this study gives a proof of the applicability of this strategy in other VS study performed for protein kinases.

Success Stories

Improvements in docking algorithms and the increasing number of scoring functions have resulted in a large number of successful VS studies. In this section, a collection of successful screening stories is described. Besides experimental high-throughput screening, VS has emerged as a knowledge-based alternative that can be applied in drug discovery. Recently published studies have revealed that the two approaches are rather complementary than competitive. Owing to the involvement of ever increasing numbers of compounds in today's drug design projects, there is a high demand for efficient computational screening tools. Progress has been made in the quality and speed of VS methods but there is still much room for further improvement. VS offers an approach with requirements opposite to those of experimental screening, which is mainly technology-driven ignoring the structural properties of the target. Nevertheless, VS depends on factors determining binding to the target. Structural information of target proteins and generation of reasonable binding modes of the ligands can serve for prediction of binding affinities. Either structure-based or ligand-based screening can be used to scan large virtual compound libraries.

The applicability of VS generally depends on the target selected for investigation. Recently published success stories demonstrate that these two approaches can be applied simultaneously or in a screening cascade to find quality hit or lead molecules. Large databases containing hundreds of thousands or millions of compounds can be focused or filtered, therefore, e.g., compounds with a special character are enriched resulting in a database with a reduced size. As the docking programs still need large computational power and the currently used scoring functions are not sophisticated enough to operate as a sole criterion for the final hit selection from a list of hundreds of thousands of molecules, there is a need to concentrate on information in a database containing, e.g., filtered compounds. These screening cascades are generally applied and hit rates of recently published success stories provide clear evidence for their effectiveness in drug discovery projects. Considering the current drug discovery landscape, establishing more effective target identification and validation strategies appears to be as important as making progress with VS and predictions of in vitro and in vivo characteristics. Any of these areas has significant potential for computational approaches and the opportunity to streamline the discovery process. As the amount of the experimental data grows, the computational models can be developed and tuned in an easier way. The most straightforward in lead discovery if virtual and experimental approaches are complementary applied.

24

Imaging of Lung Deposition

Inhalation aerosols have been successfully used to deliver drugs to the lung for local and systemic therapeutic effects. In vivo evaluation of pharmaceutical inhalation products is achieved by gamma scintigraphic imaging of the aerosol deposited in the lung. Imaging provides direct information on the amount and location of the drug deposited in the lung after inhalation. This local bioavailability, rather than the systemic bioavailability after absorption, is pertinent to drugs that act directly on the lung. For drugs that act systemically, the deposition site affects the rate and extent of absorption. As a result, lung deposition using gamma scintigraphy has been proposed for bioequivalence studies of aerosol products. The deposition data can further be linked to the clinical response and in vitro particle size distribution, adding a new dimension to the interrelationship between them. To measure lung deposition by imaging, the aerosol must be first labeled or tagged with a suitable radionuclide. Radiolabeling techniques have been developed for current inhalation products including nebulizers, propellant-driven metered dose inhalers (MDIs), and dry powder inhalers (DPIs).

Lung imaging is achieved using a gamma camera, which creates an image of the gamma rays emitted by the radionuclide in the lung. In the past, numerous lung deposition studies on radiolabeled aerosol products have been carried out using planar imaging by which only the anterior or posterior two-dimensional view of the lung is obtained. However, as the lung is a three-dimensional object, spatial distribution of the aerosol in the lung can be best obtained using tomographic (rather than planar) imaging such as single photon emission computed tomography (SPECT), a technique for producing cross- sectional images of the radionuclide distribution in the body. This is achieved by imaging the lung at different angles (e.g., 64 or 128 images at 180 or 360°, respectively) around the thorax using a rotating gamma camera, followed by computational image reconstruction.

Radiolabeling Pharmaceutical Aerosols

It is a prerequisite that the pharmaceutical aerosols be suitably radiolabeled before any lung scintigraphic imaging can commence. Ideally, the drug can be directly radiolabeled, that is, chemically by substitution of an atom in the drug molecule with a radioactive isotope. This can be achieved using positron emitters such as C-11, N-13, and O-15 atoms. Positrons are positively charged electrons, which, when combined with an electron, produce two gamma rays with equal energy (511 keV) emitted at 180° to each other. Theoretically, as C, N, and O atoms are present in all organic molecules, they can be used to label virtually any drug. In reality, the use of these atoms is limited by their short half-lives (20, 10, and 2 min for C-11, N-13, and O-15 atoms, respectively) relative to the time taken for manipulating the drug (including organic synthesis for radiolabeling and successive processing for product characteristics assurance such as particle size distribution of the aerosol particles). Furthermore, to produce these positron emitters, it is necessary to have a nearby cyclotron facility, which means that the process involves extra cost. So far, only three antiasthmatic compounds have been successfully radio- labeled by positron emitters: ipratropium bromide (Br-77), triamcinolone acetonide (C-11), and fluticasone proprionate (F-18). As Br-77 will dissociate from ipratropium in water, tracking ipratropium in the body still requires proper labeling of the molecule itself with a positron emitter. This is indicative of the difficulties of direct radiolabeling.

Because of the aforementioned limitation, gamma emitters have been employed to radiolabel the drug indirectly for gamma scintigraphy. In this case, the radiolabel associates with the drug by physical means instead of chemically incorporating into the drug molecule via covalent bonds. Hence, instead of being a direct chemical approach, it is indirect radiolabeling. Technetium-99m is the most commonly used pure gamma emitter for indirect radio labeling of pharmaceutical aerosols. The gamma ray of ^{99m}Tc has sufficient energy (140 keV) to penetrate body tissues without significant absorption or scattering, but when it reaches the detector of the gamma camera, it is absorbed and converted into light photons, thus optimal for gamma camera imaging. The half-life of ^{99m}Tc is 6 hr, which is long enough for handling and imaging, but not too long to increase the radiation dose to the subject unnecessarily. As a result, ^{99m}Tc is used for the majority of nuclear medicine imaging studies. Once inhaled into the lung, ^{99m}Tc can have a much shorter biological half-life, depending on the physical form. As diethylenetriamine pentaacetic acid or DTPA complex, it will be absorbed rapidly from the lung into systemic circulation, followed by glomerular filtration in the kidney to the bladder where it is excreted in the urine, and the whole process can take less than 2 hr, if the subject drinks plenty of water.

Regardless of the type of aerosol products to be radiolabeled, a fundamental requirement in radiolabeling aerosol products is that the radiolabel must associate with the drug in such a way that not only the radiolabel distribution matches the drug distribution, but also that the radiolabel distribution matches that of the unlabeled aerosol product.

Nebulizer Solutions

Nebulizer solutions are by far the simplest among the aerosol products, and radiolabeling is achieved by simply mixing the radionuclide with the drug solution. As the radionuclide and the drug are uniformly distributed in the solution and provided that no precipitation of the ingredients occurred, each nebulized aerosol droplet would contain both radioactivity and drug in proportion to the droplet size. Technetium-99m, complexing with DTPA or human serum albumin, is widely used as the radionuclide. Sodium pertechnetate is not suitable as the free anion, like iodide, has a high affinity for the thyroid. Lung deposition of nebulized salines and drug solutions including nedocromil sodium, salbutamol, fenoterol, ipratropium bromide, carbenicillin, pentamidine isethionate, flunisolide, liposomes containing beclomethasone dipropionate, interferon gamma, and cyclosporine have been studied using this radiolabeling technique of mixing the radionuclide with the drug solution.

Propellant-Driven MDIs

Historically, there are three major methods of radiolabeling suspension MDIs, developed by Few, Short, and Thomson, Newman et al., and Kohler, Fleischer, Matthys. The first two were initially developed for polymeric particles but were later modified for drugs.

Early in 1970, Few, Short, and Thomson radio- labeled polystyrene particles for a mucociliary clearance study. The radiolabeled aerosols were produced by a spinning-disk generator. The technique involves the key steps of extracting sodium pertechnetate ($Na^{99m}TcO_4$) into chloroform as tetraphenylarsonium (TPA) pertechnetate, followed by evaporation of the chloroform. A solution of polystyrene is added to the radioactive residue and dispersed. This technique has subsequently been adopted by other workers for radiolabeling pharmaceutical MDIs of sodium cromoglycate. It is important to note that in this technique, the complexing agent TPA chloride is classified as poisonous. Although the actual amount of the compound inhaled is in the nanogram range, safety to the researchers and the subjects inhaling the aerosols has to be carefully ensured.

Another way to radiolabel the pharmaceutical MDI is to use Teflon particles with a size distribution similar to that of the drug of interest. This was carried out in 1981 by Newman et al., who employed Teflon particles of mean size 2 ± 0.4 μm to mimic the MDI aerosols of bronchodilators. Hence, the Teflon particles were used as a surrogate for the drug. The Teflon particles were almost monodisperse and were produced by a spinning-disk aerosol generator. However, this approach is limited by the physicochemical characteristics of the Teflon particles being different from those of the drug particles. Furthermore, the aerosol particle size distribution of the Teflon may not match that of the drug. By coadministering a physical mixture of the radiolabeled Teflon particles with the drug salbutamol, the lung deposition and clinical response had been monitored simultaneously.

The first attempt to radiolabel drug particles (instead of polymers like polystyrene or Teflon particles) for pharmaceutical aerosols was carried out on fenoterol and salbutamol by Kohler, Fleischer, and Matthys. However, it was later found that their method would change the particle size distribution of the labeled aerosol, resulting in a coarser aerosol than the unlabeled product. After subsequent improvement by Summers et al., this method has become widely used for radiolabeling MDIs. It is preferred over other methods, as it does not involve extraction with TPA chloride and chloroform.

It is worth noting that each of the above-mentioned radiolabeling methods can be further modified for the study need. For example, the drug particles can be suspended in the organic phase containing the radiolabel and spray-dried, followed by reconstitution in the propellants, as has been carried out on salbutamol sulfate.

Although the radiolabeling methods have been widely used, the mechanism of association between the radiolabel and the drug particles has been studied only recently. The study by Farr on MDI systems indicated that in the chlorinated fluorocarbons (CFC) formulation, the radiolabel $^{99m}TcO_4^-$, being hydrophilic, would associate with hydrophilic domains including the surface of hydrophilic drug particles and the interior of surfactant reverse micelles. There is a need to extend the study to other systems, such as hydrophobic drugs and non-CFC propellants.

DPI

A method of wide application to radiolabeling dry powders is by adsorbing the radiolabel on the particles in a suitable liquid. The drug particles are wetted with a non-solvent containing the radiolabel, followed by evaporation of the solvent, leaving the radiolabel on the surface of the drug particles. This method has been applied to radiolabel terbutaline sulfate, budesonide, and formoterol. Factors influencing the radiolabeling of dry powder formulations include the physicochemical nature of the drug, choice of non-solvent for the drug, solubility of radiolabel in the non-solvent, moisture level, electrostatic charge, and the number of processing steps. Unfortunately, the details still remain largely as proprietary information and are not available in the literature. For example, exactly how the spherical agglomerates of budesonide powder are to be wetted with the ^{99m}Tc solution to ensure reproducible radiolabeling has not been reported.

Alternatively, a method resembling can be used, provided that the drug (e.g., terbutaline sulfate) to be radiolabeled does not dissolve in $CHC1_3$. After the filtrate (the $CHCl_3$ phase containing the ^{99m}Tc-TPA) is collected and added to the drug powder, the $CHCl_3$ is then evaporated (e.g., at 70°C), leaving the radiolabel with the powder. The powder is ready for filling into the DPI. Bronchodilators (salbutamol and terbultaline sulfate) and prophylactics (nedocromil sodium) for asthma along with lactose carriers have been successfully labeled by this technique for lung deposition studies.

An earlier method of radiolabeling dry powders (mainly sodium cromoglycate) involved spray-drying. The basic principle can be considered the same as the one for MDIs in that radiolabeled particles were produced by evaporation of radiolabel-containing atomized droplets. The method is straight-forward, but suffers the limitation that the spray-dried particles may not be physicochemically the same as those in the commercial products, because milling rather than spray-drying is normally used for micronization of the drug particles. Spray-drying, following ^{99m}Tc adsorption to the surface of the particles, has also been used to prepare radiolabeled cromoglycic acid and nedrocromil powders.

Technegas is another form of ^{99m}Tc, which can be used to radiolabel drug particles. Sodium pertechnetate is combined with carbon to form nanoparticles, which primarily has been used for lung ventilation studies. Recently researchers have adsorbed Technegas onto the surface of DPI particles to use in lung deposition studies. This technique offers the ability to achieve high levels of specific activity (MBq/mg) for the powder along with fast processing times (e.g., 10 min). However, there is still some concern over the long-term safety of administering carbon nanoparticles to the various sites of the lung.

The exact mechanism of association between the radiolabel and the drug particles is unknown and is generally regarded as a surface-coating phenomenon. However, the surface is proportional to the square of the particle size, whereas the volume (drug mass) is proportional to the cube of the particle size. It follows that to have a match between the radiolabel and drug mass in the aerosol, the radiolabeled particles must exist as agglomerates rather than as single particles.

Measuring the subjects' inhalation patterns during a scintigraphic study can be important, especially considering that many DPIs are dependent on inspiratory flow for aerosol generation. This can be measured using an inline spirometer or calibrated flowmeter connected to oscilloscope. The critical flow parameters that may affect the aerosol generation are peak flow rate, total volume of inhalation, initial acceleration, and time of inhalation. These parameters are becoming more commonly measured to help explain any variation or flow dependency. Depending on the study aims, controlling the patterns with restriction valves may be needed to obtain consistent flow profiles.

Quality Control of Aerosols

It is imperative that the radiolabeling process be sufficiently validated before the aerosols are administered to human subjects. This includes identifying the purity and form of the radiolabel if complex extractions are performed. As mentioned previously, it is important to ensure that the particle size distribution of the radiolabeled aerosol is similar to that of the unlabeled aerosol, which is most commonly accessed using an impaction method to determine the aerodynamic size. Depending on the process, it may also be necessary to perform the quality check on the day of study prior to inhalation of the aerosol. Dose uniformity is important for MDIs and reservoir DPIs; thus knowledge of the dosing needs to be established. Assessment of the physical characteristics such as particle morphology and crystallinity, which can affect dispersion of dry powders, is required to ensure that the radiolabeling process has not altered these parameters.

Microbial contamination of aerosol products is of major concern, as contaminated aerosols entering the human airways may lead to infection. This is especially important when aqueous solutions or compressed air are used in the labeling process. Autoclaving and using hospital grade disinfectants on equipment used in the radiolabeling process along with a suitable environment (good manufacturing practice or cleanroom facility) may help to minimize the risk of contamination. The use of inlet air filters on spray drying equipment is also recommended. External testing laboratories are able to test the aerosol product against the British Pharmacopoeia or other regulatory standards for microbial requirements on inhalation products. Yeast, mould, and total viable aerobic count must all be less then 10^2 cfu/g with no pathogens present.

Radiotracer Imaging of Lung Deposition

Nuclear medicine scintigraphic imaging provides a powerful tool for studying drug delivery and the use of the gamma camera for the non-invasive measurement of aerosol deposition and clearance is well established. The gamma camera allows the formation of an image of the radiotracer distribution in the patient or subject. The gamma camera detector consists of a collimator in front of a scintillating crystal, which is coupled to an array photomultiplier tubes and then the gamma camera electronics and computer. The collimator acts like a lens and only allows gamma rays within a specified angle to reach the scintillation crystal, which converts the energy of the gamma rays to light photons. The light photons are converted to electrical signals by the photomultiplier tubes. Electronic processing of the signals from the photomultiplier tube then provides position information of the detected gamma ray, which is used to build up an image of the radiotracer distribution in the subject in computer memory. The image formed by the gamma camera is a compression of the three-dimensional radiotracer distribution into a two-dimensional image and is usually referred to as planar imaging. Planar imaging is well established for lung deposition studies, being considered the "industry standard" and method of choice, and indeed has provided valuable insight into the performance of aerosols and aerosol delivery devices as well as interventions and pathologies that affect lung aerosol clearance through, for example, mucociliary clearance. However, compressing the three-dimensional radioaerosol distribution in the lungs into a two-dimensional image is a major drawback. This limits the ability to assess regional distribution of the aerosols in the lungs, and this may become particularly critical if the lung deposition data are to be used for bioequivalence comparisons.

Images of the three-dimensional tracer distribution in the lungs can be produced by SPECT. Single photon emission computed tomography involves taking typically 60–120 projection images at regular angular increments, while the gamma camera is rotating around the patient covering 360°. The projection images are then reconstructed into transverse slices that provide images of the three-dimensional aerosol distribution in the lungs. The stack of transverse slices reconstructed from the SPECT projections describes the volumetric distribution of the radiotracer in the lungs and can be reformatted into coronal, sagittal, or other oblique sections as required. Coronal slices as shown in Fig. 1 are most commonly employed, as they provide intuitive comparison with anterior and posterior planar imaging. Single photon emission computed tomography has been used to measure lung deposition in a number of studies, and SPECT has proved superior to planar imaging in discriminating between deposition in lung parenchyma, large and small airways and for assessing regional aerosol distribution.

Positron emission tomography (PET) is another tomographic technique using radiotracers, labeled with positron emitters. Positron emitters include ^{13}N, ^{15}O, ^{11}C, and ^{18}F, sometimes referred to the elements of life, and these radioisotopes are particularly suitable for incorporating into the drug molecule, thus allowing not only the deposition of the drug, but also its absorption and clearance from the lungs to be studied. However, as mentioned earlier, owing to the short half- life of positron emitters (^{13}N—10 min, ^{15}O—2 min, ^{11}C—20 min, and ^{18}F—110 min), ready access to a close by cyclotron and radiochemistry facility is required. This has restricted the wide spread use of the PET in aerosol studies. However, with the rapid growth of PET cyclotrons to meet the demand of the rapid expansion of clinical PET, access to this technology has improved considerably.

Quantification of Aerosol Deposition and Clearance

Assessment of aerosols and aerosol delivery devices requires accurate estimations of not only was the activity deposited in the lungs, but also in other regions such as oropharynx and stomach. For clearance measurements, such as mucociliary clearance, absolute estimates of activity are not required. Instead, the method should be able to confirm initial deposition of the aerosol to, primarily, the ciliated airways and provide good differentiation between central and peripheral regions to allow their respective clearances to be determined. Acquisition frame has to be sufficiently fast to allow clearance to be accurately followed, particularly during the fast initial clearance of aerosols from the lungs.

Estimation of in vivo activity for both planar and SPECT studies requires corrections for both attenuation and scatter. Attenuation occurs when gamma rays are absorbed by body tissue before reaching the gamma camera detector. This causes a reduction in detected activity, which depends on the amount of tissue between the source of the gamma photons and the detector. Gamma rays lose part of their energy and change direction owing to Compton interactions in the tissue, which is referred to as scatter. Scatter causes mispositioning of the detected counts and blurring in the image, as well as loss in quantitative accuracy as it causes a relative increase in detected photons in areas with increased amounts of tissue between the source of the photons and the detector.

Attenuation correction requires estimates of the amount of the tissue and its density between the gamma emitting source and the detector. Because of the heterogeneous nature of the thorax (lungs, bone, and soft-tissue) with quite different densities and attenuating properties, uniform attenuation cannot be assumed in the thorax. Thus for proper attenuation correction, attenuation has to be measured. Attenuation information can be obtained by a transmission scan with an external gamma-emitting source, or can be derived from anatomical imaging such as CT or MRI. To avoid uncertainty in the alignment between the emission and attenuation data, transmission data is ideally acquired simultaneously with the emission data, which also avoids extending the study time associated with a separate transmission data acquisition. A number of simultaneous emission/transmission techniques have been implemented for SPECT including scanning line source and fan beam collimators. For planar imaging, simultaneous emission/transmission scanning is not usually performed. Attenuation is assessed by measuring transmission using a sheet source of activity or introducing a known amount of activity into the lungs by intravenous injection of labeled particles that lodge in the capillaries of the lungs.

A number of different scatter correction techniques have also been developed, including methods based on multiple energy windows, as well as based on the transmission data and Monte Carlo modeling techniques. All of these can be applied to SPECT data, but planar imaging scatter correction is limited to the multiple energy window techniques. Attenuation correction is essential for quantitative aerosol deposition measurement, but scatter correction can sometimes be avoided by suitable phantom calibration of activity measurement. Planar activity quantification techniques have to make assumptions about the distribution of activity as a function of depth. Use of geometric mean of anterior and posterior images reduces but does not eliminate the dependence of activity estimation on the three-dimensional distribution entirely. For planar aerosol deposition studies, it is usually assumed that activity is distributed uniformly throughout the lungs and errors can be introduced when this assumption does not hold, for instance, for aerosols with pronounced central airway depositions. As SPECT provides images of the three-dimensional activity distribution, no such assumptions are required.

Planar vs. SPECT

While it is acknowledged that SPECT has the potential for better assessment of regional aerosol distribution, the main drawbacks attributed to SPECT are high radiation dose and long image acquisition times. This can potentially lead to significant clearance of the aerosols from the lungs during the SPECT study, confounding interpretation of total and regional lung deposition.

A survey of planar and SPECT imaging studies found that similar radiation doses were associated with planar than with SPECT studies. The radiation detriment to the subject from a given study is quantified by the effective dose, which not only depends on the amount of radioactivity in the lungs, but also depends on the total inhaled radioaerosol activity. The total inhaled amount of activity was approximately 50 MBq on each occasion, but the fraction delivered to the lungs differed substantially between the studies. The effective dose was 0.3 mSv on each occasion based on total administer activity of 50 MBq of ^{99m}Tc-DTPA for a total effective dose of 0.9 mSv for the three studies. It has been customary in planar studies to inhale radioaerosols until a set count rate of about 2000 cps is reached in the lungs. To achieve a count rate of about 2000 cps with the camera used for this SPECT study, approximately 40 MBq of activity would need to be deposited in the lungs. Based on the fractions delivered to the lungs, total inhaled activity would have to be 100, 190, and 565 MBq for the three studies respectively, resulting in effective doses of 0.6, 1.1, and 3.4 mSv, respectively for a total effective dose of 5 mSv from the three studies. Hence careful consideration to radiation dose must not only be given to SPECT studies but also to planar studies.

Activities >10 MBq deposited in the lungs provide adequate SPECT images of the lungs with a 2 min SPECT acquisition protocol described below. The use of less than 5 MBq still allowed the activity in the lungs to be accurately quantified. This allows the limiting of total inhaled activity to about 50–100 MBq for SPECT studies when an appreciable fraction (>10%) of the radioaerosol deposits in the lungs. The effective dose associated with that is 0.3–0.6mSv for ^{99m}Tc-DTPA and 0.6–1.3 mSv for ^{99m}Tc-pertechnetate. For comparison, most clinical nuclear medicine studies and diagnostic radiology procedures are associated with effective doses of several to 10s of mSv, and radiation dose from natural sources of background radiation is about 2–3 mSv in a year, depending on the geographical location. While the effective dose associated with SPECT studies is small, there is considerable scope for reducing inhaled activity below 10 MBq and as low as 1 MBq. Thus if a low dose planar study provides the required information, then use of a higher dose SPECT study would need to be questioned. Conversely, if a low dose planar study does not provide all the required information, but a moderate dose SPECT study does, a SPECT study is advised, as a suboptimal planar study exposes the subject to unnecessary radiation.

Traditionally, lung SPECT studies have been associated with long acquisition times of 15–30 min. Significant clearance of the radiolabel from the lungs may occur, during the SPECT study, through absorption or mucociliary clearance, particularly for radiotracers with fast clearance, such as ^{99m}Tc-pertechnetate, with lung half-clearance times of only about 10-15 min. Clearance potential not only leads to an underestimation of activity deposited in the lungs, but also reconstruction artifacts.

Current generation multidetector gamma camera systems allow complete SPECT studies to be collected in as little as 10 sec and have been used for quantifying tracer uptake and clearance for a range of applications. Application of fast, dynamic SPECT has also been demonstrated in the lungs, with SPECT frame rates of 1 min for aerosol deposition and clearance studies and as low as 30 sec for measuring the wash-out of ^{133}Xe from the lungs. Even at these fast SPECT frame rates, adequate SPECT images can be obtained while maintaining a low radiation dose to the subject. Thus these techniques have overcome the limitation of long SPECT study times and make them suitable for SPECT measurement of aerosol deposition and clearance. However, multidetector SPECT cameras are recommended to achieve these short study times. With the widespread clinical use of dual detector systems, this should not be a major issue.

Quantitative SPECT regimes are well established and rely on fewer assumptions about, e.g., three-dimensional activity distribution than planar activity quantitation approaches. While phantom studies can be used to assess accuracy of activity quantitation, these may not entirely reflect the accuracy achieved in human subjects. Mass balance calculations, where the initial activity loaded into the delivery device is compared to the activity in the subject estimated by the imaging technique plus the residual activities in the device and exhalation filter, can provide a good indication of the in vivo activity quantitation. With our quantitative fast SPECT technique, the recovered activity as a percentage of initial device activity was 102 ± 7% (n = 40) for a range of different protocols using both liquid and dry powder aerosols. Thus the accuracy of SPECT is at least as good as the "around 10%" quoted for planar studies. It has been suggested that the accuracy of planar activity estimation may be affected by differences in central distribution vs. peripheral distribution. No such distribution effect has been observed with our SPECT studies. In addition, careful attention has to be paid to attenuation and scatter correction with planar imaging to avoid large errors. It is unclear at this stage whether SPECT offers any significant advantage over planar imaging for total, as distinct from regional, activity quantitation as both techniques appear to provide quantitation with an acceptable accuracy.

Data Analysis

Image processing

No or limited processing of planar images is required before they can be analyzed with region of interested analysis. Formation of geometric mean images from anterior and posterior views reduces the dependence of the activity distribution with depth and improves quantitation. In addition attenuation correction factors have to be estimated according to the selected validated method for activity quantitation. In contrast, the acquired SPECT projections have to be reconstructed before volume of interests can be defined. Quantitative SPECT reconstruction with attenuation and scatter correction is required if aerosol deposition is to be quantitated. The main algorithms used for SPECT image reconstruction are filtered back projection and iterative reconstruction. The main advantage of filtered back projection is its computational efficiency and speed. This not only causes artifacts in the image, but can also bias the activity quantitation. Iterative reconstruction techniques avoid the streak artifacts and also can easily incorporate attenuation and scatter correction as part of the reconstruction. The main disadvantage of higher computational burden and long reconstruction times has been largely eliminated by the development of accelerated algorithms and the speed of current generation nuclear medicine computers. Further advantages of iterative reconstruction are improved noise properties and more control over noise, which is particularly important for the fast SPECT acquisition times proposed for aerosol studies. Thus iterative reconstruction is the clear method of choice for fast lung SPECT studies.

Drawing of the Lung Region

Assessment of regional lung aerosol deposition mandates reliable and reproducible definition of a region over the right lung for planar studies. As variations in aerosol deposition precludes using the aerosol image for lung region of interest (ROI) definition, either a ventilation image using ^{81m}Kr or ^{133}Xe or a transmission image is used to manually draw the right lung ROI which is then superimposed on the aerosol deposition image. The whole lung region can then be further subdivided into apex and basal regions, or for estimation of the penetration index (PI), into central, peripheral, and intermediate regions. However, there is no consensus on how the size and shape of the regions should be defined, and both rectangular and lung shape regions have been used in the past. Peripheral regions should contain more small airways, while in the central region, large, conducting airways should dominate to allow assessment of relative aerosol deposition in the small and large airways. In planar imaging, there is considerable overlapping of lung structures, and hence planar imaging only provides a crude and insensitive measure of peripheral vs. central airway deposition. However, the PI from planar images has proven to be a useful index for detecting marked differences in deposition patterns, particularly as the subjects act as their own controls.

Early regional analysis of SPECT data has been limited to applying planar image definition techniques to a central, thick coronal slice extracted from the SPECT data. However, this does not take full advantage of the information contained in the SPECT data. Automated definition of the right lung volume of interest from the simultaneously collected transmission data has been achieved using thresholding and morphological operators. Alternatively, coregistered anatomical imaging has been proposed to define the right lung volume outline. The lung volume of interest can then be divided into concentric shells, which can be related to airway generations. Central and peripheral lung regions are then defined by combining appropriate number of inner and outer shells, respectively. As has been demonstrated, this approach has proven to be more sensitive to detecting changes in regional aerosol deposition than planar imaging.

Future Directions of Lung Deposition Studies

Planar imaging will continue to provide useful information about aerosol deposition and clearance and will be sufficient for a range of applications. Fast SPECT has been shown to be feasible for aerosol studies and is likely to provide additional insight and information about aerosols and delivery devices. With the large expansion of clinical PET, PET applications to aerosols, particularly labeling of the active drug molecules and following their fate in vivo is likely to grow. Most PET scanners recently installed are combined PET/CT system, taking full advantage of the complementary information provided by the coregistered functional and anatomical information. A hybrid SPECT/CT system, with a low end CT, has been available from one manufacturer for a number of years. Recently, two more gamma camera manufacturers have announced SPECT/CT systems with high end, multi- slice CTs. The CT images from these scanners not only provide information for attenuation correction, but also show great potential for more precisely defining and characterizing regional lung deposition, provided an additional radiation dose from the CT can be obtained.

Radiolabeling of nebulizer solutions, propellant-driven metered-dose inhalers, and dry-powder inhalers is generally well documented. For some dry-powder inhalers the procedure may still be lacking sufficient details to ensure reproducible radiolabeling. Deposition of radiolabeled aerosols in the lung has been mainly measured by planar imaging. Tomographic imaging using SPECT can provide three-dimensional information about the spatial distribution of the aerosol in the lung. The recent development of the fast dynamic SPECT has made it the method of choice for aerosol imaging.

25

Radiochemical Methods of Analysis

In nuclear medicine, drugs containing radioactive metals, metal complexes, and metal conjugates are used for diagnosis and therapy of various diseases. Radioactive materials used as pharmaceuticals are not only small organic and inorganic molecules but are also macromolecules such as monoclonal antibodies and antibody fragments that are attached to radioactive metals. Nuclear medicine has become a $12 billion medical industry, and more than one-third of the hospitals in the United States currently use radioisotopes for such procedures. It is anticipated that diagnostic procedures in the United States are likely to exceed 20 million by the end of 2000. The successful use of radiochemicals needs a basic understanding of radiation, radioactivity, and the nature and characteristics of instruments to detect and quantitate radiation. This article addresses these applications related to radioactivity and radiochemical methods of measurement.

Atomic Structure, Nuclear Stability, and Radioactivity

Atomic physics describes the structure of atoms in complex mathematical terms of quantum mechanics. However, the model of the atom as described by Niels Bohr in 1913 is very simple, pictorial, and more than adequate for a basic understanding of the phenomenon of radioactivity. Bohr's planetary model of the atom consists of a dense positively charged nucleus surrounded by negatively charged electrons (e) in orbits of well-defined energy states. The nucleus consists of positively charged protons and neutral particles called neutrons. The protons and neutrons are held together by very a strong nuclear force of attraction, effective at very close distances (approximately 10^{-13} cm). These strong forces for each nucleus are computed in terms of binding energy. The electroneutrality of the atom is maintained by the orbital electrons, which are equal in number to that of the protons. This number is called the atomic number, *Z*. The masses of the atoms (*A*) and other particles are described in terms of atomic mass units (amu). The amu is defined as 1/12th the mass of a carbon atom with atomic mass of 12.0000. Any configuration of protons and neutrons is called a nuclide. There are three nuclides of the element hydrogen with atomic number 1.

The notation is used to indicate the nuclide of an element. The three nuclides of hydrogen are called isotopes of hydrogen. Tritium with an *N*/*Z* ratio of two is unstable. When the *N*/*Z* ratio becomes higher, the nucleus become unstable and results in the disintegration of the nucleus so as to achieve a stable *N*/*Z* ratio and therefore a stable nucleus. This process is called radioactive decay. This radioactive process can be spontaneous in some naturally occurring nuclides; then these elements are said to be naturally radioactive. When such instability is brought about by bombarding stable nuclides with high-energy particles, it is called *artificial radioactivity*. Of nearly 3000 known nuclides of elements, which are either man-made or natural, 287 nuclides of 83 elements are stable; the rest are unstable to varying degrees. The unstable nuclides disintegrate to form stable nuclides with release of energy and nuclear particles. Binding energy and nuclear stability are found to be dependent on the ratio of number of neutrons to protons (*N/Z* or *n/p* ratio). To be stable, at least one proton is required. The most stable heavy nuclide is, with 83 protons and 126 neutrons ($N/Z = 1.5$). In general, when the *N/Z* ratio is greater than 1.6, the radioactive nuclide readjusts to a stable ratio of *N/Z* with the release of energy and particles of matter. The three nuclides of hydrogen are called isotopes. Other members of the nuclide family are isobars and isotones.

Radioactive Decay

Different radioactive species undergo disintegration at different rates. The rate of this decay or activity is characteristic of the individual nuclide and is proportional to the number of radioactive nuclides present at the beginning of this time interval. The proportionality constant is called the decay constant and is denoted by λ. The decay constant is a measure of the probability that a certain radioactive nucleus will disintegrate within a specified time interval. These disintegrations are characteristic of the nuclide and are unaffected by pressure, temperature, concentration, and other physical or chemical properties of the radionuclide. This rate constant is conveniently denoted in terms of $t_{1/2}$, or halflife. The halflife of a radionuclide is the time required for the sample activity to decrease to half its initial value. $t_{1/2}$ is related to rate constant (λ) as follows:

$$\lambda = 0.6932/t_{1/2}$$

In fact, less than 1% will be radioactive in seven halflives, and after 10 halflives, greater than 99.9% of the radioactive nuclide will have lost its activity. The halflife refers to that of a pure nuclide. In a sample containing mixtures of disintegrating radionuclides, the total activity is the sum of the separate activities. From a plot of relative activity against time, the individual halflives can be computed. However, in practice, this can be realized for mixtures containing 3 or <3 nuclides. Other commonly used terms in nuclear medicine and pharmacy are average (mean) halflife, biological halflife, and effective halflife. Average half-life is the mean lifetime of a nuclide, and it is equal to $1.44 \times t_{1/2}$. Biologic halflife, tb, is the time required for the body to eliminate half the administered dose by normal biological process of elimination. Effective halflife (t_{eff}) is a measure of how fast the body eliminates the radioactive material by the combination of biological elimination and radioactive decay:

$$1/t_{eff} = 1/t_b + 1/t_{1/2}$$

Unit of Activity

The fundamental SI unit of activity is the Becquerel (Bq). One Bq is equal to one disintegration per second (dps). Because this is a very small unit, it is more often expressed in kilobequerels or kBq. However, the older historical unit of activity C_i is normally used for radio- pharmaceuticals. The Curie was defined in terms of the number of disintegrations per second of 1 g of ^{226}Ra and is equal to 3.7×10^{10} dps. Other commonly used units are millicurie and microcurie (mC_i and μC_i). The unit of C_i represents absolute activity (A). However, relative activity R is proportional to the efficiency of the counting device. The device reports in counts per minute.

$R = qA$; q = efficiency quotient. Sometimes specific activity, in terms of radioactivity per unit mass of an element or radiolabeled compound or unit volume of solution is also specified. In these case, the mass or volume should be clearly specified.

Decay Processes

The radioactive decay process involves the emission of radiation, which is dependent on the mode of decay of the particular radionuclide. Radiation resulting from any decay process can be classified as alpha (α), beta (β), gamma rays (γ), and/or other emissions.

α-Particles

Alpha (*α*)-particles are doubly charged, highly energetic helium nucleus. *α*-Particles originate in the nuclei of heavier atoms. The emission involving *α*-Particles is the most efficient process for a radionuclide to attain stability because the nuclide loses both charge and mass. Because *α*-Particles are very heavy (7400 times of that of an electron) and doubly charged, they attract electrons from the surrounding medium when they pass through a medium. This results in the ionization of the medium. An *α*-Particle loses energy, slows down, and finally becomes a helium nucleus. In each ionization process, it loses 34 eV per event. For example, a loss of 3.4 MeV of energy causes 100,000 ionization events. These particles travel very short distances, called the range. Because they are extremely efficient in ionizing, they lose energy very rapidly. This range is approximate 4 cm in air and a few thousandths of a centimeter in biological tissues. Because of this tremendous amount of energy transfer, *α*-Particles can cause extensive damage to organs and tissues when they are exposed to this radiation. Generally, *α*-Particles arise during the natural decay of elements with a *Z* value greater than 83. A typical alpha decay process is represented below:

$$^{238}_{92}U \rightarrow {}^{234}_{90}Th + {}^{4}_{2}He + \text{Energy}$$

β-Particles

A *β*-Particle is a high-velocity nucleon ejected out of a decaying nucleus. *β*-Particles have the rest mass (0.000548amu) of an electron. If it is negatively charged, it is called a negatron and if positively charged, it is called apositron. In common usage, *β*-Particle emission refers to the negatron (β^-) and β^+-Emission is called positron emission. For example, the decay of $^{32}_{15}P$ to $^{32}_{15}S$ results in the emission of β^-, antineutrino, and release of energy. The difference in the masses of the two nuclides, 0.001836 amu (31.965675 for P – 31.9638390 for S), results in the release of energy equivalent to 1.70 MeV. Part of this energy is used up in the ejection of particles, and the remaining is used in the release of antineutrino. Because no other energy is emitted, ^{32}P is called a pure *β*-Emitter. Sometimes some portion of the energy difference may be retained in the nucleus, and consequently the nuclide resides in a nuclear excited state. The excited nucleus may lose the excess energy and return to the stable ground state in the form of electromagnetic radiation (gamma-rays). *β*-Particles are emitted with variable energy from zero to the maximum of the difference in energy between the parent and daughter nucleus. The variability in energy arises from the distribution of energy between the *β*-Particle and the antineutrino.

Negatively charged *β*-Particles are emitted when the radionuclide has more neutrons than required by the number of protons for stability. Sometimes more than one *β*-Particle may be emitted. For example, ^{131}I decays with the emission of six *β*-Particles and 14 *γ*-Rays of different energies:

$$^{131}_{53}I \rightarrow {}^{131}_{54}Xe + \beta^- + \beta^- + \gamma$$
$$+ \text{ antineutrino} + \text{Energy}$$

Nearly 100% of all these decay processes correspond to *β*-Particles of energy 0.61 MeV and *γ*-Radiations of energy 0.364 MeV. The decay to form stable nuclides may involve the formation of many unstable intermediate radionuclides. For example, the decay of $^{127}_{50}Sn$ to $^{127}_{53}I$, shown below, involves the formation of a number of intermediate nuclides:

$$^{127}_{50}Sn \rightarrow {}^{127}_{51}Sb \rightarrow {}^{127}_{52}Te \rightarrow {}^{127}_{53}I$$

In general, β^-- and β^+-Particles penetrate deep into the medium; however, they do not cause damage to tissues and organs. Radionuclides that decay by *β*-Particle emissions are used very extensively in nuclear medicine for diagnostic and therapeutic applications. Positron-emitting nuclides are used in nuclear medicine for diagnostic purposes. β^+-Emitting radionuclides are under active study for use in radiotherapy. An example of a decay process involving emissions of positrons follows:

$$^{15}_{8}O \rightarrow {}^{15}_{7}N + {}^{0}_{1}\beta^+$$

γ-*Rays* (γ)

During the disintegration of the nucleus, part of the energy is used in the creation of excited-state radionuclide. In the excited state, the nuclide is unstable. The release of energy while the excited nucleus returns to the ground state appears as electromagnetic radiation. These radiations are called γ-Rays. γ-Emission is common when the difference between the excited state and the lowest energy ground state nucleus is greater than 100 keV. Because γ-Emission iselectromagnetic radiation, there is no change in the neutron number or mass number or atomic number. Therefore, invariably, γ-Radiation is always preceded by a nuclear decay reaction involving emission of α, β^-, β^+ particles.

γ-Rays are high-energy electromagnetic radiation such as X-Rays with no electrical charge. γ-Rays are different from X-Rays in that they differ with respect to their origin. X-Rays originate from orbital electrons, whereas γ-Rays originate from the decay of a nuclide. The γ-Rays also ionize the medium by striking orbital electrons with high energy and by knocking the electrons out of the atom. These ejected electrons cause secondary ionization referred to as indirect ionization. The degree of penetration of γ-Rays is extremely high. There are at least seven different processes by which γ-Rays can interact with matter. However, the processes associated with γ-Ray interaction or production, which are pharmaceutically relevant, are electron capture, isomeric transition, and internal conversion. These are briefly discussed below.

Electron capture is a decay process in which an orbital electron loses energy and becomes absorbed into the nucleus. As a result, outer-shell electrons jump to fill the inner-shell vacancy resulting in an electron orbit reshuffling. This process result in the release of X-Rays, and these electrons are subsequently absorbed and result in the release of weakly bound orbital electrons. These are called Auger electrons. When the decay process involves in positron emission, it is almost always followed by electron capture. As a result of nuclear reaction, an excited radionuclide (with energy > 100 keV) loses energy by de-excitation:

$^{125}{}_{53}I$

Electron Capture ——— EC

$^{125}{}_{52}Te$

More often, these occur in multiple steps with the release of γ-Ray photons of multiple energy. Thus, the resulting γ-Ray spectrum is unique to the decaying radionuclide; this uniqueness, therefore, is used to identify the unknown nuclide. γ-Rays with no mass and charge can penetrate into matter and bring about other chemical reactions in the system. γ-Rays are widely used in nuclear medicine.

An excited radionuclide may remain in several excited states before reaching ground state. However, transitions can occur within these excited states with the emission of γ-Rays. These transitions are called isomeric transitions. When these isomeric transitions are significantly long-lived, these are called metastable states. An example of the decay process is shown below. (↘-increase in Z, ↙-(left arrow) decrease in Z)

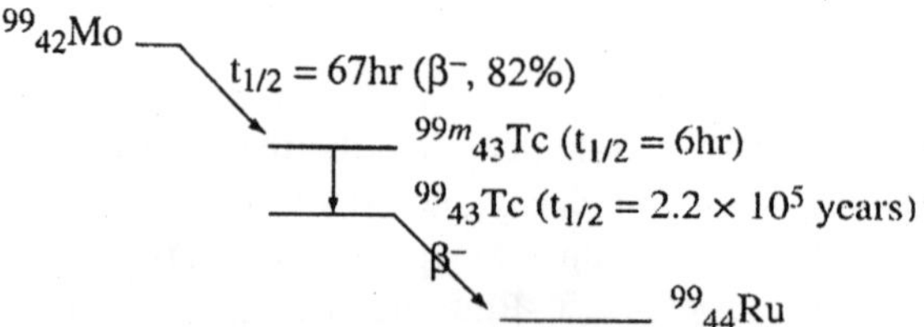

A process alternative to isomeric transition is called internal conversion (IC). In some cases, the γ-energy is absorbed by a K-shell (inner) electron. This electron is ejected out with lower energy. This ejected electron is the internal conversion electron, and the process is called internal conversion. Some diagnostic and therapeutic radionuclides with corresponding half lives are given below.

Diagnostic raidonuclides. ($t^1/_2$ in units as indicated are given in parentheses.) $t^1/_2$ hours: ^{67}Cu (62.0); ^{67}Ga (78.3); ^{90}Y (64.1); ^{117}In (67.9); ^{99m}Tc (6); ^{201}Tl (72) {β-particles}-*t* min; ^{11}C (20.4); ^{13}N (10.1); ^{15}O (2.0); ^{18}F (1.9); ^{68}Ga (68.0); and ^{82}Rb (1.25) {β^+}.

Therapeutic radionuclides. $t^1/_2$ days: D; ^{32}P(14.3); ^{47}Sc (3.4); ^{67}Cu (2.6); ^{64}Cu (0.5); ^{90}Y (2.7); ^{105}Rh (1.5); ^{111}Ag (7.5); ^{117m}SN (13.6); ^{131}I (8.0); ^{149}Pm (2.2); ^{153}Sm (1.9); ^{166}Ho (1.1); ^{177}Lu (6.7); ^{186}Re (3.8); ^{188}Re (0.7).

Radiation Detection and Measurement

Interaction of Radiation with Matter, Ionization Chamber, and GM Counters

The detection and quantitation of nuclear radiation are based on its interaction with material contained in the detector. Ionization of the gas particles in the medium and scattering are the two most common types of interaction of radiation with matter. Radiation causes darkening of photographic emulsion, ionization of a gas or a mixture of gases, or fluorescent scintillation. In radiology, exposure and observation of the photographic film are most commonly used. When α-Particles with high kinetic energies impinge on gases enclosed in a chamber, they produce approximately 40,000 ($\pm$ 10,000) ion pairs per cm. The range of α-particles is short (approximately 6 cm in air and 2 μM in lead); β-Particles have longer and irregular paths and produce approximately 100–700 ion pairs per cm. A typical ionization chamber, consists of a sealed tube containing helium, neon, or gas–air mixtures placed in a space between two electrodes. The incoming particles create ion pairs; the ions are separated and collected at the electrodes of opposite charge. Electrons are collected at the anode. The number of such ions collected at each electrode is also a function of the applied voltage across the electrodes. If the response is measured in terms of pulse height (proportional to the number of electrons collected), a plot of this value against applied voltage will exhibit a characteristic response. The different regions are explained below. Region I is called the recombination region. In this region, ion pairs produced increase linearly as a function of applied voltage (< 100V) as recombination is proportionately decreased. This is not a useful region for measurement. In region II (100–400V), pulse height attains a plateau because all ions formed are collected. This region is used in ionization chambers to measure energies of γ-Rays and X-Rays. This region is also used for identification of α- and β-Particles because the height at which plateau occurs is characteristic of the nature of the particle. Dose meters and dose rate meters, which measure high-intensity radiation fields, operate in this region. In region III (400–800 V), the number of pulses produced is proportional to the intensity of radiation. The size of the pulses counted gives a measure of the primary ionization produced. In this region, the

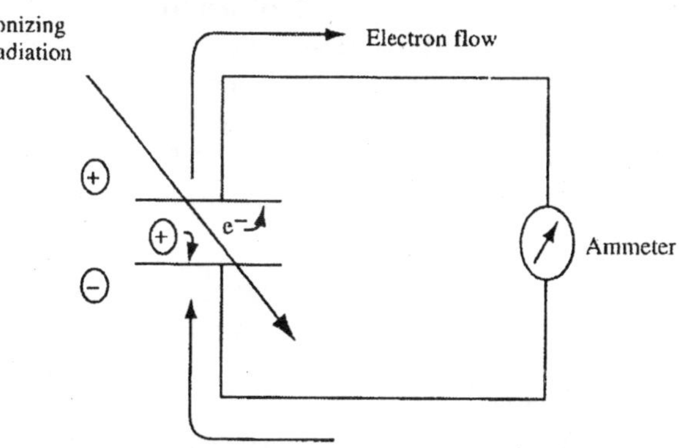

Fig. 25.1. Block diagram of a simple air ionization chamber.

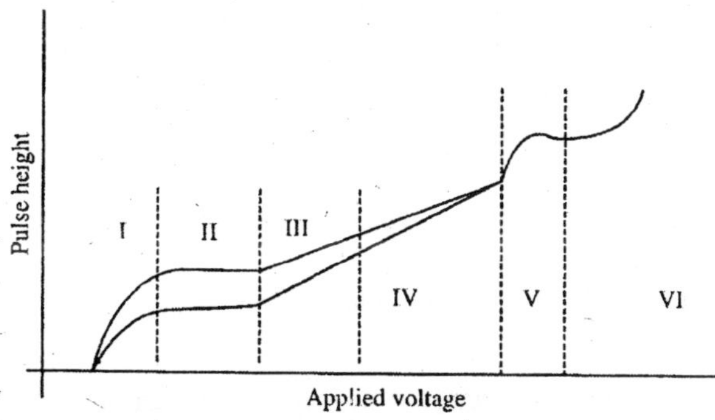

Fig. 25.2. Pulse higher versus applied voltage response.

primary electrons are accelerated with high gain in energy. This high energy causes additional secondary electrons to be generated as a result of interaction with gases in the ionization chamber. These secondary electrons cause further ionization. The net effect is pulse amplification; the size of the amplification is of the order of 100–10,000 times that of the size of the ions initially produced in the ionization chamber.

Region IV (applied voltage 800–1000V) is limited proportional region and is not important for purposes of detection. When the applied voltage is between 1000 and 1500 V, the size of the pulse is no longer proportional to the initiating event. However, each pulse corresponds to a single event. The counters that operate in this region are called Geiger–Mueller counters or GM counters. The GM counters are very sensitive. Because of the high gain involved, these are used primarily in regions where the radioactivity is of very low intensity, (e.g., radioactive contamination). The readings are given in milli-, micro-, or Roentgens/h or in counts per minute. In the GM counter, ionization produced spreads to the entire gas. Therefore, the counter may not respond to a succeeding second incoming pulse before a recovery time of approximately 100– 300 μs. This dead time for recovery is unusually high compared with the dead time for the proportional counter, which is approximately 1 μs. Secondly, because a fixed amount of gas is present in the chamber, the purity of the gas in the chamber decreases. Therefore, the GM counter has to be calibrated frequently, using standard ^{226}Ra or ^{137}Cs sources per Nuclear Regulatory Commission (NRC) requirements. Above an applied voltage of 1500 V, continuous discharge occurs, and this is not useful for any measurement.

Scintillation Detectors

When radiation interacts with certain substances called fluors or phosphors, it produces a flash of light called scintillation. The scintillation is then detected using a sensing element, amplified, sorted, and recorded by counting. The scintillation-detecting instruments include well counters, scanners, thyroid probes, and scintillation cameras called Auger cameras. In addition, all these instruments consist of a collimator (excluding well counters), photomultipliers, a high-voltage power supply, an amplifier, a gain control unit, a pulse height analyzer, and instruments or computers for appropriate display modes. The scintillation cameras also contain coordinate-positioning (x,y) circuits.

Solid-state detectors

These detectors are made of semiconducting materials. In these detectors, solid-state electrodes are made from Li doped with Si or Ge. The resolution is approximately 1–2 keV for 1 MeV γ-Rays and sometimes provides a greater than 10-fold improvement over NaI (Tl) scintillation detectors, described below. These are commercially available and more often used in research-grade instruments.

Liquid Scintillators

The sample radionuclide is dissolved in a liquid scintillator called the scintillation cocktail. It consists of two principal components. The first is a primary solvent such as toluene, xylene, or 1,2,4-Trimethylbenzene (pseudocumene). The second component is the fluor solute, 2,5-Diphenyloxazole (PPO) that emits UV light at ~380 nm. The cocktail may also contain one or more the following:

1. A secondary solvent such as dioxane to improve solubility of aqueous samples or surfactants such as sodium dodecylbenzenesulfonate as emulsifier.
2. A secondary scintillator to shift the wavelength of photons emitted (~380 nm) to the wavelength response of some photomultiplier tubes (PMT, ~420 nm).
3. One or more adjuvants for purposes of suspending or solubilizing biological tissues.

Photomultiplier (PM) tubes

The PM tube has a light-sensitive electrode called the photocathode. It emit electrons when photons strike it. The electrons are then accelerated from the photocathode to the anode of PM tube by the application of approximately 1000 V in steps of approximately 100 V by a series of electrodes called the dynodes. In the PM tube, secondary electrons are produced, resulting in pulses of 10^5 to 10^8 electrons. Typically a photo- tube with 10 dynodes delivers approximately 410 electrons. This gain or amplification is dependent on the dynode voltages.

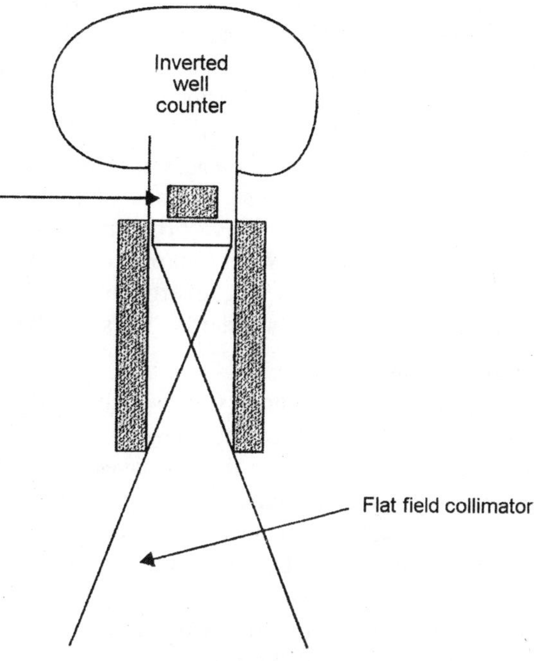

Fig. 25.3. A typical well counter used in nuclear medicine.

Preamplifier

Even though such a large number of secondary electrons are generated, these are not adequate to generate enough current. The voltage pulse is amplifed by a factor of 4–5 by the preamplifier without loss of power. The preamplifier also provides the driving force necessary to prevent loss in the several feet of connecting cables.

Linear amplifier

The pulses received from preamplifier have wide variation in energies of the particles. The gain in the amplifier is of the order of 8000 such that a 1 mV signal is amplified to approximately 8 V while still maintaining the proportionality of the energy delivered by the particle (more often γ-Ray) to the detectors. The amplified pulse is then delivered to pulse height analyzer.

Pulse height analyzers (PHA)

The pulses that emerge from the amplifier usually have different amplitudes owing to differences in energies. These analyzers are essentially energy sorters. Single-channel PHAs count pulses of a given amplitude, whereas multichannel analyzers (MCAs) scan whole energy range and record the pulses in each channel. For example, by using an MCA, γ-Ray spectrum can be recorded and, thus, these instruments that use MCAs are called γ-Ray spectrometers. MCAs may have as many as 4000 channels.

X- Y-positioning circuits

These are unique to scintillation cameras, known as Auger cameras, used in nuclear medicine studies. Approximately 19–91 PMTs are mounted on a Na(Tl) crystal used in the camera. These crystals are typically- thick. The number of PMTs, which are optically coupled to the back of the crystal, is determined by the size and shape of the crystal. A maximum amount of light will be received by the PMT nearest to the point of interaction compared with the other PMTs, which are positioned differently. The amount of light received in these PMTs is proportional to the solid angle subtended by the PMT. Therefore, X-Y-positioning of the camera has to be controlled and known so that X–Y-coordinate of the γ-Ray interaction can be assessed accurately. These data are stored in a computer and then processed or recorded on Polaroid or X-Ray films.

Efficiency of detection in scintillation detectors

In gas-filled as well as scintillation detectors, the observed count rate is typically less than the actual decay rate of the radionuclide. The efficiency of detection may differ from particle to particle under identical conditions using the same type of detector. The factors that affect the efficiency of detection are operating voltage, resolving time, geometry of the instrument used in relation to the position of the sample with respect to the detector, scaler, energy resolution, absorption by cells, and sometimes constituents of the sample itself. For example, the scintillation cocktail sometimes reduces counts considerably. This effect is known as quenching. For accurate measurements of radioactivity, appropriate correction for quenching is required.

Frequent calibration of the instruments with the use of appropriate standards is required to make suitable allowances for decreases in the efficiency of the instruments. Such calibration standards are available from the National Institute of Standards and Technology (NIST). Other sources traceable to NIST standards through active program of participation in comparison measurements also provide such standards. The United States Pharmacopeia (USP) also provides nuclear decay data for new calibration standard. USP 24 lists $t^1/_2$, energy of photons, and number of photons per disintegrations, for the following radionuclide standards: ^{137}Cs, ^{137m}Ba, ^{22}Na, ^{60}Co, ^{57}Co, ^{54}Mn, ^{109}Cd, ^{109}Ag, and ^{129}I.

Tomographic Imagers

Tomography is a process in which three-dimensional images are constructed using a large number of two- dimensional slices of images from an object. Computed tomography uses rigorous mathematical algorithms to reconstruct these images. When radionuclide emissions are used, it is called emission tomography. Two common techniques are now used to obtain images using emission tomography, namely, single photon emission computed tomography (SPECT) and positron emission tomography (PET). In SPECT, γ-Emitting nuclides are used, whereas in PET, positron-emitting nuclides are used. In the SPECT system, an object is photographed using many Auger cameras at a number of small angles (between 3 and 10°) around the object. The total span may be between 0 and 180° or between 0 and 360°. Because the rotating cameras provide two-dimensional digital images, these are stored as 64 × 64 matrix (for 180° span) or as 128 × 128 matrix (for 360° span) digital information. The Auger cameras use NaI (Tl) crystals in the detector heads. In PET, positron-emitting radionuclides are used. Each positron emitted from these radionuclides travels through tissues, deposits energy, and finally is annihilated by interaction with an electron. The annihilation results in the formation of two photons traveling in opposite directions (180° apart) with energy of 0.511 MeV. Two Auger cameras are placed 180° apart but at the same distance from the object. Each camera detects a photon at the same time. By appropriately moving cameras in pairs, the data are collected over many angles and stored in 64 × 64 or 128 × 128 matrix. Thus, this electronic collimation brought about by simultaneous detection increases sensitivity and reduces the need for use of collimators as in SPECT. Additional advantages of PET include easy availability of radionuclides with short halflives of isotopes of elements commonly found in organic molecules (such as F, N, C, and O).

Analysis of Radiochemicals

Radiochemical methods of analysis are considerably more sensitive than other chemical methods. Most spectral methods can quantitate at the parts-per-million (ppm) level, whereas atomic absorption and some HPLC methods with UV, fluorescence, and electrochemical methods can quantitate at the parts-perbillion (ppb) levels. By controlling the specific activity levels, it is possible to attain quantitation levels lower than ppb levels of elements by radiochemical analyses. Radiochemical analysis, inmost cases, can be done without separation of the analyte. Radionuclides are identified based on the characteristic decay and the energy of the particles as described in detection procedures presented above. Radiochemical methods of analysis include tracer methods, activation analysis, and radioimmunoassay techniques.

Tracers and Tracer Methods of Analysis

Radiochemical tracers or radiotracers are compounds labeled with radioisotopes. For tracer methods, the compound to be measured or a suitable reagent is radiolabeled. A measurement of the redistribution of tracer within such a sample–reagent reaction system provides the required quantitative analytical information. Major advantages of tracer methods are high sensitivity, simplicity, and speed. Radiotracers are more commonly used for following mechanisms of biological and/or chemical processes or if there is need to eliminate complicated separation procedures, especially in biological processes.

Isotopic dilution analysis

In isotope dilution analysis, a known amount of radio- labeled compound with known specific activity is spiked to a known amount of an unknown mixture containing the same compound made up of stable isotopes. Then, the components of the radiotracer-diluted samples are mixed thoroughly to form a homogeneous mixture. This istopically diluted mixture, with known levels of dilution, is then suitably treated to isolate a small amount of the desired constituent. The radioactive isotope content of the isolated portion is determined by measuring its specific activity. From the specific activities of the tracer before and after dilution, the concentration of the component in the mixture can then be calculated. The major advantage is that these isolation procedures need not be quantitative; however, it is necessary that the compound isolated should be pure enough for an activity determination. Isotope dilution analyses are used for determination of inorganic trace elements and for the determination of organic compounds in biological systems. If separations are required and the radioisotope concentration is not adequate to bring about separation, dilutions can be accomplished by using a non-radioactive compound (or carrier) with similar chemical behavior. For example, if radio strontium is to be precipitated and it is in low amounts such that it cannot be quantitatively precipitated, it can be coprecipitated along with a calcium salt by the addition of calcium before precipitation. An alternative procedure to isotope dilution, reverse or inverse isotope dilution, can be used to determine the quantity of radioactive compound by dilution with an inactive compound. This procedure is applicable when a system contains an unknown amount of isotopically labeled substance of known specific activity.

Radioisotope exchage

For understanding mechanisms and kinetics of organic or biological reactions, non-radioactive atoms in molecules or ions are allowed to exchange with appropriate radiolabeled compound. After chemical exchange between a labeled compound and the test sample (the chemical form of the element being different in the two solutions, e.g., iodine in CH_3I vs $^{131}I^-$ in labeled sodium iodide), the specific activity of the element becomes the same in the sample and reagent. A measured decrease in the activity of the reagent or increase in the activity of the sample can then be related to the amount of element present in the sample. Isotopic exchange methods of analysis are very sensitive, rapid, and specific. Isotopic exchange plays a very important role in pharmacokinetic studies. For example, a drug molecule may be labeled with tritium to follow the drug distribution. Exchange of tritium with an unlabeled compound or with a water molecule in the vicinity may lead to erroneous interpretation of the drug distribution if suitable precautions are not taken to avoid potential isotopic exchange reactions.

Radiotracers as radiopharmaceuticals: Methods for radiopharmaceutical analysis

When radiolabeled compounds (radiotracers) are used for diagnostic and therapeutic purposes, it is called a radiopharmaceutical. A radiopharmaceutical should be easily produced, inexpensive, readily available, have relatively short halflife, and preferably should be a γ-Emitter with an energy between 30 and 300 keV. Such a γ-Emitting nuclide should invariably decay by electron capture or isomeric transition. When positron-emitting nuclides are used, they must have specific localization in the desired organ or tissue and should not result in undue radiation exposure. Radiotracers, used as pharmaceuticals, are produced in one of two ways: either as a product of nuclear fission reactions or as a product of nuclear reactions induced by high-energy accelerator particles or neutrons. Particle accelerators are instruments that cause nuclear reactions by bombarding target nuclides with highly accelerated and energized particles such as protons, deutrons, and electrons. For production of radiopharmaceuticals, on-site accelerators called cyclotrons are used. For production of positron-emitting radionculides linear accelerators are used. Readily transportable instruments, which serve as sources for short-lived radionuclides, are called *generators*. Typically, in a generator, a long-lived parent nuclide is allowed to decay to a short-lived daughter radionuclide. Using differences in chemical properties, the daughter nuclide is separated from the parent.

A radiopharmaceutical is a radioactive chemical used as a pharmaceutical. Therefore, as pharmaceuticals, they should have proper ionic strength, pH, isotonicity, and osmolarity. In addition to chemical purity, radionuclide purity and radiochemical purity also have to be demonstrated. The radionuclide purity refers to the ratio of the amount of radioactivity corresponding to that of desired radionuclide to the total amount of radioactivity owing to other isotopes and other isotopic impurities. Radionuclide purity is determined by measuring halflives and other characteristics of radiation of the radionuclide. Radiochemical purity refers to the fraction of total radioactivity in the desired form. Radiochemical impurities are general chemical impurities formed by the chemical as a result of decomposition of the chemical entity, whereas all the resulting impurities may still be radioactive. Potential decomposition pathways are the same as for any other pharmaceutical. Examples include acid and base hydrolysis products, oxidized and reduced species, additional radiolysis products, and photochemical and thermal decomposition products of the chemical. For example in many ^{99m}Tc-labeled complexes, free unreacted $^{99m}TcO_4^-$ and hydrolyzed ^{99m}Tc are radiochemical impurities. A number of analytical methods can be used to detect and determine radiochemical impurities. For example, when separating the impurities from radiochemical compound of interest using HPLC, if a radiochemical detector is used, all the radioactive impurities that are separated can be quantitated, and radiochemical purity can be ascertained. These include but are not limited to distillation, precipitation, paper, thin layer, gel chromatography, HPLC, ion exchange, solvent extraction, and other separation and purification techniques. The techniques and principles of these techniques are the same as for any other pharmaceutical.

Activation analysis

Activation analysis is a process in which a target trace element in a sample matrix is irradiated with particles in a nuclear reactor. As a result, an activated radionuclide is formed. The characteristic particles or γ-Rays emitted are used for qualitative identification and, more often, for quantitative measurement. The most common activation analysis is neutron activation analysis (NAA). In this technique, a sample containing the element is irradiated with neutrons in a reactor. After irradiation, γ-Emissions ensue from the decaying radionuclide. These are quantitated by using appropriate semiconductor radiation detectors. Detecting γ-Rays of a specific energy identifies the radionuclide. These particular energy values correspond to unique energies characteristic of the decaying radionuclides. For example, when ^{24}Na decays to ^{24}Mg, the γ-Rays released have unique energies of 1.268 and 2.754 MeV. A plot of γ-Ray counts versus energy yields a γ-Ray spectrum; the area under the curve is proportional to the radioactivity of the sample. The rate at which γ-Rays are emitted is proportional to the concentration of the radionuclide. When a large number of elements in a single sample matrix are analyzed using appropriate instruments for quantitation, without separation of the elements, it is called instrumental neutron activation analysis. When there is spectral interference in the sample matrix and if chemical separation is carried out to isolate the element, it is called radiochemical neutron activation analysis. When other charged particles are generated for analysis by activation, it is called charged particle activation analysis (CPAA). CPAA is applied to the determination of elemental concentration in surface layers. All methods of activation analysis are very accurate and sensitive, and a precision of approximately 2% RSD is easily attainable. Detection limits in parts per per billion or lower, depending on the element and sample matrix, are easily attainable. As many as 60 different elements that can form radionuclide can be analyzed using NAA.

Radioimmunoassay

Radioimmunoassay (RIA) is a technique based on the formation of antigen–antibody complex. This technique essentially involves the application of isotope dilution analysis. An antigen is typically a protein of molecular weight greater than 10,000 that stimulates the production of antibody in an animal body. The antigen subsequently binds with the antibody. Antigen is usually measured in the patient's sample, and the antigen becomes the analyte. To an antibody, a mixture of labeled and unlabeled antigen is added in excess such that the quantity of antibody needed to bind is allowed to be insufficient. As a result, both types of antigen compete with the limited amount of antibody in the sample. The reaction in an RIA mixture can be described as follows.

$$\begin{matrix} Ag^* \\ \quad \end{matrix} + Ab \underset{k_2}{\overset{k_1}{\rightleftharpoons}} \begin{matrix} Ag^* - Ab + Ag \\ Ag - Ag + Ag \end{matrix}$$
$$Ag$$

k_1 and k_2 are rate constants; equilibrium constant $K = k_1/k_2$.

To a constant amount of labeled antigen and antibody, increasing amounts of unlabeled antibody are added. The initial amount added is still in excess of the antibody needed for binding. As a result of competing reactions of the labeled and unlabeled antigen, the greater the concentration of the unlabeled antigen added, the less is the amount of bound labeled complex (Ag^*–Ab complex) and hence greater is the free (unbound) antigen. After incubation to equilibrium at a specified temperature and time, unique to the system, separation of the free labeled Ag^*, the fraction of the bound labeled antigen is determined by measuring the activity of the radioactive nuclide. By plotting the percent of bound labeled antigen versus the concentration of antigen added, the concentration of the unknown antigen can be determined. Several radionuclides such as ^{14}C, ^{3}H, ^{131}I , ^{32}P, ^{75}Se, ^{59}Fe, ^{99}Mo, and ^{57}Co have been used for RIA. However, ^{125}I is the most commonly used radionuclide for RIA. The earliest method of separation included electrophoresis and chromatography. However, today RIA kits are marketed by commercial manufacturers with detailed description of the principles of the method, methods of use, sensitivity, precision, and limitations of use for specific uses. The RIA methods are very rapid, sensitive, specific, and inexpensive, especially for large biological samples in complex sample matrices.

The RIA technique is applied in assays of hormones, steroids, peptides, aminoglycosides such as to bramycin and gentamycin, insulin, many immunoglobulins, different types of viral heptitis, plasma catecholamines, angiotension-converting enzymes, many vitamins including vitamine $B_{12,}$ human growth hormones, many folate derivatives, and others. Many commercially available RIA kits, unique to each kit, contain series of standards with known concentrations of unlabeled antigen, a vial of suitable labeled antigen, a vial of antibody solution, and appropriate precipitants or other analytical aides.

RADIATION SAFETY

When radiation energy is absorbed by tissues, depending on the dose received, rupture of chemical bonds occurs that causes damage to cells and tissues. Such damage may not be clinically apparent even for years if the absorbed dose is small. Radiation damage is measured in terms of absorbed dose. Dose is defined as the energy imparted to a material per unit mass. The SI unit of dose is called Gray, or Gy (joules/Kg). The traditional unit is rad. One Gy = 100 rads. However, the effectiveness of all radiations is not the same. The effectiveness is dependent on the nature of the particle, the thickness of the tissue or organ, and the characteristics of the material or organ to which such a dose is administered. Thus, to account for such differences in effectiveness, another term, called dose equivalent, is used. The SI unit of dose equivalent is Sievert, which is numerically equivalent to Gy multiplied by the appropriate weighting factor corresponding to biological tissue or organ. For example, the weighting factor (W_R) for many tissues is 0.3, whereas it is 0.03 for bone surfaces. The radiation weighting factor is also dependent on the energy of the particles. For example, for neutrons with less than 10 keV, W_R, = 5, whereas it is equal to 20 for neutrons greater than 100 keV.

For purposes of administered dose of a radiopharmaceutical, the package insert contains a table that lists dosage for the "average" patient as a function of administered activity. This information may be used for calculation of radiation dose. If needed, a medical physicist will calculate administered dose based on Medical Internal Radiation Dose (MIRD) committee recommendations.

External exposure to ionizing radiation as a result of occupation is measured using dosimeters. Three different types of dose monitors are commercially available. They are pocket dosimeters, film badges, and thermoluminescent detectors (TLDs). Pocket dosimeters are GM counting-based digital dosimeters, which provide immediate reading. Film badges are the least expensive and most popular. Using appropriate filters in the film holder, accurate readings to exposure to different particles can be measured. The major disadvantage with film badges is the waiting period required for developing and processing films. In TLDs, the radiation received is stored in holders containing crystals of LiFor manganese-activated calcium fluoride. Subsequently, during measurement, the crystals are heated to required temperatures such that they emit light. When measured, the emitted light provides a measure of absorbed dose.

Regulatory Requirements

The regulations of various advisory groups and government organizations have to be met in handling, use, and disposal of radioactive material and radio- pharmaceuticals. These include the FDA, NRC, Department of Transportation (DOT), Environmental Protection Agency (EPA), and Occupational Safety and Health Administration (OSHA). Of these, the FDA regulates safety, stability, efficacy, and toxicity of the radiopharmaceuticals; NRC regulates all reactor-produced by-products regarding use, handling, disposal, and radiation safety and protection of workers and the public using the facilities. Title 10 of the Code of Federal Regulations, 10 CFR 20, contains the regulations for radiation protection, whereas 10 CFR 35 addresses medical uses of radioactive materials. Title 49, 49 CFR, addresses packaging and transportation of radioactive materials. In addition, all USP requirements have to be met for a radiopharmaceutical.

The International Committee on Radiation Protection (ICRP) and the National Committee on Radiation Protection (NCRP) provide radiation dose recommendations for adoption to other regulatory agencies. The NRC requires that licensees follow the ALARA philosophy regarding radiation exposure. ALARA is an acronym for as low as reasonably achievable. Under the ALARA concept, when radiation exposure of a worker exceeds 1 0% of the allowed occupational limit, an investigation is required. If it exceeds 30%, investigation and corrective action are necessary per NRC requirements. As with any other pharmaceutical, radiotracers used as pharmaceuticals are subject to all regulatory requirements. The radiopharmaceutical manufacturer must, at a minimum, satisfy the requirements of the NRC and the FDA.

INDEX

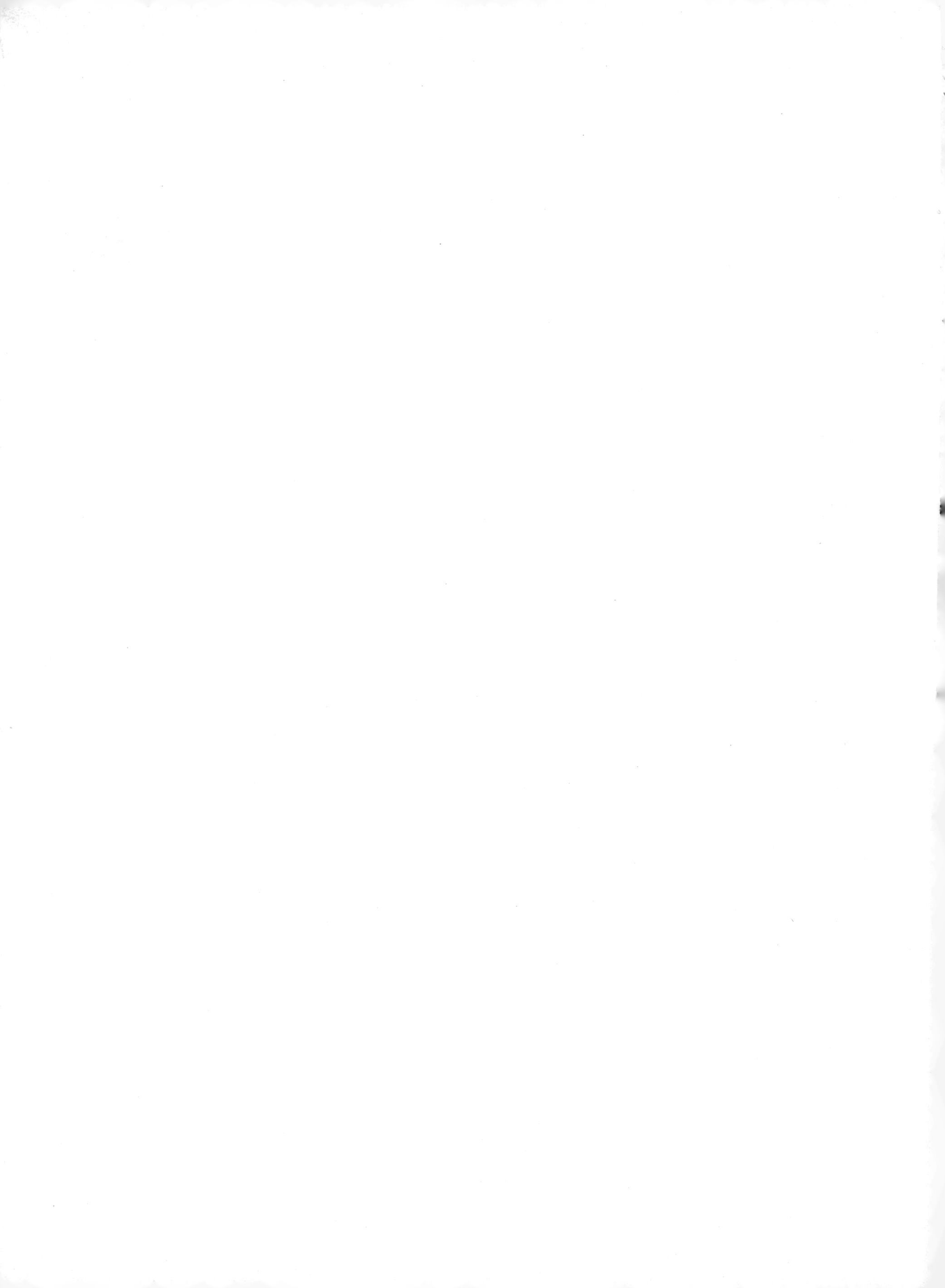